D1758670

Intraoperative Neurophysiological Monitoring

Third Edition

Intraoperative
Neurophysiological Monitoring

Third Edition

Aage R. Møller, PhD (DMedSci)

The University of Texas at Dallas
Dallas, TX

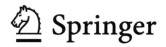 Springer

Aage R. Møller, PhD (DMedSci)
The University of Texas at Dallas
School of Brain and Behavioral Sciences
800 W. Campbell Road
Richardson, TX 75080 USA
amoller@utdallas.edu

ISBN 978-1-4419-7435-8   e-ISBN 978-1-4419-7436-5
DOI 10.1007/978-1-4419-7436-5
Springer New York Dordrecht Heidelberg London

© Springer Science+Business Media, LLC 2011
All rights reserved. This work may not be translated or copied in whole or in part without the written permission of the publisher (Springer Science+Business Media, LLC, 233 Spring Street, New York, NY 10013, USA), except for brief excerpts in connection with reviews or scholarly analysis. Use in connection with any form of information storage and retrieval, electronic adaptation, computer software, or by similar or dissimilar methodology now known or hereafter developed is forbidden.
The use in this publication of trade names, trademarks, service marks, and similar terms, even if they are not identified as such, is not to be taken as an expression of opinion as to whether or not they are subject to proprietary rights.
While the advice and information in this book are believed to be true and accurate at the date of going to press, neither the authors nor the editors nor the publisher can accept any legal responsibility for any errors or omissions that may be made. The publisher makes no warranty, express or implied, with respect to the material contained herein.

Printed on acid-free paper

Springer is part of Springer Science+Business Media (www.springer.com)

Preface

This book is based on three earlier books: Aage R. Møller: *Evoked Potentials in Intraoperative Monitoring* published in 1988 by Williams and Wilkens; and more directly by Aage R. Møller: *Intraoperative Neurophysiologic Monitoring* published in 1995 by Gordon and Breach under the imprint of Harwood Academic Publishers. This was followed by a Second Edition, published in 2006 by Humana Press. While the general organization of the book is preserved, the Third Edition of the book represents an expansion and extensive rewriting of the 2006 book. In particular, the coverage related to the monitoring of the spinal motor system and deep brain stimulation has been extended and new parts have been added. The description of the anatomical and physiological basis for these techniques has been largely rewritten, and many practical aspects of such monitoring have been added. The section on blood supply to the spinal cord has been extended. The chapters on peripheral nerves have been updated and extended. Anesthesia is now covered in more detail. Chapters on monitoring of sensory systems and monitoring in skull base surgery have also been revised. The section on techniques used in the operating room is also updated and many parts have been rewritten. This edition of the book describes many uses of intraoperative neurophysiology other than monitoring.

GENERAL OUTLINE

Chapter 1 is a general introduction to intraoperative neurophysiology and monitoring with some historical background. The general principles of intraoperative monitoring are discussed in Part I where Chap. 2 describes the basis for intraoperative monitoring. Chapter 3 discusses the various forms of electrical activity that can be recorded from nerve fibers and nerve cells; near-field activity from nerves, nuclei, and muscles that is recorded with monopolar and bipolar electrodes. This chapter also discusses far-field potentials and the responses from injured nerves and nuclei. Chapter 4 discusses practical aspects of recording evoked potentials from nerves, nuclei, and muscles including a discussion of various stimulus techniques.

Part II covers sensory systems. Chapter 5 describes the anatomy and physiology of the somatosensory, auditory, and visual systems. Monitoring of the somatosensory system is covered in Chap. 6; Chap. 7 concerns monitoring of the auditory system and Chap. 8 concerns monitoring of the visual system.

Part III discusses motor systems, beginning in Chap. 9 with a thorough description of the anatomy and basic physiology of the two main systems, the lateral and medial systems. Practical aspects of monitoring the spinal motor and brainstem motor systems are covered in Chaps. 10 and 11, respectively.

Part IV is devoted to peripheral nerves; Chap. 12 describes the anatomy and physiology and Chap. 13 discusses practical aspects of monitoring peripheral nerves.

Part V discusses different ways that intraoperative electrophysiological recordings can guide the surgeon in an operation, thus the use of neurophysiology in the operating room. Chapter 14 discusses methods to identify motor and sensory nerves and map the spinal cord and the floor of the fourth ventricle. Chapter 15 describes methods that can guide the surgeon in an operation such as MVD operations for HFS, placement of electrodes for DBS, and for removing lesions in the thalamus and basal ganglia. Intraoperative diagnosis of peripheral nerve disorders is also discussed in this chapter.

Part VI discusses practical aspects of intraoperative monitoring. Chapter 16 discusses anesthesia and how it can affect the use of intraoperative neurophysiologic techniques in the operating room. Chapter 17 discusses general matters regarding intraoperative monitoring

and neurophysiological recordings in anesthetized patients such as how to reduce the risk of
mistakes and how to reduce the effect of electrical interference of recorded neuroelectric
potentials. Chapter 18 discusses equipment and
data analysis related to intraoperative monitoring including electrical stimulation of nervous
tissue. The final chapter, Chap. 19, discusses
the importance of evaluation of the benefits
from the use of intraoperative neurophysiologic
monitoring to the patient, the surgeon, and the
field of surgery in general.

Aage R. Møller

Acknowledgments

I have had valuable help from many individuals in writing this book. I have had valuable discussions with Jay Shils, David MacDonald, Tod Sloan, and Leo Happel.

Jerry Crawford was immensely helpful by editing the manuscript; he provided many valuable suggestions. Mary Lee and Lola McCartney helped with graphic works. Paige Wahl transcribed many of the revisions of the manuscript and she copy edited the page proof.

I would not have been able to write this book without the support from the School of Behavioral and Brain Sciences at The University of Texas at Dallas.

Last, but not least I want to thank my wife, Margareta B. Møller, MD, DMedSci., for her support during writing of this book.

Aage R. Møller
Dallas June 2010

Contents

1

Introduction

Surgery may generally be regarded as a risk-filled method for treating diseases, and many forms of surgery have a potential for causing injury to the nervous system. Since such injuries may not be detected by visual inspection of the operative field by the surgeon, they may occur and progress without the surgeon's knowledge. Intraoperative neurophysiological monitoring involves the use of neurophysiological recordings for detecting changes in the function of the nervous system that are caused by surgically induced insults while the changes are still reversible.

Intraoperative neurophysiological monitoring relates to the spirit of the Hippocratic Oath, namely, "Do no harm." We may not be able to relieve suffering from illness, but we should at least not harm the patient in our attempts to relieve the patient from illness. Intraoperative neurophysiological monitoring provides an example in medicine and surgery of improvements accomplished specifically by reducing failures, and thus, improving performance by reducing failures, a principle that is now regarded with great importance in the design of complex applications, such as in military wargaming and in space exploration.

Intraoperative neurophysiological monitoring is an inexpensive and effective method that provides real time monitoring of function, which can reduce the risk of permanent postoperative deficits in many different operations where nervous tissue is being manipulated. The benefits to the patient and to the surgeon of using appropriate neurophysiological monitoring methods during operations in which neural tissue is at risk of being injured are well recognized

and intraoperative neurophysiological monitoring is now widely practiced in many hospitals in connection with such operations. Individuals on the neurophysiological monitoring team are now accepted as members of the operating room team.

While the greatest benefit of intraoperative neurophysiological monitoring is that it provides the possibility to reduce the risk of postoperative neurological deficits, it can also be of great value to the surgeon by providing other information about the effects of the surgeon's manipulations that is not otherwise available. Intraoperative recordings of neuroelectric potentials can help the surgeon identify specific neural structures, making it possible to determine the location of neural blockage on a nerve. Intraoperative neurophysiological recordings can often help the surgeon carry out the operation, and in some cases, it can determine when the therapeutic goal of the operation has been achieved. Intraoperative neurophysiological monitoring can often give the surgeon a justified, increased feeling of security.

While monitoring of patients' vital signs in the operating room has been done for many years, monitoring the function of the nervous system is a relatively new addition to the operating room, and it has a wide range of applications.

During the late 1970s and early 1980s, electrophysiological methods in the operating room came into use within some university health centers and a few large hospitals. It soon after became evident that standard laboratory techniques transplanted to the operating room could reduce the risk of inadvertently injuring neural tissue and, thereby reduce the risk of permanent neurological deficits. This new use of standard laboratory techniques became known as intraoperative neurophysiological monitoring.

From: *Intraoperative Neurophysiological Monitoring: Third Edition*,
By A.R. Møller, DOI 10.1007/978-1-4419-7436-5_1,
© Springer Science+Business Media, LLC 2011

Orthopedic surgery was one of the first specialties to make systematic use of intraoperative neurophysiological monitoring, particularly in operations involving the spine. In the 1970s, work by Dr. Richard Brown, a neurophysiologist, reduced the risk of damage to the spinal cord during scoliosis operations by using the recordings of somatosensory evoked potentials (1, 2).

While it is assumed that the era of intraoperative neurophysiological monitoring started in the late 1970s, electrophysiological methods were used in the operating room in a few hospitals for the purpose of reducing the risk of permanent neurological deficits even before that time. In the early 1960s, monitoring of the facial nerve was performed to reduce the risks of facial paresis or palsy after operations for vestibular schwannoma (3, 4). Leonid Malis, a neurosurgeon who pioneered the use of microneurosurgical techniques, used the recordings of evoked potentials from the sensory cortex in his neurosurgical operations. Dr. Malis, fascinated by the development of microneurosurgery, stated later that microneurosurgery had made intraoperative monitoring unnecessary, (5) although others expressed the opposite opinion in support of the usefulness of intraoperative monitoring (6).

Monitoring of auditory Techniques of intraoperative monitoring for spinal cord function: Their past, present and future directions (ABR) was also one of the earliest applications of intraoperative neurophysiological monitoring in the neurosurgical operating room. It was used first in microvascular decompression (MVD) operations for hemifacial spasm (HFS) and trigeminal neuralgia pioneered by Betty Grundy (7) and Peter Raudzens (8) in the early 1980s and others (9, 10) thereafter. Direct recordings from the exposed intracranial structures, such as the eighth cranial nerve and the cochlear nucleus, decreased the time to get an interpretable record (11, 12). Such recordings had been used earlier for research purposes (13).

Later, intraoperative monitoring of the function of the auditory nerve came into general use by neurosurgeons, and its use spread to other surgical specialties, such as otoneurological surgery.

In the 1980s, intraoperative neurophysiological monitoring was introduced in operations for large skull base tumors (14–16). Monitoring in such operations could involve many cranial nerves depending on the location of the tumor.

Intraoperative neurophysiological monitoring got its own society in the USA (the American Society for Neurophysiological Monitoring, ASNM) and soon after the establishment of ASNM, there followed the creation of certification processes, established by the American Board for Neurophysiologic Monitoring (ABNM), which certifies Diplomats of the American Board for Neurophysiologic Monitoring (DABNM). The Certification of Neurophysiologic Intraoperative Monitoring (CNIM) is provided through the American Board of Registration of Electroencephalographic and Evoked Potential Technologists (ABRET).

Methods for the monitoring of spinal motor systems advanced during the 1990s with the development of techniques using magnetic (17) and electrical stimulation (18) of the motor cortex and stimulation of the spinal cord (19). Methods that provided satisfactory anesthesia and, at the same time permitted activation of motor system by stimulation of the motor cortex were developed (20, 21).

We are now seeing the beginning of an era of treatment of certain movement disorders and severe pain that moves away from the use of medications and towards the use of procedures, such as deep brain stimulation (DBS), that aim treatment at specific structures of the CNS. Other forms of functional intervention using neuromodulation of various kinds are coming into increasing use. Common for these methods is their dependence on intraoperative neurophysiology. Thus, using neurophysiological methods is as critical for the placement of electrodes for DBS as it is for selective lesioning of brain tissue for treating movement disorders and severe pain.

The obvious advantage of such procedures as DBS and selective lesions is that the treatment is directed specifically to structures that are involved in producing the symptoms while other general medical (pharmaceutical) treatments, even when applied in accordance with the best known experience, are much less specific and often have severe side effects and limited beneficial effects. While any licensed physician can prescribe any drug, even such drugs that have complex actions and known and unknown side effects, procedures, such as DBS, can only be done, at least adequately, by teams of experts, which include members with a thorough understanding of neuroscience and pathophysiology of the disorders that are to be treated.

There is little doubt that the use of procedures, such as DBS expands to include disorders that are currently treated with medication alone. The treatments using neuromodulation increase and become broadened and consequently, increase the demands on neurosurgeons who perform these procedures as well as neurophysiologists who are providing the neurophysiological guidance for proper placement of such stimulating electrodes.

Research in the operating room can uncover new knowledge about normal and pathological conditions and provide immediate improvement of treatment, including the reduction of postoperative deficits, but no direct benefit to patients is expected. However, experience has taught us that even basic research can provide (unexpected) immediate as well as long-term benefits to patient treatment.

There are several advantages of doing research in the operating room. To begin with, humans are different from animals, but the results of research in the operating room are directly applicable to humans. Secondly, it is easier to study the physiology of diseased systems in humans than trying to make animal models of diseases.

Research in the operating room has a longer history than intraoperative neurophysiological monitoring. One of the first surgeons–scientists who understood the value of research in the neurosurgical operating room was Wilder Penfield (1891–1976), who founded the Montreal Neurological Institute in 1934. Penfield, a neurosurgeon with a

solid background in neurophysiology, was inspired by neurophysiologist Sherrington during a Rhodes scholarship to Oxford, England. He later stated, "Brain surgery is a terrible profession. If I did not feel it will become different in my lifetime, I should hate it." (1921). Penfield may be regarded as the founder of intraoperative neurophysiological research, and he did groundbreaking work in many areas of neuroscience. His work on the somatosensory system is especially recognized (22, 23). In the 1950s, he used electrical stimulation to find epileptic foci, and in connection with these operations, he conducted extensive studies of the temporal lobe, especially with regard to memory.

Other neurosurgeons have followed Penfield's tradition. George A. Ojemann contributed much to understanding pathologies related to the temporal lobe as well as conducting basic research on memory and large individual variations of the brain. Like Penfield, he operated upon many patients for epilepsy, and during those operations, he mapped the temporal lobe and studied the centers for memory and speech using electrical current to inactivate specific regions of the brain in patients who were awake and were able to respond and perform memory tasks. Dr. Ojemann, working with Dr. Otto Creutzfeldt from Germany, studied neuronal activity during face recognition, and their studies also contributed to the development of the use of microelectrodes in recordings from the human brain.

A neurologist, Dr. Gaston Celesia (24, 25), mapped the auditory cortex in humans and studied somatosensory evoked potentials from the thalamus and primary somatosensory cortex (26). Other investigators have studied other structures, such as the dorsal column nuclei, the cochlear nucleus, and the inferior colliculus, in patients undergoing neurosurgical operations where these structures became exposed (27–30). The methods used to record evoked potentials from the surface of the cochlear nucleus by inserting an electrode into the lateral recess of the fourth ventricle (28, 31) became a useful method for monitoring the integrity of the auditory nerve in operations for vestibular schwannoma where the preservation of hearing was attempted (*32*) as well as in MVD operations for trigeminal neuralgia, HFS, and disabling positional vertigo.

Studies of the neural generators of the auditory brainstem response (ABR) have likewise benefited from recordings from structures that became exposed during neurosurgical operations. Recordings from the auditory nerve were first published in 1981 by two groups, one in Japan (Isao Hashimoto, neurosurgeon) (*33*), and one in the USA (*13*), which showed that the auditory nerve is the generator of two vertex positive deflections in the auditory brainstem-evoked responses, while the auditory nerve in small animals is the generator of only one (major) peak (*34–36*).

The neurosurgeon Fred Lenz has studied the responses from nerve cells in the thalamus in awake humans using microelectrodes and mapped the thalamus with regard to the involvement in painful stimulation as well as in response to innocuous somatosensory stimulation (*37–39*).

Electrophysiological studies of patients undergoing MVD operations for HFS have supported the hypothesis that the anatomical location of the physiological abnormalities that cause the symptoms of HFS is central to the location of vascular contact with the facial nerve (the facial motonucleus) involving mechanisms similar to the kindling phenomenon (*40*) described by Goddard and Wada (*41, 42*) and was not primarily caused by ephaptic transmission at the location of the vascular contact that caused the symptoms as another hypothesis had postulated. The findings extend our understanding of how activation of neural plasticity can cause symptoms of disease (*43*). These studies showed that a specific sign, the abnormal muscle response (or lateral spread response), disappears when the offending blood vessel is moved off the facial nerve (*44*), and that technique is now widely used in such operations as a guide to the surgeon in finding the vessel that is the culprit and in effectively decompressing the facial nerve. It has increased the success rate of the operation, decreased the operating time, and

reduced the risk that a reoperation would be necessary. This is again an example of how studies undertaken for pure, basic science purposes can result in practical methods that can improve specific kinds of treatment.

These examples show clearly that there is no sharp border between basic and applied research. The method used for studies of neural generators for the ABR came into use for monitoring the auditory nerve. Research on speech and language centers in the brain has proven to be important for epilepsy operations. Research on HFS provided better outcomes of MVD operations.

While it has been difficult to use exact scientific methods for assessing the benefits of intraoperative neurophysiological monitoring, it is my opinion, based on many years of experience, that the skill of the surgeon together with good use of electrophysiology in the operating room can benefit the patient who is undergoing surgery, and it can benefit many future patients by the progress in treatment that an effective collaboration between surgeons and neurophysiologists promotes.

REFERENCES

1. Nash CL, RA Lorig, LA Schatzinger et al (1977) Spinal cord monitoring during operative treatment of the spine. Clin Orthop 126:100–5.
2. Brown RH and CL Nash (1979) Current status of spinal cord monitoring. Spine 4:466–78.
3. Hilger J (1964) Facial nerve stimulator. Trans Am Acad Ophthalmol Otolaryngol 68:74–6.
4. Kurze T (1964) Microtechniques in neurological surgery. Clin Neurosurg 11:128–37.
5. Malis LI (1995) Intra-operative monitoring is not essential. Clin Neurosurg 42:203–13.
6. Sekhar LN, G Bejjani, P Nora et al (1995) Neurophysiologic monitoring during cranial base surgery: is it necessary? Clin Neurosurg 42:180–202.
7. Grundy B (1983) Intraoperative monitoring of sensory evoked potentials. Anesthesiology 58:72–87.
8. Raudzens PA (1982) Intraoperative monitoring of evoked potentials. Ann N Y Acad Sci 388:308–26.

9. Friedman WA, BJ Kaplan, D Gravenstein et al (1985) Intraoperative brain-stem auditory evoked potentials during posterior fossa microvascular decompression. J Neurosurg 62:552–7.

10. Linden R, C Tator, C Benedict et al (1988) Electro-physiological monitoring during acoutic neuroma and other posterior fossa surgery. Le J des Sci Neurol 15:73–81.

11. Møller AR and PJ Jannetta (1983) Monitoring auditory functions during cranial nerve microvascular decompression operations by direct recording from the eighth nerve. J Neurosurg 59:493–9.

12. Silverstein H, H Norrell and S Hyman (1984) Simultaneous use of CO2 laser with continuous monitoring of eighth cranial nerve action potential during acoustic neuroma surgery. Otolaryngol Head Neck Surg 92:80–4.

13. Møller AR and PJ Jannetta (1981) Compound action potentials recorded intracranially from the auditory nerve in man. Exp Neurol 74:862–74.

14. Møller AR (1987) Electrophysiological monitoring of cranial nerves in operations in the skull base, in *Tumors of the Cranial Base: Diagnosis and Treatment*, LN Sekhar and VL Schramm Jr, Editors. Futura Publishing Co: Mt. Kisco, New York. 123–32.

15. Sekhar LN and AR Møller (1986) Operative management of tumors involving the cavernous sinus. J Neurosurg 64:879–89.

16. Yingling C and J Gardi (1992) Intraoperative monitoring of facial and cochlear nerves during acoustic neuroma surgery. Otolaryngol Clin North Am 25:413–48.

17. Barker AT, R Jalinous and IL Freeston (1985) Non-invasive magnetic stimulation of the human motor cortex. Lancet 1:1106–7.

18. Marsden CD, PA Merton and HB Morton (1983) Direct electrical stimulation of corticospinal pathways through the intact scalp in human subjects. Adv Neurol 39:387–91.

19. Deletis V (1993) Intraoperative monitoring of the functional integrety of the motor pathways, in *Advances in Neurology: Electrical and Magnetic Stimulation of the Brain*, O Devinsky, A Beric and M Dogali, Editors. Raven Press: New York. 201–14.

20. Sloan TB and EJ Heyer (2002) Anesthesia for intraoperative neurophysiologic monitoring of the spinal cord. J Clin Neurophysiol 19:430–43.

21. Sloan T (2002) Anesthesia and motor evoked potential monitoring, in *Neurophysiology in Neurosurgery*, V Deletis and JL Shils, Editors. Elsevier Science: Amsterdam. 451–74.

22. Penfield W and E Boldrey (1937) Somatic motor and sensory representation in the cerebral cortex of man as studied by electrical stimulation. Brain 60:389–443.

23. Penfield W and T Rasmussen (1950) *The Cerebral Cortex of Man: A Clinical Study of Localization of Function*. Macmillan: New York.

24. Celesia GG, RJ Broughton, T Rasmussen et al (1968) Auditory evoked responses from the exposed human cortex. Electroencephalogr Clin Neurophysiol 24:458–66.

25. Celesia GG and F Puletti (1969) Auditory cortical areas of man. Neurology 19:211–20.

26. Celesia GG (1979) Somatosensory evoked potentials recorded directly from human thalamus and Sm I cortical area. Archives of Neurology 36:399–405.

27. Møller AR, PJ Jannetta and HD Jho (1990) Recordings from human dorsal column nuclei using stimulation of the lower limb. Neurosurgery 26:291–9.

28. Møller AR and PJ Jannetta (1983) Auditory evoked potentials recorded from the cochlear nucleus and its vicinity in man. J Neurosurg 59:1013–8.

29. Hashimoto I (1982) Auditory evoked potentials from the humans midbrain: Slow brain stem responses. Electroencephalogr Clin Neurophysiol 53:652–7.

30. Møller AR and PJ Jannetta (1982) Evoked potentials from the inferior colliculus in man. Electroencephalogr Clin Neurophysiol 53:612–20.

31. Kuroki A and AR Møller (1995) Microsurgical anatomy around the foramen of Luschka with reference to intraoperative recording of auditory evoked potentials from the cochlear nuclei. J Neurosurg 82:933–9.

32. Møller AR, HD Jho and PJ Jannetta (1994) Preservation of hearing in operations on acoustic tumors: An alternative to recording BAEP. Neurosurgery 34:688–93.

33. Hashimoto I, Y Ishiyama, T Yoshimoto et al (1981) Brainstem auditory evoked potentials recorded directly from human brain stem and thalamus. Brain 104:841–59.

34. Møller AR and JE Burgess (1986) Neural generators of the brain stem auditory evoked potentials (BAEPs) in the rhesus monkey. Electroencephalogr Clin Neurophysiol 65:361–72.

35. Spire JP, GJ Dohrmann and PS Prieto (1982) Correlation of brainstem evoked response with direct acoustic nerve potential, J Courjon,

F Manguiere and M Reval, Editors. Vol. 32. Raven Press: New York.

36. Martin WH, H Pratt and JW Schwegler (1995) The origin of the human auditory brainstem response wave II. Electroencephalogr Clin Neurophysiol 96:357–70.

37. Greenspan JD, RR Lee and FA Lenz (1999) Pain sensitivity alterations as a function of lesion localization in the parasylvian cortex. Pain 81:273–82.

38. Lenz FA and PM Dougherty (1995) Pain processing in the ventrocaudal nucleus of the human thalamus, in *Pain and the Brain*, B Bromm and JE Desmedt, Editors. Raven Press: New York. 175–85.

39. Lenz FA, JI Lee, IM Garonzik et al (2000) Plasticity of pain-related neuronal activity in the human thalamus. Prog Brain Res 129: 253–73.

40. Møller AR and PJ Jannetta (1984) On the origin of synkinesis in hemifacial spasm: Results of intracranial recordings. J Neurosurg 61:569–76.

41. Goddard GV (1964) Amygdaloid stimulation and learning in the rat. J Comp Physiol Psychol 58:23–30.

42. Wada JA (1981) *Kindling 2*. Raven Press: New York.

43. Møller AR (2008) Neural plasticity: For good and bad. Prog Theor Phys 173:48–65.

44. Møller AR and PJ Jannetta (1985) Microvascular decompression in hemifacial spasm: Intraoperative electrophysiological observations. Neurosurgery 16:612–8.

PART I

PRINCIPLES OF INTRAOPERATIVE NEUROPHYSIOLOGICAL MONITORING

The basic principles of recording and stimulation of the nervous system used in intraoperative neurophysiological monitoring resemble techniques used in the clinical diagnostic laboratory with some very important differences. The electrical potentials that are recorded from the nervous system in the operating room must be interpreted immediately and are recorded under circumstances of interference of various kinds.

This means that the person who does intraoperative neurophysiological monitoring must be knowledgeable about the function of the neurological systems that are monitored, how electrical potentials are generated by the nervous system, and how such potentials change as a result of pathologies that occur because of surgical manipulations.

This section provides basic information about the principles of intraoperative neurophysiological monitoring. Chapter 2 discusses the basis for neurophysiological monitoring and intraoperative neurophysiology. Chapter 3 describes how electrical activity is generated in the nervous system and how such electrical activity can be recorded and used as the basis for detecting injuries to specific parts of the peripheral and central nervous system. Chapter 4 provides practical information about recording of neuroelectric potentials from the nervous system and how to stimulate the nervous system in anesthetized patients. This chapter also discusses how to record very small electrical potentials in an electrically hostile environment such as the operating room.

2

Basis of Intraoperative Neurophysiological Monitoring

INTRODUCTION

Intraoperative neurophysiological monitoring is often associated with reducing the risk of postoperative neurological deficits in operations where the nervous system is at risk of being permanently injured. While the main use of electrophysiological methods in the operating room may be for reducing the risk of postoperative neurological deficits,

electrophysiological methods are now in increasing use for other purposes. For example, electrophysiological methods are now regarded a necessity for guidance in placement of electrodes for deep brain stimulation (DBP) or for making lesions in specific structures for treating movement disorders and pain. Intraoperative electrophysiological recordings can also help the surgeon in carrying out other surgical procedures. Finding specific neural tissue such as cranial nerves or specific regions of the cerebral cortex are examples of tasks that are included in the subspecialty of intraoperative neurophysiological

From: *Intraoperative Neurophysiological Monitoring: Third Edition*,
By A.R. Møller, DOI 10.1007/978-1-4419-7436-5_2,
© Springer Science+Business Media, LLC 2011

monitoring. Neurophysiological methods are increasingly used for diagnostic support in operations such as those involving peripheral nerves. In certain operations, intraoperative neurophysiology can increase the likelihood of achieving the therapeutical goal of an operation. Intraoperative neurophysiological recordings have shown to be of help identifying the offending blood vessel in a cranial nerve disorder (hemifacial spasm, HFS).

REDUCING THE RISK OF NEUROLOGICAL DEFICITS

The use of intraoperative neurophysiological monitoring to reduce the risk of loss of function in portions of the nervous system is based on the observation that the function of neural structures usually changes in a measurable way before being permanently damaged. Reversing the surgical manipulation that caused the change within a certain time will result in a recovery to normal or near normal function, whereas if no intervention is taken, there will be a risk of permanent postoperative neurological deficit.

Surgical manipulations such as stretching, compressing, or heating from electrocoagulation are insults that can injure neural tissue. Ischemia, caused by impairment of blood supply due to surgical manipulations or intentional clamping of arteries, may also result in permanent (ischemic) injury to neural structures causing a risk of noticeable postoperative neural deficits.

The effect of such insults represents a continuum; at one end, function decreases during the time of the insult, and at the other end of this continuum, nervous tissue is permanently damaged, and normal function never recovers and results in permanent postoperative deficits. Between these extremes, there is a large range over which recovery may occur either totally or partially. Thus, up to a certain degree of injury, there can be total recovery, but thereafter, the neural function may be affected for some time. Following a more severe injury, the recovery of normal function not only takes a longer time,

but the final recovery would be partial with the degree of recovery depending on the nature, degree, and duration of the insult.

Injuries acquired during operations that result in a permanent neurologic deficit will most likely reduce the quality of life for the patient for many years to come and maybe for a lifetime. It is, therefore, important that the person who is responsible for interpreting the results of monitoring is aware that the neurophysiologist has a great degree of responsibility, together with the surgeon and the anesthesiologist, in reducing the risk of injury to the patient during the operation.

Techniques for Reducing Postoperative Neurological Deficits

The general principle of intraoperative neurophysiological monitoring is to apply a stimulus and then to record the electrical response from specific neural structures along the neural pathway that are at risk of being injured. This can be performed by recording near-field evoked potentials by placing a recording electrode on a specific neural structure that becomes exposed during the operation, or, as more commonly done, by recording far-field evoked potentials from, for instance, electrodes placed on the surface of the scalp.

Intraoperative neurophysiological monitoring that is done for the purpose of reducing the risk of postoperative neurological deficits makes use of relatively standard and well-developed methods for stimulation and recordings of electrical activity in the nervous system. Most of the methods that are used in intraoperative neurophysiological monitoring are similar to those that have been used in the physiologic laboratory and in the clinical testing laboratory for many years.

Sensory System. Intraoperative neurophysiological monitoring of the function of sensory systems has been widely practiced since the middle of the 1980s. The earliest uses of intraoperative neurophysiological monitoring of sensory systems were modeled after the clinical practice of recording sensory evoked potentials for diagnostic purposes.

Sensory systems are monitored by applying an appropriate stimulus and recording the response from the ascending neural pathway, usually by placing recording electrodes on the surface of the scalp to pick up evoked far-field potentials from nerve tracts and nuclei in the brain (far-field responses).

It has been mainly somatosensory evoked potentials (SSEP) and auditory brainstem responses (ABR) that have been recorded in the operating room for monitoring the function of these sensory systems for the purpose of reducing the risk of postoperative neurological deficits. Visual evoked potentials (VEP) are also monitored in some operations. When intraoperative neurophysiological monitoring was introduced, it was first SSEP that were monitored routinely (1), followed by ABR (2–4).

While the technique used for recording sensory evoked potentials in the operating room is similar to that used in the clinical diagnostic laboratory, there are important differences. In the operating room, it is only changes in the recorded potentials that occur during the operation that are of interest, while in the clinical testing laboratory, the deviation from normal values (laboratory standard) are important measures.

Another important difference is that results obtained in the operating room must be interpreted instantly, which places different demands on the personnel who are responsible for intraoperative neurophysiological monitoring than those working in the clinical laboratory. In the operating room, it is sometimes possible to record evoked potentials directly from neural structures of sensory pathways (near-field responses) when such structures are exposed during an operation.

The use of evoked potentials in intraoperative neurophysiological monitoring for the purpose of reducing the risk of postoperative permanent sensory deficits is based on the following:

1. Electrical potentials can be recorded in response to a stimulus.

2. These potentials change in a noticeable way before permanent damage occurs from surgical manipulations of heating from electrocoagulation.
3. Proper surgical intervention, such as reversal of the manipulation that caused the change, will reduce the risk that the observed change in function develops into a permanent neurological deficit or, at least, will reduce the degree of the postoperative deficits.

Motor Systems. Intraoperative neurophysiological monitoring of the facial nerve was probably the first motor system that was monitored (5, 6). Systematic monitoring came later (7, 8). The introduction of skull base surgery in the beginning of the 1980s (9) caused an increased demand for monitoring of other cranial systems, and the use of monitoring for many cranial motor nerves spread rapidly (10, 11). Intraoperative neurophysiological monitoring of spinal motor systems was delayed because of technical difficulties, mainly in eliciting recordable evoked motor responses to stimulation of the motor cortex in anesthetized patients. After these technical obstacles in activating descending spinal motor pathways were resolved in the 1990s, intraoperative neurophysiological monitoring of spinal motor systems gained widespread use (12). Monitoring of cranial nerve motor systems commonly relies on electrical stimulation of specific cranial motor nerves while recording electromyographic (EMG) potentials from muscles that are innervated by the motor nerves in question. Monitoring of spinal motor systems makes use of stimulation of the motor cortex (or cortices) by transcranial electrical stimulation or (rarely) by transcranial magnetic stimulation while recording directly from the descending motor pathways of the spinal cord or EMG potentials from specific muscles (Chaps. 10 and 11).

Peripheral Nerves. Monitoring of motor nerves is often accomplished by observing the electrical activity that can be recorded from one or more of the muscles that are innervated by the motor nerve or motor system that is to be monitored (evoked EMG potentials). The respective motor nerve may be stimulated electrically or by the electrical current that is induced by a strong magnetic impulse (magnetic stimulation). Recordings of muscle activity that is elicited by mechanical stimulation of a motor nerve or by injury to a motor nerve are important parts of many forms of monitoring of the motor system. Such muscle activity is monitored by the continuous recording of EMG potentials ("free running EMG"). When such activity is made audible, it can provide important feedback to the surgeon, and the surgeon can then modify his/her operative technique accordingly.

Monitoring peripheral nerves intraoperatively may be done by electrically stimulating the nerve in question at one point and recording compound action potentials (CAP) at a different location. Changes in neural conduction that may occur between these two locations will result in changes in the latency of the CAP and/or in the waveform and amplitude of the CAP. The latency of the CAP is inversely related to conduction velocity, and decreased conduction velocity is a typical sign of injury to a nerve. The latency of the recorded CAP typically increases as a result of many kinds of insults to a nerve and its waveform changes.

Interpretation of Neuroelectric Potentials

The success of intraoperative neurophysiological monitoring depends greatly on the correct interpretation of the recorded neuroelectric potentials. In most situations, the usefulness of intraoperative neurophysiological monitoring depends on the person who watches the display, makes the interpretation, and decides what information should be given to the surgeon. It is, therefore, imperative for success in intraoperative neurophysiological monitoring that the person who is responsible for the monitoring be well trained. It is also important that he/she is familiar with the different steps in the operation, the kind of anesthesia used, and well informed in advance about the patient who is to be monitored.

It is important that information about changes in recorded potentials be presented to the surgeon in a way that contributes specific descriptive details that the surgeon will find useful and actionable. Surgeons are not neurophysiologists, and the knowledge about neurophysiology varies among surgeons. Neurophysiologists who provide results of monitoring to the surgeon must, therefore, present their skilled interpretation of the recorded potentials. The surgeon may not always appreciate data, such as latency values, because the surgeon may not understand what such data represent. Monitoring is of no value if the surgeon does not take action accordingly. If the surgeon does not understand what the information provided by the neurophysiologist means, then there is little chance that he/she will take appropriate action.

Correct and prompt interpretation of changes in the waveforms of the recorded potentials is essential for such monitoring to be useful. The far-field potentials, such as ABR, SSEP, and VEP, are often complex and consist of a series of peaks and troughs that represent the electrical activity that is generated by successively activated nerve tracts and nuclei of the ascending neural pathways of the sensory system. Exact descriptions of the implications of the changes in such potentials that may occur as a result of various kinds of surgical insults, therefore, requires thorough knowledge about the anatomy and physiology of the systems that are monitored and how the recorded potentials are generated.

The most reliable indicators of changes in neural function are changes (increases) in the latencies of specific components of sensory evoked potentials, but surgically induced insults to nervous tissue often cause changes in the amplitude of sensory evoked potentials as well.

It must be remembered that the recorded sensory evoked potentials do not measure the function (or changes in function) of the sensory system that is being tested. For example, there is no direct relationship between the change in the ABR and the change in the patient's hearing threshold or change in speech discrimination. This is one reason why it has been difficult to establish guidelines for how much evoked potentials may vary during an operation without presenting a noticeable risk for postoperative deficits.

Interpretation of sensory evoked potentials is based on knowledge about the anatomical location of the generators of the individual components of SSEP, ABR, and VEP in relation to the structures that are being manipulated in a specific operation. Interpretation of sensory evoked potentials also depends on the processing of the recorded potentials; for example, filters or filtering techniques of various kinds that are used affect the waveform of the potentials.

The amplitude of these sensory evoked potentials is smaller than the background noise (ongoing brain activity such as electroencephalographic potentials) and electrical noise that enters recording amplifiers from the environment (see Chap. 18). It is, therefore, necessary to use signal averaging to enhance the signal-to-noise ratio of far-field potentials such as sensory evoked potentials. Signal averaging (adding the responses to many stimuli) is based on the assumption that the responses to every stimulus are identical and that they always occur at the same time following stimulation. Since the sensory evoked potentials that are recorded in the operating room are likely to change during the time that responses are being averaged, the averaging process may produce unpredictable results.

These matters are important to take into consideration when interpreting sensory evoked potentials. Signal averaging and filtering are discussed in detail in Chap. 18. This chapter also discusses different ways to reduce the time necessary to obtain an interpretable recording. The specific techniques that are suitable for intraoperative neurophysiological monitoring of the auditory, somatosensory, and visual systems are dealt with in detail in Part II (Chaps. 6, 7, and 8, respectively).

In some instance, it is possible to record evoked potentials from the structures that actually generate the recorded potentials in question (near-field potentials). Such potentials often have sufficiently large amplitudes allowing observation of the potentials directly without

signal averaging. If it is possible to base the intraoperative neurophysiological monitoring on recording of evoked potentials directly from an active neural structure (nerve, nerve tract, or nucleus), little or no signal averaging may be necessary because the amplitudes of such potentials are much larger than those of far-field potentials such as the ABR and SSEP. Such near-field potentials can often be viewed in real time on a computer screen or after only a few responses have been averaged. These matters are also discussed in detail in the chapters on sensory evoked potentials (Part II).

The design of the monitoring system, the way the recorded potentials are processed, and the way the recorded potentials are displayed are important factors in facilitating proper interpretation of the recorded neuroelectric potentials (see Chap. 17). The proper choice of stimulus parameters and the selection of the location along the nervous pathways where the responses are recorded also facilitate prompt interpretation of recorded neuroelectric potentials.

When recording EMG potentials, it is often advantageous to make the recorded response audible (7, 13) so that the neurophysiologist who is responsible for the monitoring and the surgeon can hear the response and make his or her own interpretation. Still, the possibilities to present the recorded potentials directly to the surgeon are currently few, and it is questionable whether it would be advantageous. Few surgeons are physiologists, and most surgeons prefer the results of monitoring to be presented in a descriptive form rather than raw data.

The importance of being able to detect a change in function as soon as possible cannot be emphasized enough. Prompt interpretation of changes in recorded potentials makes it possible for the surgeon to accurately identify the step in the operation that caused the change, which is a prerequisite for proper and prompt surgical intervention and thus, the ability to reduce the risk of postoperative neurological deficits!

Correct identification of the step in an operation that entails a risk of complications may make it possible to modify the way such an operation is carried out in the future and to reduce the risk of complications in subsequent operations. In this way, intraoperative neurophysiological monitoring may also contribute to the development of safer operating methods by making it possible to identify which steps in an operation may cause neurologic deficits, and it thereby, naturally, plays an important role in teaching surgical residents and fellows.

When to Inform the Surgeon

It has been debated extensively whether the surgeon should be informed of all changes in the recorded electrical activity that could be regarded as caused by surgical manipulations or only when such changes reach a level that indicate a noticeable risk for permanent neurological deficits. The dilemma is thus: should the information that is gained be used only as a warning (alarm) that implies that if no intervention is made there is a likelihood that the patient will get a permanent postoperative neurological deficit, or should all information about changes in function be conveyed to the surgeon?

If only information that is presumed to indicate a high risk of neurological deficits is given to the surgeon, then it must be known how large a change in the recorded neuroelectric potentials can be permitted without causing any (detectable) permanent damage. So far, this question has largely remained unanswered. The degree of the change, the nature of the change, and the length of time that the adverse effect has persisted are all factors that are likely to affect the outcome, and the effect of these factors on the risk of postoperative neurological deficits is largely unknown. Individual variation in susceptibility to surgical insults to the nervous system and many other factors affect the risk of neurological deficits in mostly unknown ways and degrees. An individual's disposition, the patient's homeostatic condition, and perhaps the effect of anesthesia on the patient are likely to affect the susceptibility to surgically induced injuries. This all means that it is not possible to define general rules about the level of changes in recorded potentials that

does not have any (small) likelihood of causing permanent effects, and thus, it is not possible to know what changes are "safe."

If the surgeon is given information about any noticeable change in the recorded potentials that may be related to his/her action, it is not necessary to know how large a change in recorded potentials can be permitted to occur before any action is taken to reverse the change. Such information is in itself important because it tells the surgeon that the functions of specific structures have been affected. The surgeon can use such information in the planning and the decision making of how to proceed with the operation. This means that changes in the recorded potentials that are larger than the (small) normal variations typically seen in these recordings should be reported to the surgeon if there is reasonable certainty that these changes are related to surgical manipulations. In that way, intraoperative neurophysiological monitoring provides information rather than warnings. Some authors find that the best use of intraoperative neurophysiological monitoring is for the purpose of decreasing the risk of neurological deficits.

If the surgeon is made aware of any change in the recorded potentials that is larger than those normally occurring, it can help the surgeon to carry out the operation in an optimal way with as little risk of adverse effect on neural function as possible. Providing such information gives the surgeon the option of altering his or her course of action in a wide range of time. If the change in the recorded potentials is small, it is likely that the surgeon would be able to reverse the effect by a slight change in the surgical approach or by avoiding further manipulation of the neural tissue affected. Alternatively, the surgeon may choose not to alter technique if the surgical manipulations that caused the changes in the recorded neurophysiological potentials are essential to carrying out the operation in the anticipated way. However, even in such a case, the knowledge that the surgical procedure is affecting neural function in a measurable way is valuable to the surgeon, and continuous monitoring of the change allows the surgeon the ability to modify or not modify the procedure because monitoring has identified which step in the operation caused the change in function.

Other authors have expressed that it is desirable to have general rules (alarm criteria) about the size of changes in the recorded potentials that are allowed and that only when the changes reach such levels should the surgeon be informed. However, if information about a change in the recorded potentials is withheld until the change in the recorded electrical potentials have reached such "alarm" levels, it would be difficult for the surgeon to determine which step in the surgical procedure caused the adverse effect, and thus, it would not be possible for the surgeon to intervene appropriately because he or she would not know which step in the procedure had caused the change. In such a situation, the surgeon would not have had the freedom of delaying his or her action to reverse the change because the problem the change signaled had already reached dangerous levels.

When conveying information about early changes in the recorded potentials, it is important that it be made clear to the surgeon that such information represents guidance details, as opposed to a warning, that the surgical manipulations are likely to result in a high risk of serious consequences if appropriate action is not taken promptly by the surgeon. Warnings are justified, if, for instance, there is a sudden large change in the evoked potentials or if the surgeon has disregarded the need to reverse a manipulation that has caused a slow change in the recorded electrical potentials.

Some patients will likely experience neurological deficits when changes in recorded potentials during an operation are below such alarm levels. The more knowledge that is gathered about the effect of mechanical manipulation on nerves, the more it seems apparent that even slight changes in measures of electrical activity (such as the CAP) may be signs of permanent injury. However, studies that relate changes in evoked potentials to morphological changes and changes in postoperative function are still rare. Thus, relatively little is known quantitatively about the degree to which a nerve can be stretched, heated, or deprived of oxygen before a permanent injury results, but there is no doubt that different nerves respond in different ways to injury due to mechanical manipulations or heat. Even less is known about the relationship between changes in sensory and motor evoked potentials and deficits from deprivation of oxygen.

Presenting information about changes in the recorded neuroelectric potentials as soon as they reach a level where they are detectable also has an educational benefit in that it tells the surgeon precisely which steps in an operation might result in neurologic deficit. It is often possible on the basis of such knowledge to modify an operation to avoid similar injuries in future operations.

The surgeon should be informed of the possibility of a surgically induced injury even in cases in which the change (or total disappearance of the recorded potentials) could be caused by equipment or electrode malfunction. Thus, only after assuming that the problem is biological in nature can equipment failure be considered as a possible cause of the change. Some authors have advocated that if sudden large changes occur, technical problems should be ruled out before the surgeon is notified. Other authors are of the opinion that the surgeon must be informed immediately, and then the neurophysiologist can check the equipment. Technical problems are rare, and if the observed change is caused by equipment failure after the surgeon was informed the only loss would be a few minutes of the surgeon's time. If, on the other hand, the observed change was caused by some major functional change, precious time would have been wasted if the surgeon's action was delayed by the search of a technical cause.

False Alarms

The question of false-positive and false-negative responses in intraoperative neurophysiological monitoring has been extensively debated. In some of these discussions, a false-positive response meant that the surgeon was alerted to a situation that would not have led to any noticeable risk of neurological deficits if no action had been taken.

Before discussing false-positive and false-negative responses in intraoperative neurophysiological monitoring, the meaning of false-positive and false-negative responses should be clarified. A typical example of a false-positive result of a test for a specific disease occurs when the test showed the presence of a disease while there was, in fact, no disease present. Using the same analogy, a false-negative test would mean that the test failed to show that a certain individual, in fact, had the specific disease. In the clinic or in screening of individuals without symptoms, false-negative results are more serious than false-positive results. False-positive results may lead to an incorrect diagnosis or unnecessary treatment, while false-negative results may have the dire consequence of no treatment being given for an existing disease.

These definitions cannot be transposed directly to the field of intraoperative neurophysiological monitoring. One reason is that the purpose of intraoperative neurophysiological monitoring is not to detect when a certain surgical manipulation will cause a permanent neurological deficit. Instead, the purpose is to provide information that a (noticeable) risk of permanent neurological deficit may occur. In fact, in most cases when intraoperative neurophysiological monitoring shows changes in function that indicate a risk of causing neurological deficits, no permanent deficits occur. There are no serious consequences associated with these kinds of false-positive responses in intraoperative neurophysiological monitoring.

A situation in which the surgeon was mistakenly alerted to a change in the recorded potentials that was afterward shown to be a result of a technical fault or a harmless change in the nervous system rather than being caused by surgical manipulations may be regarded as a true false-positive response.

The occurrences of false-negative results, which mean that a serious risk has occurred without being noticed, indicate a failure in reaching the goal of intraoperative neurophysiological

monitoring, and these failures may have serious consequences.

The conventional definition of false-positive and false-negative results can, therefore, not be applied to intraoperative neurophysiological monitoring because the purpose of monitoring is to identify signs that have a certain risk of leading to such deficits if no action is taken, not to identify individuals with neurological deficits.

Nonsurgical Causes of Changes in Recorded Potentials

Alerting the surgeon as soon as a change occurs implies a faint possibility that a change in evoked potentials may be caused by technical problems that affected some part of the equipment that is used or by a loss of contact of one or more of the electrodes that are used. The characteristics of changes caused by technical problems are usually so different from those of changes in the function of some part of the nervous system caused by injury from surgical manipulations that these two phenomena can easily be distinguished by an experienced neurophysiologist. It is possible that a total loss of recorded potentials can be caused by a technical failure, but it could also be caused by a major failure in the part of the nervous system that is being monitored. However, if such an event should occur, it is much better to first assume that the cause is biologic and to promptly alert the surgeon.

Equipment trouble-shooting activities are secondary actions. In general, when something unusual happens it is advisable to alert the surgeon promptly that something serious may have happened instead of beginning to check the equipment and electrodes. It is highly unlikely that a technical failure will occur and cause a change in the recorded potentials that may be confused with a biological cause for the change. The neurophysiologist should explain to the surgeon that a potentially serious event has occurred, and then after alerting the surgeon, check the equipment and the electrodes for malfunction. The surgeon should not wait for the completion of this equipment check. Instead, he/she should immediately begin his/her own investigation to ascertain whether a surgically induced injury has occurred. If it is discovered that the change in the recorded potentials was caused by equipment malfunction, the surgeon can then be notified, and thus, the only loss that the incident would have caused was a few minutes of the surgeon's time. If such an occurrence is regarded as a "false alarm", then the price for tolerating such "false alarms," namely, that the operation may be delayed unnecessarily for a brief time, seems small compared with what could occur if the equipment was checked before alerting the surgeon.

If the cause of the change in the recorded neuroelectric potentials was indeed a result of an injury that was caused by surgical manipulation of neural structures, and appropriate action was not taken immediately by the surgeon, precious time would have been lost. This would occur if the neurophysiologist had assumed that the cause of the change was technical in nature. Not only would the opportunity to identify the cause of the change be missed by taking the time to check the equipment first, but such a delay could also have allowed the change in function to progress, thus increasing the risk of a permanent neurological deficit. The opportunity to properly reverse the cause of the observed change in the recorded neuroelectric potentials may be lost if action is delayed while searching for technical problems.

In accepting this way of performing intraoperative neurophysiological monitoring, it must also be assumed that everything is done that can be done to keep technical failures that may mimic surgically induced changes in the recorded potentials to an absolute minimum. Actually, high-quality equipment very seldomly malfunctions, and if needle electrodes are used in the way described in the following chapters and care is taken when placing the electrodes, incidents of electrode failure will be rare.

There are factors other than surgical manipulations or equipment failure that can cause changes in the waveform of the recorded potentials, for example, changes in the level of anesthesia, a change in the patient's blood pressure, or change in the patient's body temperature.

It is, therefore, important that the person who is responsible for the intraoperative neurophysiological monitoring be knowledgeable about how these factors may affect the neuroelectric potentials that are being recorded. The physiologist should maintain consistent and frequent communication with the anesthesiologist to keep informed about any changes in the level of anesthesia and changes in the anesthesia regimen that may affect the electrophysiological parameters that are to be monitored.

How to Evaluate Neurological Deficits

To assess the success in avoiding neurological deficits, it is important that patients are properly examined and tested both pre- and postoperatively so that changes can be verified quantitatively. In some cases, an injury is detectable only by specific neurologic testing, while in other cases, injury causes impaired sensory function that is noticeable by the patient. Other patients may suffer alterations in neural function that are noticeable to the patient as well as to others in everyday situations. It is, therefore, important that careful objective testing and examination of the patient be performed before and after operations to make accurate quantitative assessments of sensory or neurological deficits.

There is no doubt that the degree to which different types of neurological deficits affect individuals varies, but reducing the risk of any measurable or noticeable deficit as much as possible must be the goal of intraoperative neurophysiological monitoring. (See Chap. 19 for further discussion on these matters.)

AIDING THE SURGEON IN THE OPERATION

In addition to reducing the risk of neurological deficits, the use of neurophysiological techniques in the operating room (intraoperative neurophysiology) can provide information and guidance that can help the surgeon carry out the operation and make better decisions about the next step in the operation. In its simplest form, this may consist of identifying the exact anatomical location of a nerve that cannot be identified visually, or it may consist of identifying where in a peripheral nerve a block of transmission has occurred (*14*). In operations to repair peripheral nerves, intraoperative diagnosis of the nature of the injury and its exact location using neurophysiological methods have improved the outcome of such operations.

An example of a more complex role of intraoperative recording is the recording of the abnormal muscle response in patients undergoing microvascular decompression operations to relieve HFS (*15, 16*). This abnormal muscle response disappears when the facial nerve is adequately decompressed (*17*), and by observing this response, it is possible to identify the blood vessel or blood vessels that caused the symptoms of HFS, as well as to ensure that the facial nerve has been adequately decompressed.

Electrophysiological guidance for placement of lesions in the basal ganglia and the thalamus for treatment of movement disorders and pain is absolutely essential for the success of such treatment. More recently, making lesions in these structures has been replaced by electrical DBS, and electrophysiological methods are equally important for guiding the placement of electrodes for DBS (*18, 19*).

There is no doubt that implantation of electrodes for DBS and for stimulation of specific structures in the spinal cord will expand during the coming years. Such treatments are attractive in comparison with pharmacological (drug) treatments in that electrophysiological treatments are more specific and have fewer side effects than drug treatments. While a physician with a license to practice medicine can prescribe many complex medications, procedures such as electrode implantation for DBS require expertise in both surgery and neurophysiology, and intraoperative neurophysiological monitoring must be performed adequately. This means that the need for people with neurophysiological knowledge and operating room experience will be in increasing demand for the foreseeable future.

The future will see the development of many other presently unexplored areas in which intraoperative neurophysiological recordings will become an aid to the surgeon in specific operations, and the use of neurophysiological methods in the operating room will expand as a means to study normal as well as pathological functions of the nervous system.

WORKING IN THE OPERATING ROOM

Intraoperative neurophysiological monitoring should interfere minimally with other activities in the operating room. If monitoring causes more than minimal interference, there is a risk that it will not be requested as often as it should. There is so much activity in modern neurosurgical, otologic, and orthopedic operating rooms that adding activity that consumes time will naturally be met with a negative attitude from all involved and may result in the omission of intraoperative neurophysiological monitoring in certain cases. Careful planning is necessary to ensure that intraoperative neurophysiological monitoring interferes with other forms of monitoring and the use of life-support equipment as little as possible.

How to Reduce the Risk of Mistakes in Intraoperative Neurophysiological Monitoring

The importance of selecting the appropriate modality of neuroelectric potentials for monitoring purposes cannot be overemphasized, and making sure that the structures of the nervous system that are at risk are included in the monitoring is essential. Thus, monitoring SSEP elicited by stimulating the median nerve while operating on the thoracic or lumbar spine may lead to a disaster because it is the thoracic lumbar spinal portion of the somatosensory pathway that is at risk of being injured while only the cervical portion of the somatosensory pathway is being monitored.

Monitoring the wrong side of the patient's nervous system is also a serious mistake. An example of this monitoring error is presenting the sound stimulus to the ear opposite to the side on which the operation is being performed while monitoring ABR. This kind of mistake may occur when earphones are fitted in both ears and selection of which earphone to be used is controlled by the neurophysiologist. A user error may select the wrong earphone to be used. Since the ABR is not fundamentally different when elicited from the opposite side, such a mistake will not be immediately obvious, but it will naturally prevent the detection of any change in the ear or auditory nerve as a result of surgical manipulation. The possible catastrophic consequence of failing to detect any change in the recorded potentials when the auditory nerve is injured by surgical manipulation is obvious.

Generally speaking, if a mistake can be made by the action of the user (neurophysiologist), it will be made, but it may be rare. Mistakes may be tolerated, depending on the consequences and the frequency of their expected occurrence. Mistakes can only be avoided if it is physically impossible to make the mistake. Thus, only by placing an earphone solely in the ear on the operated side can the risk of stimulating the wrong ear be eliminated. If earphones are placed in each ear, the risk of making mistakes can be reduced by clearly marking the right and left earphone and only having properly trained people operate the stimulus equipment. This will reduce the risk of mistakes but not eliminate mistakes.

In a similar way, monitoring the wrong part of the spinal cord may cause serious neurologic deficits since no change in the recorded neuroelectric potentials would be noticed during the operation. When an operation involves the spinal cord distal to the cervical spine and stimulating electrodes are placed in the median nerve as well as in a nerve of the lower limb, the median nerve may mistakenly be stimulated when the intention was to elicit evoked potentials from the lower limb. It is, however, valuable to monitor median nerve SSEP because it is a check that the positioning does not injury the brachial plexus. The considerable difference between the waveform of the upper limb SSEP and that of the lower limb SSEP may

make the mistake of watching median nerve SSEP instead of lower limb SSEP during the operation more easily detectable than mistakes made eliciting ABR by stimulating the wrong ear or when eliciting SSEP from the wrong part of the spine.

Reliability of Intraoperative Neurophysiological Monitoring

Like any other new addition to the operating room armamentaria, intraoperative neurophysiological monitoring must be reliable to enjoy routine use. It is not unreasonable to assume that if intraoperative neurophysiological monitoring cannot always be carried out (and consequently, operations are performed without the aid of monitoring), it may be assumed by the surgeon that it is not necessary at all to have such monitoring.

Reliability can best be achieved if only routines that are well thought through and which have been thoroughly tested are used in the operating room. The same methods that have been found to work well over a long time should be used consistently. New routines, or modifications of old routines, should only be introduced in the operating room after thorough consideration and testing. Procedures of intraoperative neurophysiological monitoring should be kept as simple as possible. The KISS (Keep it Simple (and) Stupid or Keep it Simple and Straightforward) principle is applicable to intraoperative neurophysiological monitoring. These matters are discussed in detail in Chaps. 17 and 18.

Electrical Safety and Intraoperative Neurophysiological Monitoring

A final, but not inconsiderable, concern is that intraoperative neurophysiological monitoring should not add risks to the safety, particularly electrical safety, of any operation. Intraoperative neurophysiological monitoring requires the addition of complex electrical equipment to an operating room already crowded with a variety of complex electrical equipment. Electrical safety is naturally of great concern whenever electronic equipment is in direct galvanic contact with patients, but this is particularly true in the operating room, where many pieces of electrical equipment are operated together, often in crowded conditions, and frequently under wet conditions. The equipment and procedures used for intraoperative neurophysiological monitoring must, therefore, be chosen with consideration for the protection of the patient as well as of the personnel in the operating room from electrical hazard. Accidents can best be avoided when those who work in the operating room and who use the electronic equipment are knowledgeable about the function of the equipment and how risks of electrical hazards that are associated with specific equipment may arise. For the neurophysiologist, it is important to have a basic understanding of how electrical hazards may occur and to specifically have an understanding of the basic functions of the various pieces of equipment used in electrophysiological monitoring. The area of greatest concern in maintaining electrical safety for the patient is the placement of stimulating and recording electrodes on the patient. It is particularly important to consider the safety of the patient that is connected to equipment by electrodes placed intracranially for either recording or stimulation (for details, see Chap. 17).

HOW TO EVALUATE THE BENEFITS OF INTRAOPERATIVE NEUROPHYSIOLOGICAL MONITORING

It is the patient that can gain the most from intraoperative neurophysiological monitoring. Many of the severe postoperative neurological deficits that were common before the introduction of intraoperative neurophysiological monitoring are now rare occurrences. It is not only the use of intraoperative neurophysiological monitoring that has enabled these improvements of medical care; better surgical techniques and various technological advancements have led to significant progress as well. There is no doubt that the introduction of microneurosurgery

(and more recently, minimally invasive surgery) has made operations that affect the nervous system less brutal than they were 25 years ago, and even the last decade has seen steady improvements in reducing complications (see also Chap. 19).

Assessment of Reduction of Neurological Deficits

It has been difficult to accurately assess the value of intraoperative neurophysiological monitoring with regard to reducing the risk of postoperative neurological deficits. One of the reasons for these difficulties is that it has not been possible to apply a commonly used method, such as double-blind methods, to determine the value of intraoperative neurophysiological monitoring. Surgeons who have experienced the advantages of intraoperative neurophysiological monitoring are reluctant to deprive their patients of the benefits provided by an aid in the operation that they believe can improve the outcome. The use of historical data for comparison of outcomes before and after the introduction of monitoring has been described in a few reports, but such methods are criticized because advancements in surgical techniques other than intraoperative neurophysiological monitoring may have contributed to the observed improvement of outcomes. Even more difficult to evaluate is the increased feeling of security that surgeons note while operating with the aid of intraoperative neurophysiological monitoring.

For the sake of evaluating future benefits from monitoring, it is important that all patients who are monitored intraoperatively be evaluated objectively before and after the operation and that the results obtained during monitoring be well documented. (For more details about evaluation of the benefit from intraoperative monitoring and neurophysiology, see Chap. 19.)

Which Surgeons Benefit Most from Intraoperative Monitoring?

Surgeons at all levels of competence may benefit in one way or another from the use of intraoperative neurophysiological monitoring, but the degree and the kind of benefit depends on the experience of the surgeon in the particular kind of operation being performed. While an extremely experienced surgeon may benefit from monitoring only in unusual situations or for confirming the anatomy, a surgeon with moderate-to-extensive experience may feel more secure and may have additional help in identifying specific neural structures when using monitoring. A surgeon with moderate-to-extensive experience will also benefit from knowing when surgical manipulations have injured neural tissue. A less-experienced surgeon who has performed only a few of a specific type of operations is likely to benefit more extensively from using intraoperative neurophysiological monitoring, and surgeons at this level of experience will learn from intraoperative monitoring and, through that, improve his/her surgical skills.

Even some extremely experienced surgeons declare the benefit from neurophysiological monitoring and appreciate the increased feeling of security when operating with the assistance of monitoring. Many very experienced surgeons are in fact not willing to operate without the use of monitoring.

In fact, most surgeons can benefit from intraoperative neurophysiological monitoring mainly by its aid in reducing the risk of postoperative neurological deficits as well as by its ability to provide the surgeon with a feeling of security from knowing when neural tissue is being adversely manipulated. Most surgeons will appreciate the aid that monitoring can provide in confirming the anatomy when it deviates from normal as a result of tumors, other pathologies, or extreme variations.

RESEARCH OPPORTUNITIES

The operating room offers a wealth of research opportunities. In fact, many important discoveries about the function of the normal nervous system, as well as about the function of the pathological nervous system, have been derived from research activities within the operating room. Neurophysiological recordings are almost the only way to study the pathophysiology of many disorders. Many important discoveries were made by applying neurophysiological methods to work in the operating room, but many discoveries were made before the introduction of intraoperative neurophysiological monitoring (20, 21), and many studies were made in connection with intraoperative neurophysiological monitoring (17, 22, 23). Some studies have concerned basic research (24), other studies have been directly related to the development of better treatment and better surgical methods (17, 22, 23), and some studies have served both purposes (17, 20, 22, 24–29).

REFERENCES

1. Brown RH and CL Nash (1979) Current status of spinal cord monitoring. Spine 4:466–78.
2. Grundy B (1983) Intraoperative monitoring of sensory evoked potentials. Anesthesiology 58:72–87.
3. Grundy B (1985) Evoked potentials monitoring, in *Monitoring in Anesthesia and Critical Care Medicine*, C Blitt, Editor. Churchill-Livingstone: New York. 345–411.
4. Raudzens PA (1982) Intraoperative monitoring of evoked potentials. Ann. N. Y. Acad. Sci. 388:308–26.
5. Jako G (1965) Facial nerve monitor. Trans. Am. Acad. Ophthalmol. Otolaryngol. 69:340–2.
6. Rand RW and TL Kurze (1965) Facial nerve preservation by posterior fossa transmeatal microdissection in total removal of acoustic tumours. J. Neurol. Neurosurg. Psychiatry 28:311–6.
7. Møller AR and PJ Jannetta (1984) Preservation of facial function during removal of acoustic neuromas: use of monopolar constant voltage stimulation and EMG. J. Neurosurg. 61:757–60.
8. House J and D Brackmann (1985) Facial nerve grading system. Otolaryngol. Head Neck Surg. 93:146–67.
9. Sekhar LN and AR Møller (1986) Operative management of tumors involving the cavernous sinus. J. Neurosurg. 64:879–89.
10. Møller AR (1987) Electrophysiological monitoring of cranial nerves in operations in the skull base, in *Tumors of the Cranial Base: Diagnosis and Treatment*, LN Sekhar and VL Schramm Jr, Editors. Futura Publishing Co: Mt. Kisco, New York. 123–32.

11. Yingling C (1994) Intraoperative monitoring in skull base surgery, in *Neurotology*, RK Jackler and DE Brackmann, Editors. Mosby: St. Louis. 967–1002.

12. Deletis V (1993) Intraoperative monitoring of the functional integrety of the motor pathways, in *Advances in Neurology: Electrical and Magnetic Stimulation of the Brain*, O Devinsky, A Beric and M Dogali, Editors. Raven Press: New York. 201–14.

13. Prass RL and H Lueders (1986) Acoustic (loudspeaker) facial electromyographic monitoring. Part I. Neurosurgery 392–400.

14. Kline DG and DJ Judice (1983) Operative management of selected brachial plexus lesions. J. Neurosurg. 58:631–49.

15. Møller AR and PJ Jannetta (1987) Monitoring facial EMG during microvascular decompression operations for hemifacial spasm. J. Neurosurg. 66:681–5.

16. Haines SJ and F Torres (1991) Intraoperative monitoring of the facial nerve during decompressive surgery for hemifacial spasm. J. Neurosurg. 254–7.

17. Møller AR and PJ Jannetta (1985) Microvascular decompression in hemifacial spasm: intraoperative electrophysiological observations. Neurosurgery 16:612–8.

18. Deletis V and JL Shils (2004) *Neurophysiology in Neurosurgery*. Amsterdam: Academic Press.

19. Shils JL, M Tagliati and RL Alterman (2002) Neurophysiological monitoring during neurosurgery for movement disorders, in *Neurophysiology in Neurosurgery*, V Deletis and JL Shils, Editors. Academic Press: Amsterdam. 405–48.

20. Penfield W and E Boldrey (1937) Somatic motor and sensory representation in the cerebral cortex of man as studied by electrical stimulation. Brain 60:389–443.

21. Ojemann GA, O Creutzfeldt, E Lettich et al (1988) Neuronal activity in human lateral temporal cortex related to short-term verbal memory, naming and reading. Brain 111:1383–403.

22. Lenz FA, JO Dostrovsky, HC Kwan et al (1988) Methods for microstimulation and recording of single neurons and evoked potentials in the human central nervous system. J. Neurosurg. 68:630–4.

23. Lenz FA, HC Kwan, RL Martin et al (1994) Single unit analysis of the human ventral thalamic nuclear group. Tremor-related activity in functionally identified cells. Brain 117:531–43.

24. Lenz FA, JO Dostrovsky, RR Tasker et al (1988) Single-unit analysis of the human ventral thalamic nuclear group: somatosensory responses. J. Neurophysiol. 59:299–316.

25. Lenz FA and NN Byl (1999) Reorganization in the cutaneous core of the human thalamic principal somatic sensory nucleus (Ventral caudal) in patients with dystonia. J. Neurophysiol. 82:3204–12.

26. Ojemann GA (1988) Effect of cortical and subcortical stimulation on human language and verbal memory. Res. Publ. Assoc. Res. Nerv. Ment. Dis. 66:101–15.

27. Ojemann GA (1975) Language and the thalamus: object naming and recall during and after thalamic stimulation. Brain Lang. 2:101–20.

28. Ojemann JG, GA Ojemann and E Lettich (1992) Neuronal activity related to faces and matching in human right nondominant temporal cortex. Brain 115:1–13.

29. Penfield W and T Rasmussen (1950) *The Cerebral Cortex of Man: A Clinical Study of Localization of Function*. New York: Macmillan.

3

Generation of Electrical Activity in the Nervous System and Muscles

INTRODUCTION

To understand why and how neuroelectric potentials, such as evoked potentials, may change as a result of surgical manipulations, it is necessary to understand the basic principles underlying the generation of such neuroelectric potentials that can be recorded from various parts of the nervous system. In this book, we discuss electrical potentials that are generated in response to intentional stimulation, and we will describe how the waveform of such recorded potentials may change as a result of injury to nerves or nuclei. It is also important to

From: *Intraoperative Neurophysiological Monitoring: Third Edition*,
By A.R. Møller, DOI 10.1007/978-1-4419-7436-5_3,
© Springer Science+Business Media, LLC 2011

understand the nature of the responses that may be elicited by surgical manipulations of neural tissue and from surgically-induced injuries. Further, it is important to know where in the nervous system specific components of the recorded evoked potentials are generated, so that the exact anatomical location of an injury can be identified on the basis of changes in specific components of the electrical potentials that are being monitored.

The potentials that can be recorded from nerves and structures of the central nervous system can be divided into three large categories: unit (or multiunit), near-field, and far-field potentials.

Unit potentials are neural discharges recorded from single nerve fibers or nerve cells; multiunit potentials are recordings of discharges from small groups of nerve fibers or nerve cells. Such potentials can be either spontaneous activity that occurs without any intentional stimulation or activity evoked by some form of stimulation. Unit or multiunit responses are recorded by placing small electrodes (microelectrodes) in direct contact with or close to nerve fibers or nerve cells. Recordings of such potentials have played important roles in animal studies of the function of the nervous system. These techniques have only recently been introduced for use in the operating room.

Near-field evoked potentials are recorded by placing a much larger recording electrode directly on or close to a nerve, a nucleus or a muscle, and these potentials represent the sum of the activity in many nerve cells or fibers in one or only a few structures. It is not always possible to record near-field potentials because it is not possible to place a recording electrode directly on the structure in question; instead, one often has to rely on far-field potentials.

Far-field potentials are recorded from electrodes that are placed at a (long) distance from the structures that generate the potentials that are being recorded. While near-field potentials, such as those recorded by placing an electrode directly on a nerve, nucleus, or muscle, reflect electrical activity in that specific structure, far-field potentials are usually mixtures of potentials that are generated by several different anatomical structures.

Far-field potentials have smaller amplitudes than near-field potentials, and their waveforms are more difficult to interpret because they represent more than one generator. The generation of far-field potentials is complex, and it is not completely understood. The contribution from such different structures depends on the distance from the recording electrode(s), as well as the properties of the sources. For example, only under certain circumstances can propagated neural activity in a long nerve generate stationary peaks in potentials recorded at a distance from the nerve. The far-field potentials generated by nuclei depend on the orientation of the dendrites of the cells in the nuclei. The

contributions from different structures to recorded far-field potentials are, therefore, weighted by factors such as the distance from the source and the rate at which the amplitudes of the recorded potentials decrease with distance to the source, which depends on the properties of the source.

Components of evoked potentials often appear as a series of temporarily separated peaks and valleys because the different anatomical structures that contribute to the potentials are activated in succession. However, components of evoked potentials from different sources may overlap, depending on whether they appear with the same, or different, latencies from the stimulus that was used to evoke the response. Therefore, the waveform of far-field potentials is usually different from that of near-field potentials, and far-field potentials are generally more difficult to interpret than near-field potentials.

Because of their small amplitude, far-field evoked potentials are usually not directly discernable from the background noise that always exists when recording neuroelectric potentials; it is, therefore, necessary to add many responses using the method of signal averaging (described in Chap. 18) so that an interpretable waveform may be obtained. The use of signal averaging to enhance a signal (evoked response) that is corrupted by noise assumes that the waveforms of all the responses that are added are the same and occur in exact time relation (latency) to the stimulus. This may not be the case when the neural system that is being monitored is affected by surgical manipulation, excess heat or anoxia. The necessity to average many responses may distort the waveform if the responses being added change (slowly) over the time during which the data are being collected and averaged and, therefore, makes the averaged response difficult to interpret. This is another reason why changes in far field-evoked potentials are more difficult to interpret than are changes in near-field potentials.

In this chapter we will discuss in greater detail, the three categories of neuroelectric potentials that are often recorded in the operating room, unit or (multiunit) potentials, near-field and far-field potentials.

UNIT RESPONSES

Unit potentials reflect the activity of a single neural element or the activities from a small group of elements (multiunit recordings). Action potentials from individual nerve fibers and from nerve cells are recorded by placing microelectrodes, the tips of which may be from a few microns to a fraction of a micron in diameter, in or near individual nerve fibers. The waveform of such action potentials is always the same in a specific nerve fiber or cell body, regardless of how it has been elicited, but the waveform of the recorded potentials depends on several factors such as the relationship between the location of the recording electrode and the nerve fiber or nerve cell from which the recording is made. Information that is transmitted in a nerve fiber is coded at the rate and the time pattern of the occurrence of such action potentials. This means that it is the occurrence of nerve impulses and their frequency (rate) that is important rather than their waveform.

The action potentials of nerve fibers are the result of depolarization of a nerve fiber. Usually, the electrical potential inside a nerve fiber is about −70 millivolts (mV). When this intracellular potential becomes less negative ("depolarized"), a complex exchange of ions occurs between the interior of the nerve fiber and the surrounding fluid through the membrane. When the electrical potential inside an axon becomes sufficiently less negative than the resting potential, a nerve impulse (action potential) will be generated, and the depolarization propagates along the nerve fiber. This depolarization (and subsequent repolarization) is associated with the generation of an action potential (also known as a nerve impulse, nerve discharge, or nerve spike). In myelinated nerve fibers (such as those in mammalian sensory and motor nerves), neural propagation occurs along a nerve fiber by saltatory conduction between the nodes of Ranvier, which can be recognized as small interruptions in the myelin sheath that covers the nerve fiber. Unit potentials have the character of nerve discharges (spikes) and are recorded by fine tipped metal electrodes that are insulated except for the tip.

The main intraoperative use of recording unit potentials is to guide the surgeon in the placement of lesions in brain structures, such as the basal ganglia or thalamus, for treatment of movement disorders and pain. More recently, lesions have been replaced by the implantation of electrodes for electrical stimulation (deep brain stimulation, DBS), which have similar beneficial effects as lesions, but with the advantage of being reversible. The responses that are observed in such operations are either spontaneous activity that occurs without any intentional stimulation, such as natural stimulation of the skin (touch), or from voluntary or passive movement of the patient's limbs. For such purposes, usually multiunit recordings are made using electrodes with slightly larger tips than those used for recording of the responses from single fibers of cell bodies. These responses represent the activity of small groups of cells or fibers. (For details see Chap. 15.)

NEAR-FIELD RESPONSES

Near-field evoked potentials are defined as potentials recorded with the recording electrode(s) placed directly on the surface of a specific neurological structure such as a nerve, fiber tracts, a nucleus, or a specific part of the cerebral cortex. Such potentials reflect neural activity in many nerve fibers or cells, but typically only in a single structure. The responses are usually elicited by transient stimuli that activate many fibers of cells at about the same time. Such responses are known as compound action potentials (CAPs) because they are the sum of many action potentials. The potentials are graded potentials, and their waveforms are specific for nerves and nuclei; the waveform changes in a characteristic way when the structure, from which recordings are made, is injured. Responses recorded from fiber tracts and nuclei are the most important for intraoperative monitoring, but recordings from specific regions of the cerebral cortex are also regarded as near-field evoked potentials.

Responses from Nerves

Near-field potentials from nerves reflect the activity in many nerve fibers; hence, it is obtained as a sum of the action potentials of many nerve fibers. The CAP recorded from a nerve or fiber tract reflect the propagation of action potentials along individual nerve fibers (axons). When a depolarization is initiated at a certain point along a nerve fiber, the depolarization propagates along the nerve fiber with a (propagation) velocity that is approximately proportional to the diameter of the axons of the nerve. The relation between neural conduction velocity (in meter per sec, m/s), and fiber diameter (in micrometers, μm) is approximately 4.5 cm/ms/(μm) (1) corresponding to 4.5 cm/ms. Older data (2) indicate a slightly higher velocity: 6 cm/ms/(μm). The conduction velocity of peripheral sensory and motor nerves typically ranges from 40 to 60 m/s (4–6 cm/ms). The auditory nerve has an unusually low propagation velocity of about 20 m/s (2 cm/ms) (3). Normally, depolarization of nerve fibers is initiated at one end of a nerve fiber (peripheral end of sensory fibers and central end of motor fibers), but neural propagation can occur in both directions of a nerve fiber, and it does so with about the same conduction velocity.

Initiation of Nerve Impulses. Initiation of nerve impulses in sensory nerves normally occurs through activation of sensory receptors (4), and motor nerves are activated through motoneurons either in the spinal cord for somatic nerves or in the brainstem for cranial motor nerves (5). In the operating room, sensory nerves are almost always activated by sensory stimuli, and motor nerves may be activated by (electrical or magnetic) stimulation of the motor cortex or the brainstem. For monitoring

purpose, peripheral nerves and cranial motor nerves are also activated by electrical stimulation. Such stimulation depolarizes axons at the location of stimulation of a nerve.

Natural Stimulation. The frequency of the action potentials in individual nerve fibers (discharge rate) is a function of the strength of the sensory stimulation (4). The time pattern of the occurrence of action potentials in a fiber of a sensory nerve elicited by sensory stimulation also carries information about the sensory stimulus in the somatosensory and the auditory nerves because the discharge pattern is statistically related to the time pattern of the stimuli, which means that the probability of the occurrence of a discharge varies along the waveform of the stimulus. This neural coding of the stimulus time pattern is of particular importance in the auditory system, in which much information about sound is coded in the time pattern of the discharges in auditory nerve fibers. The deficits in speech discrimination from injuries to the auditory nerve have been assumed to be caused by corruption of the temporal coding from uneven injuries to different nerve fibers of the auditory nerve. (The ability of the auditory nervous system to use the temporal coding of sounds for interpretation of complex sounds, such as in speech, is important for the success of cochlear and cochlear nucleus prosthesis (6), although it has been shown that speech discrimination can be obtained from the (power) spectrum of speech sounds alone (7). In the visual system, the temporal pattern of nerve impulses seems to have little importance, as is also the case in the olfactory and gustatory sensory systems.

When sensory nerves are stimulated with natural stimuli, the latency of the response from a sensory nerve decreases with increasing stimulus intensity, and this dependence exists over a large range of stimulus intensities.

One reason for this stimulus-dependent latency is the neural transduction in sensory cells (such as the hair cells in the auditory system) where the excitatory postsynaptic potential (EPSP) rises from below threshold at a rate that increases with increasing stimulus intensity, and the EPSP, thereby, reaches the threshold faster when the stimulus intensity is high, as compared to when it is low (8). Another reason for stimulus-dependent latency is the nonlinear properties of the sensory organs such as the cochlea (see Chap. 4) (9).

Electrical Stimulation. While sound stimuli (click sounds) are the most common stimulation for monitoring the auditory system, electrical stimulation of peripheral nerves is the most common way to stimulate the somatosensory system for monitoring and intraoperative diagnosis of peripheral nerves. Electrical stimulation is also in general use for stimulation of the motor cortex for monitoring motor systems (transcranial electrical stimulation).

The electrical stimulation that is used to depolarize the fibers of a peripheral nerve consists of brief (0.1–0.2 ms) electrical current impulses that are passed through the nerve that is to be stimulated. A negative current is excitatory because it causes the interior of the axons to become less negative, thus causing depolarization. This may sound paradoxical, but in fact, a negative electrical current flowing through the cross-section of a nerve fiber will cause the outside area of that nerve fiber to become more negative than the inside area, and the interior of the axon will become more positive (less negative) than its outer surface; thus depolarization occurs.

When a nerve is stimulated by placing two electrodes on the same nerve, a small distance apart, the negative electrode (cathode) is the active stimulating electrode, and the positive (anode) electrode may block propagation of nerve impulses (known as anodal block) so that depolarization will only propagate in one direction, namely away from the negative electrode.

The amount of electrical current that is necessary to depolarize the axons of a peripheral nerve and initiate nerve impulses depends on the properties of the individual nerve fibers. Large diameter axons have lower thresholds than nerve fibers with small diameters. The

threshold for depolarization also depends on the duration of the electrical impulses that are used to stimulate a nerve. Current intensity and current duration are inversely related. The necessary current to activate nerve fibers decreases when the duration of the current impulses is increased. This relationship holds until a point is reached (asymptotically) where further increases in duration have little effect on the current needed to reach threshold for depolarization. This phenomenon occurs at shorter durations for large fibers than for axons of smaller diameter. The diameters of axons of a peripheral nerve can vary considerably, and stimulation with impulses of a certain duration and at a certain intensity may, therefore, depolarize different populations of nerve fibers in a peripheral nerve.

When stimulating a nerve consisting of many nerve fibers, increasing the stimulus intensity does not change the way an electrical stimulus activates an individual axon, but it affects the number of axons that become depolarized. More axons will be depolarized when the stimulus strength is increased to just above the threshold of the most sensitive nerve fibers. The anatomical location of a nerve fiber in relation to the stimulating electrodes is a factor because the effectiveness of stimulation decreases with increasing distance.

When a normal peripheral nerve is electrically stimulated, supramaximal stimulation is usually desired, which means that the applied electrical stimulation should depolarize all axons of the nerve. It is a general rule for intraoperative neurophysiological monitoring to increase the stimulus current to approximately one-third above the current that produced a response with the maximal amplitude. This may require stimulus strength of 100 V (10–20 mA) when the stimulus duration is 0.1 ms, and the stimulating electrodes are located close to a peripheral nerve. Damaged or impaired nerves may require as much as 300 V (30–60 mA) in order to depolarize all fibers. In clinical settings, in which the patient is conscious, it is not possible to reach supramaximal stimulus levels because of unacceptable pain that such stimulation incurs, but that is not a limitation in the anesthetized patient.

Activation of individual nerve fibers of a peripheral nerve by electrical stimulation with short impulses is an "all-or-none" process and therefore, the latency of the response is little dependent, if at all, on the stimulus intensity. Only the number of nerve fibers that are activated depends on the stimulus intensity.

Monopolar Recording Compound Action Potentials from a Long Nerve

An electrode that is much larger than the size of individual nerve fibers records the sum of the nerve impulses of many nerve fibers (CAP). When a single electrode (monopolar) is placed on a nerve in which a depolarization has been initiated by a transient stimulation, the CAP has a triphasic shape (**Fig. 3.1**) with an initial (small) positive deflection that is followed by a large negative peak, which is then followed by a small positive peak.

In the example illustrated in **Fig. 3.1**, the potentials were recorded differentially between one electrode, which was placed on a nerve, and the other electrode – the reference electrode – that was placed at a distance from the recording electrode in the electrically conducting fluid that surrounded the nerve. This is an example of a monopolar recording of the CAP from a long nerve. The CAP occurs with a certain delay after the stimulus, which reflects the neural travel time from the location where the stimulus is applied and the location where the potentials are recorded. The latency of the negative peak depicts the time it takes for the depolarization of the nerve fibers to travel from the site of stimulation to the site of recording.

The depolarization of nerve fibers that elicited the CAP, such as that shown in **Fig. 3.1**, was initiated by electrical stimulation at a distance from the recording site. Similar depolarization could be initiated by a natural transient stimulus such as that of a receptor that is innervated by the nerve. When a click stimulus is applied to the ear, transient excitation of auditory nerve fibers occurs, and a CAP similar to the one shown in **Fig. 3.1** can be recorded from the exposed auditory nerve (see Chaps. 5 and 7).

The initial positive deflection of the CAP recorded from a long nerve occurs when the

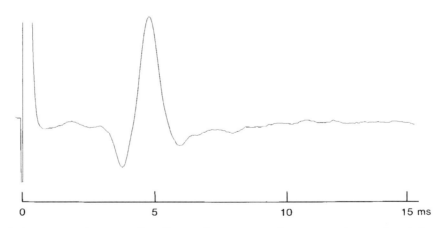

Figure 3.1: Monopolar recording from a long nerve of propagated neural activity elicited by electrical stimulation with a brief impulse of current passed through the nerve far from the location of recording. Notice the stimulus artifact at the beginning of the trace. The electrode placed on the nerve was connected to the inverting input of the amplifier, and the electrode that was placed away from the nerve was connected to the non-inverting input. This arrangement caused negativity to be shown as an upward deflection (as it is in all illustrations in this book).

depolarization in the nerve approaches the location of the recording electrode (**Fig. 3.2A**). The large negative peak is generated when the depolarized portion of the nerve is directly under the recording electrode (**Fig. 3.2B**). The small positive deflection that follows is generated when the zone of depolarization moves away from the recording electrode (**Fig. 3.2C**). The width of the negative peak is related to the length of the depolarization and the propagation velocity of the nerve. A long area of depolarization or a slowly moving region of depolarization yields a CAP with a wide negative peak.

Since recording of CAP in **Figs. 3.1** and **3.2** is done using differential recording techniques, it is the difference in the potentials recorded between two recording electrodes that is measured. To make a true monopolar recording, it must be assured that the reference electrode will not record any potential that is related to activity in the nerve. In real recording situations, this is often difficult to achieve because the reference electrode will also record evoked potentials, although of a lesser amplitude, than the active electrode will record.

Effects of Temporal Dispersion of Action Potentials. When a nerve is stimulated by an electrical impulse, and all the nerve fibers that discharge (depolarize) have identical properties so that the action potentials in all of the nerve fibers occur simultaneously, then the waveform of the CAP recorded by a monopolar recording electrode placed on a long nerve is mathematically described as the second derivative of the waveform of an action potential of an individual nerve fiber (*10*). The action potentials of different nerve fibers elicited by electrical stimulation are assumed to arrive at the site of recording simultaneously, so that the action potentials of different nerve fibers coincide. In such a situation, the amplitude of the negative peak in the CAP is a measure of the number of nerve fibers that have been activated (*11*).

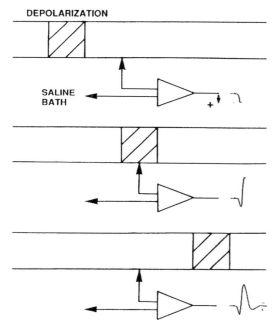

DEPOLARIZATION

SALINE BATH

Figure 3.2: Illustration of how the CAP recorded from a long nerve by a monopolar electrode develops. The nerve is being stimulated electrically at a location to the far left (not shown), and the resulting area of membrane depolarization (marked by the cross-hatched area) travels from left to right. The recorded electrical potentials that develop as the area of depolarization propagates along the nerve are shown to the right. The electrode that is placed on the nerve was connected to the inverting input to the amplifier and the inactive electrode placed in the saline bath away from the nerve was connected to the non-inverting input of the amplifier.

The situation that exists when recording from mammalian peripheral nerves is different because such nerves are composed of nerve fibers with different conduction velocities. The action potentials in individual nerve fibers, therefore, do not occur exactly at the same time at a certain point along a nerve. The shape of the CAP, therefore, depends on the distribution of the arrival time of the discharges in the different nerve fibers at the site of recording. This in turn is a function of the conduction velocity and the length of travel of nerve impulses in the fibers that make up the nerve from which the recording is made. This means that the waveform of the CAP will reflect the distribution of the differing diameters of nerve fibers (conduction velocities) and the distance between the site of stimulation and that of the recording.

Such time dispersion will broaden the recorded CAP compared to what it would have been if the action potentials in all the nerve fibers arrived at the recording site accurately aligned in time. Also, the amplitude of the CAP will be lower than it would have been if all nerve impulses traveled at the same velocity. The mathematical description of the recorded CAP in such a situation is the convolution between the waveform of an individual action potential of a nerve fiber and the distribution of action potentials in the nerve fibers that make up the respective nerve (*11*). This assumes that the waveforms of the action potentials of all nerve fibers are identical. In such a situation, it is the area under the negative peak of the CAP that is a measure of the number of nerve fibers that have been activated rather than the amplitude of the negative peak.

Depending on how great the dispersion is, the waveform of the CAP may differ from a triphasic waveform to a waveform with several peaks. If there are specific subgroups of nerve fibers in a nerve with similar conduction velocities, the activity in such subgroups may give rise to multiple peaks in the CAP. The late peaks move further away from the initial peak when recorded at a longer distance from the location of stimulation (**Fig. 3.3**). The effect on the waveform of the recorded CAP from a nerve with subgroups of nerve fibers with different conduction velocities is dependent on the size of the variations in neural conduction velocity in the individual nerve fibers, and the distance between the site of stimulation and the site of recording (**Fig. 3.3**).

Not all nerve fibers of a peripheral nerve may contribute equally to the CAP; depending on the recording situation, some nerve fibers may contribute more than others. The mathematical solution of the generation of the CAP from a peripheral nerve may, therefore, require that different weighting factors be applied to

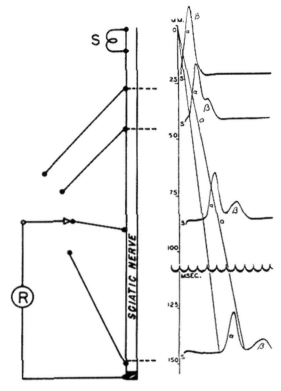

Figure 3.3: Recording of CAP from a nerve in which there are groups of fibers with different conduction velocities. Recordings at different distances from the site of electrical stimulation (*S*) are shown (Reprinted from (*12*) with the permission from Elsevier).

the contribution to the CAP from different populations of the nerve fibers that make up a peripheral nerve.

Determining the Number of Active Nerve Fibers. In the operating room, the task is not to determine the absolute number of active nerve fibers, but rather to obtain an estimate of the proportion of nerve fibers of a specific nerve that has been rendered inactive due to surgical insults. An increase in the latency of the response and/or a change in the waveform of the recorded CAP are perhaps the two most important indicators of injury to a nerve, and these measures are therefore used extensively in intraoperative monitoring as indicators of injury to a nerve and fiber tracts. Monitoring the amplitude of the CAP is also important in intraoperative monitoring because of its relation to how many fibers are activated and how close together in time the action potentials of individual nerve fibers appear.

> The area of the negative peak in the CAP offers an accurate measure of the number of nerve fibers that have been activated. Because it is the change in the number of active nerve fibers that is of interest in connection with intraoperative monitoring, measuring changes in the amplitude of the negative peak provides a sufficiently accurate measurement for most tasks in the operating room, although this measure also includes the effect of increased dispersion due to increased difference in conduction velocity of individual nerve fibers.

It is worth mentioning that a monopolar recording electrode placed on a nerve will also record potentials that are conducted passively to the recording site. This is because a nerve, in addition to conducting propagated neural activity, also conducts other kinds of activity because it is an electrical conductor. For a sensory nerve, this would mean that a monopolar recording electrode may record electrical activity that is generated in the target nucleus. This is, for example, the case when recording from the intracranial exposed auditory nerve in response to click stimulations. Such a recording includes the triphasic potentials generated by the propagated activity in the nerve and activity generated in the cochlear nucleus (see Chap. 7).

Bipolar Recording from a Nerve

Bipolar recordings from a long nerve can be realized by placing a pair of recording electrodes that are connected to the two inputs of a differential amplifier close together on the nerve in question (**Fig. 3.4**). The output of the differential amplifier will be the difference between the potentials that are recorded by each individual electrode. A bipolar recording from a nerve in which neural activity is propagated produces a waveform that differs from

DEPOLARIZATION

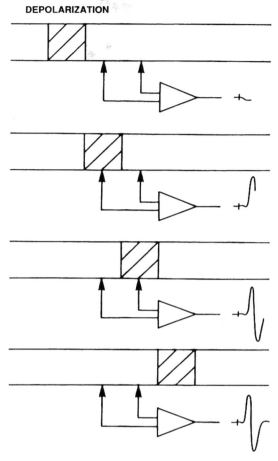

Figure 3.4: Bipolar recording from a long nerve, illustrated in the same way as the monopolar recording in **Fig. 3.2**. The two electrodes are connected to the two inputs of the differential amplifier in such a way that a negative potential at the electrode closest to the recording site (left-hand electrode) will result in an upward deflection (inverting input).

that of monopolar recordings. Two such electrodes act as two monopolar electrodes that are placed on a nerve, and the output of the amplifier is the difference between these two "monopolar" recordings. When a wave of depolarization approaches the electrode, the one closest to the depolarization will record a larger positive potential than the electrode that is further away (**Fig. 3.4**). A large negative potential will be recorded by the electrode that is close to the site of stimulation when the region of depolarization reaches the site of that electrode, and an upward (negative) deflection in the output of the differential amplifier will be produced. As the area of depolarization reaches the second electrode, the output of the amplifier will be a downward deflection because a large negative potential will be subtracted from a positive potential recorded by the electrode closest to the stimulation site. When the depolarization progresses further along the nerve, the output of the differential amplifier may show a small, upward deflection (negative potential) because the second electrode records a positive potential, while the first electrode records a smaller positive potential.

A bipolar electrode placed on a long nerve generally records only propagated neural activity. Passively conducted electrical potentials will appear at both electrodes with the same amplitude and exactly the same waveform and thus, do not generate any output of the differential amplifier that is connected to the bipolar electrodes. Propagated activity on the other hand will appear at the two electrodes with a certain time delay and, therefore, will generate a noticeable output at the differential amplifier. This means that the output of the differential amplifier (that is connected to such a pair of electrodes that are placed close together on a long nerve) would be equal to the difference between the potentials recorded by one of the electrodes and the potentials' delayed replicas, the delay being the time it takes for the propagated neural activity to travel the distance between the two electrodes. If the distance is 2 mm and the propagation velocity is 20 m/s or 20 mm/ms (as it approximately is in the intracranial portion of the auditory nerve in humans), the delay would be 1/10 ms = 100 μS. The waveform and amplitude of the recorded potentials that appear at the output of the differential

amplifier, connected at its input to a pair of electrodes, will thus depend on the distance between the two recording electrodes in relation to the length of the area of the nerve that is depolarized.

The waveform of the recorded potentials will change in a specific way when the distance between the two electrodes is varied. **Fig. 3.5** shows the waveform of a simulated bipolar recording during which the distance between the two electrodes was varied. This simulation was realized by subtracting the response recorded by a monopolar recording electrode from that same response after it had been delayed. The delay was varied to simulate different distances between two electrodes. It was assumed that a bipolar recording electrode records the difference between the potentials that are recorded at two locations along a nerve, and that the only difference between the potentials recorded by two such electrodes would be that they appear with a small difference in latency, the amount of which would be equal to the distance between the two electrodes divided by the propagation velocity.

If there is a difference between such calculated (simulated) bipolar recordings and actual bipolar recordings (**Fig. 3.5B**), it would mean that either the bipolar electrodes recorded other potentials than the propagated neural activity, or that the propagated neural activity had undergone a change while it traveled the distance between the two tips of the bipolar electrode so that it appeared with different waveforms or amplitudes at the two electrodes. The latter seems unlikely, and it may be justified to assume that any difference between actual and simulated bipolar recordings is a result of both of the bipolar recording electrodes picking up passively conducted neural activity. A difference in the actual recorded bipolar response versus that calculated on the basis of recording from only one electrode and shifting that recording in time could occur if the two electrode tips were placed on slightly different parts of the nerve (i.e., the two tips of the bipolar electrode not being properly aligned with regard to the course of the nerve fibers of the nerve), or because the two electrodes were different in size or geometry.

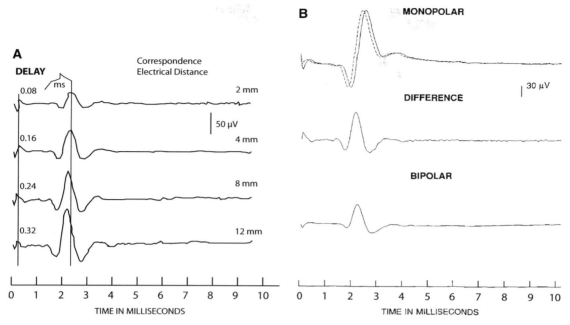

Figure 3.5: (**A**) Simulated bipolar recording from a long nerve on which the distance between the recording electrodes was varied. (**B**) Comparison between an actual bipolar recording (*lower tracing*) and a simulated bipolar recording using one of the bipolar electrode tips as a monopolar electrode (*middle tracing*). The *upper tracing* shows the monopolar recording together with a time-shifted version (*dashed lines*). The reference electrode was placed a long distance from the monopolar recording (*13*).

Unfortunately, it is often more difficult in practice to use bipolar recordings from a nerve when monitoring neural conduction intraoperatively and therefore, many operations limit the use of bipolar recording electrodes. (For more details about practical arrangements for recording from nerves, see Chap. 4.)

Responses from Muscles

Individual muscle fibers are organized into motor units, which are groups of muscle fibers that are activated by the same motor endplate. When nerve fibers of a motor nerve are activated normally or are electrically stimulated, motor endplates are activated, and the motor units that are innervated by the fibers that are activated will contract. Transmission of impulses from a motor nerve to a muscle is chemical in nature. The impulses elicit the release of a transmitter substance (acetylcholine) from the motor nerve. Acetylcholine binds to receptors on the motor endplate and initiates a series of events, which cause muscle fibers to contract and the generation of electrical events that are similar to those generated in single nerve fibers (for details in this process, see textbooks in neuroscience such as (*14*)). Because the process that occurs in the muscle endplates takes 0.5–0.7 ms, the earliest electrical activity that can be recorded from the muscle is delayed relative to the arrival of the neural activity at the muscle endplate. The electrical events that can be recorded in connection with contraction of muscles are electromyographic (EMG) potentials or compound muscle action potentials

(CMAPs). The CMAPs are equivalent to the CAP recorded from a nerve.

It is important to note that the paralyzing agents that are used in many anesthesia regimens abolish such muscle potentials. Use of such agents makes recording of EMG potentials impossible. Muscle relaxants used in connection with anesthesia are of two types: substances that block transmission in muscle endplates (the curare type of substances), and succinylcholine that causes a constant depolarization of the muscle endplates and thereby, prevents muscle contractions. Such drugs can, therefore, not be used when recordings of muscle activity are to be done as a part of intraoperative monitoring (see Chaps. 10 and 16). EMG potentials and CMAP can be recorded by placing electrodes on the surface of the skin close to the muscle, or from needle or wire hook electrodes placed in a muscle, or by surface electrodes placed on the skin over the muscles in question. The use of needle or wire hook electrodes for recording EMG potentials is usually preferred for intraoperative monitoring because it is more specific and yields larger and more stable potentials than recordings

using surface electrodes, which also are likely to include responses from several muscles. Recording from surface electrodes, therefore, makes it difficult to differentiate the responses from individual muscles compared with recording differentially from a pair of needle electrodes placed in the same muscle.

EMG recordings may be made by placing a single electrode on or in a muscle (monopolar recording) or by placing two electrodes in a specific muscle (bipolar recording). These two forms of recordings produce EMG potentials with different waveforms when a muscle is activated by a single electrical impulse applied to its motor nerve (**Fig. 3.6**).

Responses from Fiber Tracts

The neural activity that propagates in individual nerve fibers in a fiber tract in the central nervous system is similar to that in a peripheral nerve, namely, as a series of neural discharges. Recordings may be made directly from fiber tracts in the spinal cord in intraoperative neurophysiological monitoring of the motor system, such as from the corticospinal tract, which are done routinely (see Chap. 10).

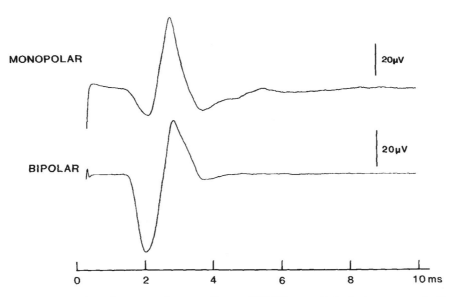

Figure 3.6: Comparison between the waveform of EMG potentials that are recorded by a single electrode (monopolar recording) and a pair of electrodes (bipolar recording).

Response from Nuclei

The near-field response from clusters of nerve cells (nuclei) is more complex than those from a nerve or a nerve tract because the nerve cells of a nucleus generate different kinds of electrical potentials. Generally, a nucleus generates two distinctly different kinds of electrical potentials when activated by a transient volley of neural activity in the nerve or fiber tract that serves as its input. One kind of potential is fast, and one is slow. When recorded by a monopolar electrode, the initial component of the response to transient activation is a sharp, positive–negative complex, which is usually followed by a slow potential (**Fig. 3.7A**). Several peaks may be riding on the slow potential (**Fig. 3.7B**). The slow potential is generated by dendrites, and the sharp peaks that are riding on that slow wave are generated by firings of cells (somaspikes). The duration of the initial sharp peaks of the response is about the same as that of the CAP recorded from a nerve (0.5–2 ms). These initial fast components are generated when neural activity in the fiber tract that serves as the input to the nucleus reaches the nucleus.

The initial, fast potentials are generated by the termination of the nerve in the nucleus, and this component shows a similar waveform no matter where on the surface of the nucleus the component is recorded (**Fig. 3.7A**). The size

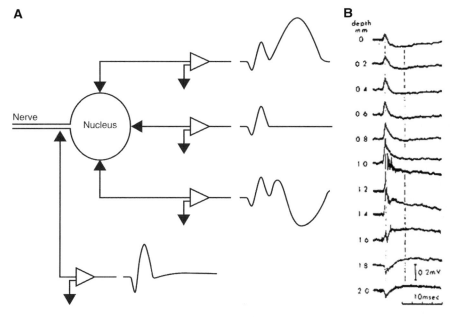

Figure 3.7: Responses that can be recorded from the surface of a nucleus. (**A**) Schematic illustration of the potentials that may be recorded from the surface of a sensory nucleus in response to transient stimulation such as a click stimulation for the auditory system. The three waveforms shown refer to recordings at different locations on the nucleus to illustrate the dipole concept for describing the potentials that are generated by a nucleus. The waveform of the response that can be recorded from the nerve that terminates in the nucleus is also shown. (**B**) Schematic illustration of the responses that may be obtained from the cunate nucleus to stimulation of the median nerve at the wrist. The recording electrode was passed through the nucleus, and the *traces to the right* show the recorded potentials at different locations (From Andersen P, Eccles JC, Schmidt RF and Yokota T. Slow potential wave produced by the cunate nucleus by cutaneous volleys and by cortical stimulation (*15*) with permission from the American Physiological Society).

and the polarity of the slow potential, however, depend on the location on a nucleus from which the slow potential is recorded (**Fig. 3.7A**). The slow potential is assumed to be generated by dendrites, and it has the property of a dipole. An electrode placed on one side of a nucleus will record a negative slow potential (top recording in **Fig. 3.7A**), while an electrode placed on the opposite side will record a positive potential. Placed in between these two locations, the electrode will record very little of the slow potential (**Fig. 3.7A**), but only the initial positive–negative deflection is seen.

When the recording electrode is placed close to cell bodies, it records a positive potential because the electrode has been placed close to a source of current. A negative potential is recorded when the electrode is placed away from the cell bodies, but close to their dendritic trees because the electrode is then close to a "current sink."

The amplitude and the distribution of the potentials on the surface of a nucleus depend on the internal organization of the nucleus. Nuclei in which there is an orderly arrangement of the cells with dendrites pointing in the same direction produce responses of higher amplitude than nuclei in which the dendrites point in different directions.

Recordings from the cuneate nucleus of the cat (*15*) have helped understand how nuclei can generate near-field potentials (**Fig. 3.7B**). An electrode is passed through a nucleus; the polarity of this slow potential will reverse at a certain point along the course of the recording electrode (**Fig. 3.7B**). This is why the generator of evoked potentials from a nucleus is often likened with that of a dipole source: positive if recordings are made from one side of the nucleus and negative if the recordings are made from the opposite side. If the recording electrode is placed at a point equidistant from these two sides of the imaginary dipole, it will not record any response because the positive and negative contributions are equal (**Fig. 3.7A**).

The description of the response from a nucleus shown in **Fig. 3.7A** applies generally to sensory nuclei (such as the cochlear nucleus and the

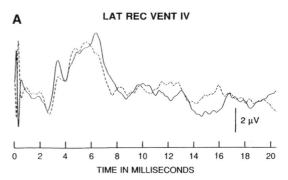

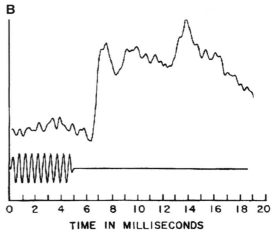

Figure 3.8: Typical response from nuclei recorded by a monopolar electrode. (**A**) The recordings obtained from the surface of the cochlear nucleus in a patient undergoing an operation to relieve HFS. The stimuli used to elicit the response were click sounds. The *solid lines* show the response to rarefaction clicks and the *interrupted line* shows the response to condensation clicks. (Reprinted from (*16*) with permission from Elsevier.) (**B**) Responses recorded from the exposed inferior colliculus in a patient operated on to remove a pineal body tumor. The responses were elicited by 2-kHz tone bursts (Reprinted from (*17*) with permission from Elsevier).

inferior colliculus in humans) in response to click stimulation are seen in **Fig. 3.8A, B**, respectively.

The sharp peaks that often are seen riding on the slow potentials in recordings from the surface of a nucleus such as those seen in **Fig. 3.8A, B** are assumed to be generated by firings of cells (somaspikes). These sharp peaks occur with longer latencies than the initial positive–negative deflection because of the delay in synaptic transmission in the nucleus.

FAR-FIELD POTENTIALS

The response that can be recorded from an electrode placed at a long distance from a nerve or a nucleus that is surrounded by an electrically conductive medium is known as a far-field response. For the purpose of intraoperative monitoring recording, far-field potentials are recorded when it is not possible to place electrodes directly on the active structures. Generally, the amplitudes of far-field potentials are much smaller than those of near-field potentials, and the waveforms of far-field potentials differ from those of near-field potentials. Far-field potentials often have contributions from several different sources. If these sources are activated sequentially, the contributions will appear in the recorded potentials with different latencies because of the delays in neural transmission. Contributions from individual sources that are activated simultaneously may not be easily discernable in the recordings because they are likely to overlap in time.

Most theories about how far-field potentials are related to the electrical activity of nerves, fiber tracts, and nuclei have been based on the concept that different neural structures can be regarded as independent generators of electrical activity in a way similar to that of a dipole. This means that nerves, fiber tracts, and nuclei, can be viewed as sources of electrical current that at any given time are positive at one anatomical location and negative at another. When this theory is applied to the electrical activity that is generated by a nerve, the dipole in question is not stationary, but moves along the nerve with the propagation of the neural activity in the nerve. The dipoles of nuclei are mainly stationary, but may change after the initial activation because different parts of a nucleus may

be activated sequentially in response to a transient stimulus.

The amplitude of the potentials that can be recorded from an electrode placed on the scalp in response to transient stimulation of a sensory system, such as the auditory system, depends not only on the strength of the dipoles that represent the neural activity in the different structures of the auditory pathways, but also on the (three dimensional) orientation of these dipoles in relation to the placement of the recording electrodes. The distance from the recording electrodes to the structures in question also plays a role, as does the electrical properties of the medium between the recording site and the active neural structures. The electrical resistance of the skull bone affects far-field potentials recorded from the brain by electrodes placed on the scalp.

While various recording techniques are discussed later in this book, some basic principles of recording far-field evoked potentials must be mentioned here. Ideally, when recording far-field potentials, one of the two recording electrodes connected to a differential amplifier should be placed as close to the source as possible (even though this location may be at a considerable distance), while the other recording electrode (often called the "reference electrode" or the "indifferent electrode") should be placed far away from the source from which the recordings are being made so that it records as little as possible of the potentials that are generated by the part of the nervous system that is being studied. When recording neural activity from the brain, the best way to achieve that is by placing the reference electrode outside the head (noncephalic reference) (*18–20*). The practice of using such a noncephalic reference makes interpretation of the potentials easier, and it provides better correspondence between the far-field potentials and the near-field potentials, thus, facilitating identification of the neural generators of the different components of far-field potentials. However, it is not always possible to achieve this ideal situation, and in many instances both of the two recording electrodes that are connected to a differential amplifier will record considerable evoked potentials from the system that is being tested, and the recording will show the difference between the potentials that appears at the two locations where the recording electrodes are placed.

Nerves and Fiber Tracts

The neural activity that is propagated in a nerve or a fiber tract does not always generate stationary peaks in a far-field recording. This is because the neural depolarization that is elicited by a single transient stimulation propagates continuously along the nerve and does not generate any stationary peaks in a far-field recording unless certain conditions are filled (*21*):

1. The propagated activity stops as it does when a nerve terminates in a nucleus.
2. A nerve is bent (*22*).
3. The electrical conductivity of the medium that surrounds the nerve in question changes (*23–25*).

Stationary peaks in far-field potentials can, therefore, be produced when a nerve or a fiber tract passes through a bony canal from one fluid-filled space to another, which, for example, occurs when the spinal cord passes through the foramen magnum or the auditory nerve where it emerges from the internal auditory meatus (porus acusticus).

Nuclei

A nucleus may be regarded as one, or several, stationary electrical dipoles with a certain orientation in space. If the neuron's dendrites are all oriented in nearly the same direction, the (slow) far-field potentials that are generated by these dendrites will be large (**Fig. 3.9**). The cerebral cortex is one example of a neural structure with a highly organized dendritic field in which large dendritic trees point in nearly the same direction (**Fig. 3.9A**), and this orientation results in the generation of a large far-field potential. The amplitudes of the far-field potentials generated by a nucleus, with dendrites pointing in all directions (**Fig. 3.9B**), will be small and may not

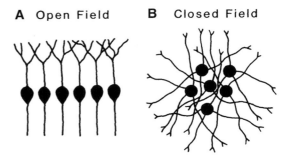

Figure 3.9: Two different types of organization of cells in a nucleus. (**A**) Open field. (**B**) Closed field. Modified from (*26*). (Reprinted with the permission from Wiley).

be measurable at all. Such a nucleus is said to have a closed electrical field (*26*). A seemingly paradoxical situation may, therefore, arise in which a nucleus, despite the fact that it may have a large near-field potential, may not contribute measurably to the far-field potentials because of its internal organization; whereas another nucleus, in which many dendrites point in the same direction, may contribute significantly to the far-field potentials, although it may produce smaller near-field potentials. In practice, it is difficult to find nuclei with an internal organization of just one such type; most nuclei have an organization that is somewhere between these two extremes.

In addition to potentials generated by dendrites, cell bodies in a nucleus may produce sharp peaks in the far-field potential when discharging (somaspikes).

EFFECT OF INSULTS TO NERVES, FIBER TRACTS AND NUCLEI

The changes in the recorded neuroelectric potentials that are caused by changes in function of specific parts of the nervous system are the basis for interpreting the results of intraoperative neurophysiological monitoring. Various forms of surgical insults to nerves and nuclei result in characteristic changes in recorded neuroelectric potentials, which can make it possible to diagnose different forms of injury.

The Injured Nerves

The responses (CAP) from injured nerves have different waveforms than those recorded from a normal nerve. It is important to understand the meaning of these differences for proper diagnosis of injuries to peripheral nerves. (Trauma to peripheral nerves is discussed in detail in Chap. 12.)

Most forms of insults to a nerve reduce its conduction velocity, thus, increasing the latency of the CAP recorded proximal to the injury when elicited by stimulation at a location that is distal to the recording site. If neural conduction in a fraction of the nerve fibers of a nerve is blocked, the amplitude of the negative peak in the CAP decreases. Similar changes in the CAP may occur when nerves are subjected to mechanical manipulation or injury from, for instance, heating such as may occur from electrocoagulation near the nerve. The magnitude of the decrease in amplitude of the negative peak is a measure of approximately how large a fraction of the nerve fibers have ceased to conduct nerve impulses. If the conduction velocity in different nerve fibers is affected differently by an insult, such as stretching or heating, temporal dispersion of the nerve impulses will occur and cause the negative peak of the CAP to become broader because the action potentials in different nerve fibers will appear at different times at the site of recording.

Stretching of a nerve can increase the conduction time (decrease the conduction velocity) of all nerve fibers or a fraction of the fibers of a nerve. The decreased conduction velocity causes the latency of the CAP to increase. The waveform of the recorded CAP may become more complex and have multiple peaks as a result of insults to a nerve if the injury causes different groups of nerve fibers to have different degrees of prolonged conduction times.

If a total conduction block in all nerve fibers in a peripheral nerve occurs between the stimulation site and the recording site, it will abolish the negative peak of the CAP that is recorded

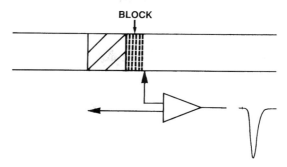

Figure 3.10: Monopolar recording from an injured nerve in which the propagation of a zone of depolarization stops before it reaches the recording electrode.

by a monopolar recording electrode because the depolarization caused by the stimulation will not pass under the recording electrode as it does normally. A total conduction block causes the initial positivity in the CAP to dominate the recorded waveform (**Fig. 3.10**). This is known as the "cut-end" potential. Likewise, a single positive deflection will be recorded if the recording electrode is placed beyond the end point of a nerve. Thus, the CAP recorded from a nerve where the neural conduction is blocked by, for instance, crushing of the nerve so that the propagation of the zone of depolarization no longer passes under the recording electrode, the waveform of the recorded potentials changes from the typical triphasic shape to a single positive deflection.

If the site of injury occurs beyond the location of the (monopolar) recording electrode, little change in the recorded potentials may be seen. Such a situation could occur, for example, when recording evoked potentials from the peripheral portion of the auditory nerve (at the ear) in response to click stimulation during operations in which the intracranial portion of the auditory nerve is being surgically manipulated. No change in the response recorded from the distal portion of a nerve is likely to be detected even after the occurrence of a severe injury to the proximal (central) portion of the nerve, or even severance of the proximal portion of the nerve (see Chap. 7).

The Injured Nuclei

Insult to nuclei can cause complex changes in the recorded evoked potentials. Synaptic transmission is more sensitive to insults such as anoxia and cooling than is the neural conduction in nerves and fiber tracts. Insults that affect synaptic transmission will cause a change in the slow potentials, but leave the fast, positive–negative deflection in the beginning of the response unchanged. Anesthetics act on synapses and may, thus, affect the function of nuclei (see Chap. 16).

REFERENCES

1. Desmedt JE and G Cheron (1980) Central somatosensory conduction in man: neural generators and interpeak latencies of the far-field components recorded from neck and right or left scalp and earlobes. Electroencephalogr. Clin. Neurophysiol. 50:382–403.
2. Gasser H (1941) The classification of nerve fibers. Ohio J. Sci. 41:145–59.
3. Møller AR, V Colletti and FG Fiorino (1994) Neural conduction velocity of the human auditory nerve: bipolar recordings from the exposed intracranial portion of the eighth nerve during vestibular nerve section. Electroencephalogr. Clin. Neurophysiol. 92:316–20.
4. Møller AR (2003) Sensory Systems: Anatomy and Physiology. Amsterdam: Academic Press.
5. Møller AR (2006) Neural Plasticity and Disorders of the Nervous System. Cambridge: Cambridge University Press.
6. Møller AR (2006) History of cochlear implants and auditory brainstem implants, in *Cochlear and Brainstem Implants*, AR Møller, Editor. Karger: Basel. 1–10.
7. Loizou PC (2006) Speech processing in vocoder-centric cochlear implants, in *Cochlear and Brainstem Implants*, AR Møller, Editor. Karger: Basel. 109–43.
8. Møller AR (1975) Latency of unit responses in the cochlear nucleus determined in two different ways. J. Neurophysiol. 38:812–21.
9. Møller AR (2000) Hearing: Its Physiology and Pathophysiology. San Diego: Academic Press.
10. Lorente de Nó R (1947) Analysis of the distribution of action currents of nerve in volume conductors. Stud. Rockefeller Inst. Med. Res. Repr. 132:384–482.
11. Goldstein Jr. MH (1960) A statistical model for interpreting neuroelectric responses. Inf. Control 3:1–17.
12. Erlanger J and HS Gasser (1937) Electrical Signs of Nervous Activity. Philadelphia: University of Pennsylvania Press.
13. Møller AR, V Colletti and F Fiorino (1994) Click evoked responses from the exposed intracranial portion of the eighth nerve during vestibular nerve section: bipolar and monopolar recordings. Electroencephalogr. Clin. Neurophysiol. 92:17–29.
14. Kandel ER, JH Schwartz and TM Jessell (2008) Principles of Neural Science. New York: Oxford University Press.
15. Andersen P, JC Eccles, RF Schmidt et al (1964) Slow potential wave produced by the cunate nucleus by cutaneous volleys and by cortical stimulation. J. Neurophys. 27:71–91.
16. Møller AR, PJ Jannetta and HD Jho (1994) Click-evoked responses from the cochlear nucleus: a study in human. Electroencephalogr. Clin. Neurophysiol. 92:215–24.
17. Møller AR and PJ Jannetta (1982) Evoked potentials from the inferior colliculus in man. Electroencephalogr. Clin. Neurophysiol. 53:612–20.
18. Cracco RQ and JB Cracco (1976) Somatosensory evoked potentials in man: farfield potentials. Electroencephalogr. Clin. Neurophysiol. 41:460–66.
19. Desmedt JE and G Cheron (1981) Non-cephalic reference recording of early somatosensory potentials to finger stimulation in adult or aging normal man: differentiation of widespread N18 and contra-lateral N20 from the prerolandic P22 and N30 components. Electroencephalogr. Clin. Neurophysiol. 52:553–70.
20. Møller AR and PJ Jannetta (1984) Neural generators of the brainstem auditory evoked potentials, in *Evoked Potentials II: The Second International Evoked Potentials Symposium*, RH Nodar and C Barber, Editors. Butterworth Publishers: Boston, MA. 137–44.
21. Kimura J, A Mitsudome, T Yamada et al (1984) Stationary peaks from moving source in far-field recordings. Electroenceph. Clin. Neurophys. 58:351–61.
22. Jewett DL, DL Deupree and D Bommannan (1990) Far field potentials generated by action potentials of isolated frog sciatic nerves in a spherical volume. Electroencephalogr. Clin. Neurophysiol. 75:105–17.

23. Kimura A, A Mitsudome, DO Beck et al (1983) Field distribution of antidromically activated digital nerve potentials: models for far-field recordings. Neurology 33:1164–9.

24. Lueders H, RP Lesser, JR Hahn et al (1983) Subcortical somatosensory evoked potentials to median nerve stimulation. Brain 106: 341–72.

25. Stegeman DF, A van Oosterom and EJ Colon (1987) Far-field evoked potential components induced by a propagating generator: computational evidence. Electroencephalogr. Clin. Neurophysiol. 67:176–87.

26. Lorente de Nó R (1947) Action potentials of the motoneurons of the hypoglossus nucleus. J. Cell Comp. Physiol. 29:207–87.

4

Practical Aspects of Recording Evoked Activity from Nerves, Fiber Tracts, and Nuclei

INTRODUCTION

Intraoperative neurophysiological monitoring employs methods and techniques similar to those currently used in the clinical neurophysiology laboratory, but there are several important differences between recording sensory evoked potentials and EMG potentials for diagnostic purposes in the clinic and for doing so in order to detect changes in neural function during an operation. The operating room is usually regarded as an electrically hostile environment, which differs

From: *Intraoperative Neurophysiological Monitoring: Third Edition*,
By A.R. Møller, DOI 10.1007/978-1-4419-7436-5_4,
© Springer Science+Business Media, LLC 2011

from the clinical neurophysiological laboratory where the recording of EMG responses and sensory evoked potentials, such as ABR, SSEP, and VEP, are usually made in electrically and acoustically shielded rooms. In the operating room, many other kinds of electronic equipment are connected to the patient. Equipment, which is used to monitor the patient's vital parameters for electrocoagulation, drilling of bone, etc., may interfere with neurophysiological monitoring. In the clinic, however, usually only the equipment used for the recordings in question is connected to the patient. Therefore, knowing how to identify and reduce electrical interference is another important matter in connection with intraoperative monitoring (discussed in detail in Chap. 17).

Another difference between work in the operating room and in the clinical physiological laboratory is related to the fact that in the operating room it is difficult to correct the placement of electrodes, earphones, and other equipment on the patient after the patient is draped. This, of course, puts great importance on the correct placement of electrodes for recording neuroelectric potentials and for electrical stimulation, as well as of other devices involved in stimulation (such as earphones), before the operation begins.

Reducing the potential for making mistakes is of critical importance when performing intraoperative neurophysiological monitoring. Since the results of monitoring must be available immediately, there are few possibilities for correcting mistakes.

Advanced planning and organization is essential for successful execution of any form of intraoperative neurophysiological monitoring. It is of significant importance that everything that is needed for monitoring is available and brought into the operating room before the operation begins, including spares of sterile items that may get contaminated during the operation. Using a checklist reduces the risks of making potential mistakes.

Everything that is needed for the monitoring to be performed should be prepared and ready well in advance of the operation. The computer, stimulators, and amplifiers should be set up for the particular recording to be made in each individual case so that the collection of data can begin immediately after the placement of the electrodes, earphones, etc.

Intraoperative neurophysiological monitoring equipment is constantly moved in and out of operating rooms, and this movement exerts strain on equipment, especially cables and connectors. It is important to bring the equipment into the operating room well in advance of the beginning of an operation so that the equipment can be checked and possible malfunctions can be corrected before it is to be used.

PREPARING THE PATIENT FOR MONITORING

When sensory evoked potentials are to be monitored, preoperative assessment of the patient's sensory functions should be obtained before the operation. If auditory evoked potentials are to be monitored, the patient must have a hearing test which includes pure tone audiograms and speech discrimination tests before the operation. If SSEP are to be monitored intraoperatively, the patient must have similar recordings of SSEP performed preoperatively. In a similar way, if motor systems are to be monitored, it must be ensured that the patients (preoperatively) have the motor functions that are to be monitored. The motor functions must be assessed before the operation.

Before the patient is brought to the operating room, it must be planned what to monitor and how to monitor, and the placement of electrodes for recording and stimulation must be planned in detail. When the patient is brought to the operating room, the monitoring team should introduce themselves and briefly explain what they are going to do and *why* which is important for the patient. It is naturally better for the monitoring team to introduce themselves to the patient the evening before the operation if the patient is in the hospital at that time.

Careful planning of the details of the intraoperative monitoring makes it possible to stimulate and record promptly when the patient has been anesthetized. In this way, the necessary setup and patient preparations are performed without interference from, or delay to, the rest of the surgical team. In some cases, it is possible to place the stimulating and recording electrodes before the patient is anesthetized.

Recording and Stimulating Electrodes

Several different types of electrodes are used for electrical stimulation and for recording of near-field and far-field potentials, and all have advantages and disadvantages. Needle electrodes and wire hooks that are applied percutaneously are often used, but surface electrodes that are applied to the skin are commonly used as well. Which type of electrode is chosen depends on factors such as safety concerns and the possibility of obtaining reliable stable recordings over a long period of time. Surface electrodes can conveniently be applied before the patient is brought to sleep. However, the electrode wires must be taped to the patient so they are not affected by moving the patient to the operating table. Needle or wire hook electrodes should not be applied before the patient is brought to sleep.

Regardless of the type of electrodes that are chosen, it is important that all electrodes stay in place throughout the entire operation because it is often not possible to gain access to the location where they were applied after the sterile drape has been placed. If recording or stimulating electrodes are to be applied after the patient has been anesthetized, it is also important that the electrodes can be applied quickly so that precious operating time is not wasted. At this time, before the operation begins, there are usually other preparations, such as shaving the head or preparing the skin, that must be performed by the operating room staff, and there is usually enough time to place even a large number of needle or wire hook electrodes in different locations while these other prepara-

tions are being made. Surface electrodes can be applied before the patient is anesthetized and even before the patient is brought into the operating room so that this task does not interfere with other activities involving the patient.

Platinum or steel needle electrodes or wire hook electrodes are suitable for recordings as well as for delivering electrical stimulation. It is important to observe the risks of acquiring potentially serious diseases in the operating room through contact with blood and accidentally acquired needle punctures. It is, therefore, recommended to use disposable needle electrodes. If platinum reusable needle electrodes are used, they must be cleaned and prepared according to the manufacturer's recommendations and handled carefully after use for the safety of the operating room personnel. Attention should also be made to the safe disposal of disposable needle and wire hook electrodes. The same precautions as are taken for hypodermic needles should be used.

When placed percutaneously to record from the body surface and secured with a good-quality plastic adhesive tape (such as, Blenderm™[1]), needle or wire hook electrodes provide stable recordings and electrical stimulation for many hours. Such electrodes are practically impossible to remove from the skin unintentionally. It is rare to have a needle electrode dislodge accidentally during an operation. The impedance of such electrodes may be slightly higher than that of some types of surface electrodes. Usually, this does not create any problems, and the impedance of needle or hook wire electrodes rarely increases noticeably during an operation.

The most common malfunction of electrodes is caused by the electrode becoming partly or completely disengaged from the patient, which increases the electrode impedance. Electrodes that are used for recording pick up more electrical interference; therefore, a sign that the electrode is coming loose is the display of an increased noise level on a recording channel. Determination of which one of the two electrodes that are connected to a differential amplifier is faulty can be

---

[1] 3M Center, St. Paul, MN 55144-1000.

determined by using the option provided by most modern amplifiers to measure electrode impedance. A malfunctioning electrode has a higher than normal electrode impedance.

Adverse effects of using needle electrodes in the form of infection or postoperative marks on the skin are rare. Within a few days after the operation, it is usually impossible to identify the sites where the needle electrodes had been placed.

When using needle electrodes or wire hook electrodes during operations, it is important that the electrocautery equipment that is used during the procedure is of high quality and has an efficient return electrode pad placed on the patient (usually the thigh). If the return connection is faulty, any electrodes placed on the patient that are in contact with grounded (electronic) equipment may carry some of the high-frequency current that is used for electrocautery back to the electrocautery generator. This may cause burns where the electrophysiological recording electrodes are placed on the skin (and possibly lead to the destruction of the electronic recording equipment as well). The degree of skin injury is inversely related to the surface area of the electrodes, and because needle electrodes or wire hook electrodes have a much smaller surface area than surface electrodes, the burns can be expected to be more severe when needle electrodes or wire hook electrodes are used compared with surface electrodes. Nevertheless, while performing intraoperative monitoring in several thousand patients, sometimes with as many as 20 electrodes placed on the same patient, this author has never seen any burn marks from electrodes or any indication that excessive current had passed through the recording electrodes, despite the fact that the recording electrodes in nearly all of these patients were in place during the first phase of the operation, when high-powered monopolar electrocautery was used for cutting purposes.

Before the recording electrodes are applied to the patient and connected to the respective amplifiers, the power to the amplifiers should be switched on because electrical surges may result from switching recording amplifiers on.

If the patient is first connected to the amplifier and then the amplifier is turned on, these electrical surges may be harmful. In the same way, equipment should not be turned off before all electrodes have been removed from the patient.

When needle electrodes or wire hook electrodes are used, they must be removed carefully from the patient when the operation is completed in order to avoid injury to the patient's skin. This is naturally of particular importance when electrodes are placed in the face. Needle electrodes and wire hook electrodes should be removed one at a time, first removing the adhesive tape that holds them in place and then pulling the needle out while gently pulling the wire in the opposite direction in which the needle was inserted. With some experience this can be done in a short time, even in cases in which many electrodes are placed in the face or in other places on the body. Disposable needle electrodes or wire hook electrodes should be disposed of in a safe way (such as in a sharps box) in order to minimize the possibility of anyone being stuck by electrode needles that have been inserted into a patient. Reusable needles or wire hook electrodes should be dropped in a solution of sodium hypochlorite for a few minutes. It is practical to place a bucket with sodium hypochlorite solution under the operating table so that the needle electrodes can be dropped into the bucket immediately after they are removed from the patient without being touched. Afterward, the electrodes may be washed, rinsed, and then sterilized (either using an autoclave or gas sterilization) in accordance with the manufacturer's directions.

When handling needle electrodes or wire hook electrodes, it must always be assumed that any patient can have a disease, such as hepatitis B or C and HIV, etc., which can be transmitted through blood borne pathogens. The same precautions that are taken when handling hypodermic needles used for injection purposes must be taken when handling needle electrodes or wire hook electrodes. The person who places and removes needles from patients before and after intraoperative monitoring must be adequately trained in handling infected needles and informed about the protocols that must be followed.

Earphones

Earphones used when recording auditory evoked potentials can be placed while other activity involving the patient is in progress. When miniature stereo earphones are used, they should be secured in the ear with adhesive tape in a watertight fashion to prevent fluids from reaching the ear canal. The earphone should be placed so that the sound-emitting surface of the earphone faces the opening of the ear canal. Before an earphone is placed in the ear, the ear canal should be inspected. In some elderly persons, the ear canal opening is nearly a narrow slit that may occlude when an earphone is placed in the ear. A short plastic tube of a suitable diameter placed in the ear canal can hold it open before the earphone is placed in the ear.

When insert earphones are used, this is not a problem because the ear canal is kept open by the tube that is inserted in the ear canal and conducts the sound to the ear. When insert earphones are used, it is important that the tube that is inserted in the ear canal fits well and is well secured so that it is not accidentally pulled out during the operation. The person who is to apply the earphones to the patient should inspect the patient's ear beforehand to assess any special needs.

Light Stimulators

Commercially available goggles with built-in light-emitting diodes are used in the clinic, but are not suitable for use in the operating room. Protective contact lenses with light-emitting diodes are a better option for eliciting VEP in anesthetized patients. The pattern-reversal visual stimulators that are used clinically cannot be used intraoperatively because it is not possible to focus the conventionally used checkerboard pattern on the retina of a patient who is anesthetized and draped for surgery. Only flash stimulation can be used in the operating room. Other forms of light sources suitable for eliciting VEP in the operating room use fiber optic

cables to connect the light from a source to the eye. This makes it possible to use high intensity light (see Chap. 18).

Electrical Stimulation of Nervous Tissue

Electrical stimulation of peripheral nerves and cranial nerves is perhaps the most common way of activating nervous tissue for monitoring purpose. For stimulating peripheral nerves, needles are suitable as are wire hook electrodes, and for transdermal stimulation surface electrodes can be used. Intracranial stimulation can be accomplished with hand-held stimulators; either monopolar or bipolar electrodes are used, depending on how specific stimulation is anticipated. Some investigators have developed surgical instruments with built-in electrical stimulators for the purpose of detecting when specific nervous tissue is manipulated with the surgical instrument (1).

Electrical stimulation of the motor cortex is in increasing use for monitoring motor systems. The most commonly used technique is TES using electrodes placed on the scalp (see Chap. 10). The voltages used are in the ranges from 500–1,000 V, thus much higher than what is used for the stimulation of nerves, and special precautions are necessary to ensure safety. Various kinds of stimulating electrodes have been used, but "cork screw" types of electrodes are probably the most commonly used types of stimulating electrodes. Such stimulation can only be used in anesthetized patients because of the excessive pain that it would cause in an awake individual. In operations where the motor cortex is exposed, direct stimulation that requires much less voltage can be applied.

Recordings from the exposed cerebral cortex are made for identifying the location of the central sulcus. For that purpose, plastic strips with a string of four to eight electrodes or fields of 4×4 or 8×8 electrodes are used and placed directly on the exposed cerebral cortex (Chap. 14).

The stimulators that deliver constant current or (semi) constant voltage impulses should be chosen depending on the circumstances. For stimulating peripheral nerves, constant current stimulators are most suitable, and for intracranial stimulation, constant voltage stimulators are most suitable. (The choice of stimulator type is discussed in detail in Chap. 18).

Magnetic Stimulation of Nervous Tissue

Magnetic stimulation is used to stimulate peripheral nerves or CNS structures, such as the cerebral cortex (transcranial magnetic stimulation, TMS). Magnetic stimulation involves applying an impulse or a train of impulses of a strong magnetic field to the structure in question and is accomplished by placing a coil through which a strong electrical current is passed over the structure that is to be stimulated. It is not the magnetic field that causes the activation of neural tissue, but rather the induced electrical current. Magnetic stimulation has advantages over electrical stimulation in that it can activate nerve and brain tissue noninvasively (extracranial) and without causing any pain. Disadvantages, such as the equipment being bulky, difficulties of generating trains of impulses, and effect on metallic objects nearby, has almost eliminated its use in the operating room.

DISPLAY OF RESULTS

Modern equipment offers a wealth of different ways of displaying evoked potentials, such as "water fall" or "stack" displays, that show successive records stacked on top of each other. Various forms of trend analysis, such as the change in amplitude and latency of specified components, are also often included in commercially available equipment. However, probably the most useful way of displaying evoked potentials is a single curve that is superimposed on a similar recording obtained at the beginning of the operation (baseline).

It is practical to use auto-scaling of the recorded potentials so that the averaged potentials can be viewed on a full screen in order to detect changes in the amplitudes of the evoked potentials. When auto-scaling is used, the amplitude must be displayed numerically on the screen so that the amplitude of the baseline

recording can be compared with the amplitudes of the averaged potentials that are recorded during the operation. (Using auto-scaling makes the waveform of the recorded potentials appear on the screen as if it always had the same amplitude.)

RECORDING OF NEAR-FIELD POTENTIALS

Near-field potentials can almost always be recorded from muscles and peripheral nerves while near-field potentials from the central nervous system can only be recorded intraoperatively in special situations. Therefore, evoked potentials from the central nervous system are normally recorded at a distance from the sources, thus "far-field" potentials.

Recording from Muscles

Recording of electromyographic potentials is now the most common way of recording responses from muscles, although other methods that make use of the measurements of movement of muscles have also been in use (2–5). Recordings of EMG potentials provide accurate information about which muscle is being activated, and such recordings make it possible to detect muscle contractions that are too small to be detected visually. EMG potential recordings also offer a quantitative way to assess not only if a specific muscle is activated or not, but it also assesses the degree to which the muscle is activated. EMG recordings permit accurate measurement of latencies, thus, making it possible to determine neural conduction velocities (and particular, changes in neural conduction velocity) during an operation. EMG recordings thereby make it possible to assess neural conduction in motor nerves and to detect conduction blocks in portions of nerves.

Continuous monitoring of neural activity in motor nerves by recording EMG activity from muscles innervated by both spinal and cranial motor nerves is useful for detecting the effects of surgical manipulations of motor nerves. Monitoring of EMG activity can also detect muscle activity elicited by mechanical stimulation of motor nerves and neural activity that may occur as a result of injury to the respective motor nerve. Detection of such mechanically-evoked EMG activity or activity caused by injury makes it possible to alert the surgeon so that the particular manipulation can be stopped. Such information can also help to avoid a similar injury in the remaining course of the operation and in future operations.

Making the recorded EMG activity audible is important because it can relate information about manipulations of motor nerves to the surgeon directly. The character of the sounds that EMG signals emit provides important information about the nature of the effects of surgical manipulations on the function of the motor nerve. Listening to the EMG sounds helps distinguish between severe injury and benign stimulation of a motor nerve. Making the muscle responses audible can alert the neurophysiologist without the necessity of continuously monitoring a computer screen, and it makes it possible for the surgeon to hear the continuous muscle activity that often results from surgical manipulation of a motor nerve (such as the facial nerve), which may indicate that the manipulation is causing injury to the nerve. Making EMG activity audible provides rapid feed-back to the surgeon about surgical manipulation that may be harmful to a nerve.

Rapid feedback to the surgeon is also important when mapping the surgical field with an electrical stimulating handheld electrode to determine where a motor nerve is located. Such mapping of the surgical field is important when removing tumors that adhere to a motor nerve. It may be even more important for finding regions of a tumor that do not contain a motor nerve so that the tumor can be removed safely one section after another without the fear of injuring a nerve.

Some commercial equipment have the option of allowing the EMG signal to trigger a tone signal intended to warn that the amplitude of the EMG potentials has exceeded some preset value. However, the unprocessed EMG signal contains much information that such

tone signals cannot communicate. Having EMG activity trigger tone signals may also be confusing because other equipment in the operating room often generates similar "beeps," and it may be difficult to distinguish EMG-elicited "beeps" from that of equipment such as that used by the anesthesia team.

Electrodes that are used for recording EMG potentials from superficial muscles may be needle electrodes, wire hook electrodes, or surface electrodes. Needle electrodes or wire hook electrodes tend to provide more stable recordings over a longer time than surface electrodes. Needle electrodes can be placed more precisely than surface electrodes, and needle electrodes can reach muscles that are located beneath the body surface such as, for example, the extraocular muscles (Chap. 11).

Monitoring the Function of Peripheral Nerves

In the operating room, the most common way of monitoring the function of peripheral nerves involves electrical stimulation of the nerves and recording of the CAPs from the nerves in question. Needle electrodes are suitable for both purposes. When recording from nerves that are surgically exposed, other kinds of stimulating and recording electrodes may be used (see Chap. 13).

Recordings from Fiber Tracts, Nuclei, and the Cerebral Cortex

For intraoperative monitoring, near-field potentials have been recorded from the intracranial portion of the auditory nerve, the cochlear nucleus, the cerebral cortex, and from the surface of the spinal cord to record from the corticospinal tract. Such recordings can be made by placing a single electrode on the structure in question, which allows the recording of evoked potentials from specific portions of the nervous system without including the recordings of potentials from other parts of that same system that may also respond to the stimulus. Using bipolar recording electrodes provides more spatial specificity than using monopolar recording electrodes. However, it is not always practical or possible to place a bipolar recording electrode on the structure from which recording is to be made.

Electrodes for intracranial stimulation and recording are placed by the surgeon, and the tasks of the monitoring team are, therefore, reduced to make sure that electrodes are available and transferred to the sterile field at the time they are to be placed by the surgeon and that the recording electrode is properly connected to the amplifier via the electrode box. Although the electrodes and a part of their connecting wires are located within the sterile field, the electrode box that is used to connect the electrodes to the amplifier is outside the sterile field. The wires connecting the intracranial electrodes to the electrode box must be carried in and out of the sterile field in a safe way. It is important that the wires are secured well so that the intracranial electrodes cannot be disengaged from the wound by an accidental pull of the wires that connect them to their respective electronic equipment.

The parts of these electrodes that have been in contact with the patient must be discarded, but all other parts may be cleaned carefully at the end of the operation and sterilized (gas) before being used again.

RECORDING OF FAR-FIELD POTENTIALS

Far-field evoked potentials are recorded from electrodes placed on the surface of the body. Sensory evoked potentials, such as ABR and SSEP, are commonly recorded modalities for intraoperative monitoring, while VEP are monitored in fewer operations. Such potentials typically contain responses from many different sources, which make interpretation more difficult than near-field potentials. Of practical importance is the fact that far-field potentials have a much smaller amplitude than near-field potentials; more important, however, is that the amplitude is often smaller than that of the background activity, thus a low SNR. This requires the use of signal processing methods,

such as signal averaging and filtering, to increase the SNR sufficiently to make it possible to interpret the recorded potentials (Chap. 18).

Placement of Recording Electrodes

The interpretation of far-field evoked potentials depends on the electrode placement. Far-field sensory evoked potentials are traditionally recorded differentially from two electrodes that both record the evoked potentials in question, although to a different degree; these kinds of recordings contribute to the difficulties in interpreting sensory evoked far-field potentials. Interpretation of far-field sensory evoked potentials are also complicated by the fact that several neural generators contribute to the response, and some of these components may overlap in time. Electrodes placed at different locations on the scalp record the various components differently, not only because of the different distances to the individual sources, but also more so because of the orientation of the dipoles of these sources. These matters are discussed in more detail in Chaps. 6, 7, and 8.

A few investigators have used electrode placement where the evoked potential that is recorded with one of the two electrodes is negligible (noncephalic reference). Recorded in this way, sensory evoked potentials are easier to interpret.

It is practical to always use the same electrode montage for a particular type of monitoring.

ELECTRICAL INTERFERENCE

One of the greatest differences between recording neuroelectric potentials in the operating room and the clinical physiology laboratory is the presence of many sources of electrical and magnetic interference in the operating room. Some forms of such electrical interferences can be reduced with appropriate measures while other kinds of interference cannot be reduced so their effect on recordings of electrical potentials from the nervous system and muscles must be reduced by other means, such as signal averaging and filtering (see Chap. 17).

There are two main kinds of electrical interference that appear in an operating room. One kind is always present in a specific operating room while the other kind occurs only occasionally.

Continuous Electrical Interference

Continuous interference signals should be reduced as much as possible at the source and should be done well in advance of doing actual intraoperative monitoring. Ideally, the operating room should be examined when it is not in use and without any time constraints, such as late afternoon the day before monitoring is scheduled in an operating room in which the monitoring team does not have the experience of monitoring (as described in Chap. 17).

Interference that Appears Intermittently During an Operation

Interference that can appear suddenly during an operation must be dealt with promptly. Its source must be identified and the interference eliminated with as short a delay as possible because monitoring cannot be done while the interference exist. The operation is not going to stop and that means that the patient does not have the protection of intraoperative monitoring until the interference is eliminated and recordings resume. Intermittent interference may be caused by any one of the numerous pieces of equipment used by the anesthesia team. For example, switching on a blood warmer that had not been used previously in the operation can generate interference. Another example of intermittent interference during the course of an operation is biological interference. Intraoperative monitoring of neuroelectric potentials involves the level of anesthesia of the patient, which may vary during an operation and can fall so low that spontaneous muscle contractions occur. Such muscle contractions cause interference in the recorded neuroelectric potentials if the EMG potentials are picked up by the electrodes used to record the evoked potentials.

If intraoperative monitoring is going to be successful, it is necessary to identify the sources and the natures of interferences within a very short time. It is, therefore, important that the neurophysiologist observe not only the averaged potentials, but also directly observe the recorded potentials continuously, and that he/she be able to distinguish between external electrical interference and interference that is of a biological origin, such as muscle activity. Promptly remedying problems related to suddenly appearing interference is one of the most challenging tasks of a monitoring team. It is important that the person who does the neurophysiological monitoring has enough experience to be able to quickly identify the source of the interference.

The use of electrocoagulation is an example of a strong intermittent kind of electrical interference that in most cases makes it impossible to do recordings of neuroelectric potentials. It cannot be avoided, and the only way to reduce its effect is to exclude recordings when electrocoagulation is done. The fact that the electrical interference almost invariably exceeds the dynamic range of the amplifiers used to record sensory evoked potentials may make it necessary to take special precautions in addition to the normally used artifact rejection options that are included in equipment to be used in the operating room (Chap. 17).

HOW TO ACHIEVE OPTIMAL RECORDINGS

Several factors affect the time it takes to obtain an interpretable record and there are many ways to shorten the time needed to obtain an interpretable recording of sensory evoked potentials and other small amplitude evoked potentials. The following list summarizes the factors that are important for obtaining a clean interpretable record in as short a time as possible:

1. Decrease the electrical interference that reaches the recording electrodes.
2. Use optimal stimulus repetition rate.
3. Use optimal stimulus strength.

4. Use optimal filtering of the recorded potentials.
5. Use optimal placement of recording electrodes.
6. Use quality control that does not require replicating records.

Decrease the Electrical Interference that Reaches the Recording Electrodes

Electrical interference increases the time it takes to obtain an interpretable recording of sensory evoked potentials, and it can influence many other kinds of recordings. The background signal noise can be electrical interference and/or biological signals, such as EMG potentials, from nearby muscles. Also, ongoing brain activity (electroencephalographic, EEG activity) is a source of interference that can obscure evoked potentials when recording from electrodes placed on the head. Reducing electrical interference that reaches the recording amplifiers is, therefore, very important, especially when monitoring sensory evoked potentials. There are many sources of such interference in the modern operating room. Sources of interference and ways to reduce the effect of electrical interference on the recordings that are done for monitoring sensory systems and other kinds of recordings are discussed in detail in Chap. 17.

Selection of Stimulus and Recording Parameters

Optimizing stimulation, the selection of optimal recording parameters, and the reduction of electrical interference are all factors that can increase the SNR of the recorded responses and, thereby, shorten the time it takes to obtain an interpretable record when signal averaging is used such as for the recording of far-field sensory evoked potentials. However, these factors have received less attention than deserved.

We discuss how to select the optimal stimulus and recording parameters in the chapters that cover monitoring of the different sensory systems (Chaps. 6, 7, and 8).

Optimal Processing of Recorded Responses

It would be ideal to be able to record responses that are clearly discernable from that of the background signal noise that always exists in recordings taken in the operating room so that the responses may be interpreted directly when recorded. Normally though, special processing of the recorded responses, such as signal averaging and/or appropriate filtering, must be performed in order to obtain an interpretable record. These matters are discussed in Chap. 18. The equipment should be set up according to such requirements, and appropriate parameters for amplification and filtering should be selected and set before the placement of electrodes on the patient.

Optimal Placement of Recording Electrodes

The amplitude of the recorded responses depends on the placement of the recording electrodes. Since it is not the level of the background noise that is important, but rather the ratio between the amplitude of the signal and the noise (SNR) that is important, the improvement of recorded evoked potentials, such as far-field sensory evoked potentials, can be achieved by increasing the amplitude of the recorded potentials. It is, therefore, important to use the optimal placement of the recording electrodes.

Quality Control of Evoked Potentials

Quality control of evoked potentials is performed in the clinical laboratory by repeating the recording to see if it replicates. This obviously implies doubling of the recording time, and since it is important to obtain an interpretable record as soon as possible when evoked potentials are used in intraoperative monitoring, other methods for quality control that do not require extra recording time have been described. These matters are discussed in Chap. 18.

In general, it is important that the recording strategy is planned ahead of the time when the operation begins and that recording and stimulation parameters are set before the patient is brought into the operating room. Baseline recording, of ABR, SSEP, or VEP should be made after the patient is anesthetized, but before the operation begins, and it is best done while the sterile drape is being placed, but before the use of electrocautery starts.

RELIABILITY OF INTRAOPERATIVE MONITORING

Another important difference between performing neurophysiological recordings in the clinical neurophysiological laboratory and in the operating room is that in the clinic, there is always time to replace an electrode that has slipped off or to repair or replace a piece of equipment if it fails to function, and if this is not possible within a reasonable time, the patient can usually be rescheduled for the test, or there could be another test room available where the test can be performed. No such possibility exists during intraoperative neurophysiological monitoring; if some equipment malfunctions, it either has to be fixed within a very short time or the operation continues without the aid of intraoperative neurophysiological monitoring. The most common problem of this type is that one or more of the electrodes used for the monitoring may stop functioning (having a high resistance). Also, the breakdown of any part of the electronic equipment used for monitoring may make it impossible to complete the intraoperative monitoring. In addition, in the operating room the sudden appearance of electrical interference, the cause of which cannot be ascertained, results in the neurophysiologist having to stop the intraoperative monitoring, whereas in the clinical laboratory such an occurrence almost never occurs because electrical interference from other equipment is not a factor.

Since any one of these problems may make continued monitoring in the operating room more difficult or impossible, it is very important that the person who is actually performing the monitoring (neurophysiologist) be prepared for a variety of problems and knows beforehand how to solve each problem. In the clinic, a technician can be called, but in the operating room there is no time for waiting on a technician to arrive. The person who is responsible for intraoperative neurophysiological monitoring must have sufficient experience and knowledge to be able to identify sources of electrical interference and to locate malfunctioning electrodes or equipment and solve the problem.

Naturally, the highest quality electronic equipment provides the most reliable service, but it is important that backup electronic equipment be available for use within a very short time. Having spare cables and electrodes available in the operating room is important, and it is wise to have redundant electrodes placed on the patient where manipulation during the operation may occur. A common factor for all such problems is that they appear when not expected.

REFERENCES

1. Kartush J and K Bouchard (1992) Intraoperative facial monitoring. Otology, neurotology, and skull base surgery, in *Neuromonitoring in Otology and Head and Neck Surgery*, J Kartush and K Bouchard, Editors. Raven Press: New York. 99–120.
2. Jako G (1965) Facial nerve monitor. Trans. Am. Acad. Ophthalmol. Otolaryngol. 69:340–2.
3. Silverstein H, E Smouha and R Jones (1988) Routine identification of the facial nerve using electrical stimualtion during otological and neurotological surgery. Laryngoscope 98:726–30.
4. Shibuya M, N Matsuga, Y Suzuki et al (1993) A newly designed nerve monitor for microneurosurgey: Bipolar constant current nerve stimualtor and movement detector with pressure sensor. Acta Neurochir. 125:173–6.
5. Sugita K and S Kobayashi (1982) Technical and instrumental improvements in the surgical treatment of acoustic neurinomas. J. Neurosurg. 57:747–52.

SENSORY SYSTEMS

Understanding the anatomy and physiology of sensory systems is a prerequisite for understanding the changes in recorded responses from sensory systems that may occur as a result of surgical manipulation. Without understanding the anatomy of the systems that are being tested during various kinds of operations and their normal physiology, it is not possible to evaluate changes that may occur during operations and relate such recordings to the potential risk of permanent postoperative deficits. The auditory and the somatosensory systems are the sensory systems that are most often monitored intraoperatively, while the visual system is monitored in operations to a lesser degree. The other sensory systems (olfaction and taste) have not been the object of intraoperative monitoring.

In addition to describing the anatomy and physiology of sensory systems (Chap. 5), this section also includes chapters that explain the technique of monitoring both far- and near-field sensory evoked potentials. Specifically, the technique of monitoring somatosensory evoked potentials (SSEP) (Chap. 6), auditory brainstem responses (ABR) (Chap. 7), and visual evoked potentials (VEP) (Chap. 8) are described.

5

Anatomy and Physiology of Sensory Systems

INTRODUCTION

The receptors and the nervous system of our five sensory systems report events that occur outside the body to the brain as well as events that occur inside the body. Some of these events create conscious awareness while others do not. Some of the activation of sensory systems produces conscious awareness, whereas other sensory activation occurs without producing any awareness. Sensory information from the body itself is known as unconscious proprioception, and this kind of sensory activation occurs in the somatosensory system. A second type of sensory activation, exteroception, is concerned with events from outside the body such as touch, vibration, heat, and cold. Hearing, vision, taste, and olfaction are also senses of events from outside the body, thus, they too are included as sensations of exteroception. When the stimuli for these senses exceed the threshold for activation, they almost always cause awareness. Proprioception, such as that which occurs in the somatosensory system, can take place without creating any awareness, or it can cause awareness, for example, of the position of a limb. Conscious proprioception provides information about orientation of the body, movements of limbs, etc. The unconscious proprioception provides feedback to the motor

From: *Intraoperative Neurophysiological Monitoring: Third Edition*,
By A.R. Møller, DOI 10.1007/978-1-4419-7436-5_5,
© Springer Science+Business Media, LLC 2011

system from receptors in muscles, tendons, and joints. This part of the somatosensory system is essential for controlling movements, and the loss of such feedback causes serious movement faults. Unconscious proprioception might be regarded as a part of the motor system rather than a part of the somatosensory system. The somatosensory system is, therefore, closely associated with the motor system.

Monitoring the sensory system is an important part of intraoperative monitoring. Knowing the anatomy and physiology of sensory systems is essential for being able to deliver high-quality intraoperative monitoring. Of our five sensory systems, the somatosensory system is probably the most important from a monitoring point of view because of its association with the motor system. It is monitored in many kinds of operations on the spine and the spinal cord. It is also monitored in aneurysm surgery associated with the middle cerebral artery. The reason that hearing is monitored is often for reducing the risk of injury to the auditory nerve, but it also plays a role for monitoring the general condition of the brainstem. Monitoring of the visual system is performed only in a few operations, such as those to resect pituitary tumors. Intraoperative monitoring of taste and olfaction has not been described.

THE SOMATOSENSORY SYSTEM

Intraoperative monitoring of somatosensory evoked potentials (SSEP) has mainly been employed in operations on the spine and the spinal cord such as operations that include fixation with instrumentation after trauma, corrective operations (for instance, scoliosis), and other operations on the spine where the spinal cord may be at risk due to surgical manipulation. Monitoring of SSEP is also essential in operations on the spinal cord, such as resection of spinal tumors, tethered cord syndrome (tissue attachment of the cord), and for syringomyelia (a cyst in the spinal cord). The spinal cord can also be at risk of being damaged in operations that affect its blood supply, which pose risks to the spinal cord from ischemia, such as in operations for aorta aneurysms. Compromised blood supply to the part of the spinal cord that generates the SSEP (mainly the dorsal part) can be detected by monitoring SSEP. Ischemia to parts of the brain that is involved in the generation of SSEP can also be detected by monitoring SSEP.

The somatosensory system includes the sense of touch, vibration, heat, cold, and pain, and not to forget, unconscious and conscious proprioception from muscles, tendons, and joints. This part of the somatosensory system is essential for normal motor function, which depends on proper feedback provided by the proprioceptive system.

This part of this chapter describes the anatomy and physiology of the somatosensory system that is important as a basis for intraoperative recordings of SSEP for monitoring the integrity of the somatosensory nervous system.

Sensory Receptors

The normal input to the somatosensory system is mechanical stimulation of receptors in the skin, muscles, tendons, and joints. This means that the somatosensory system has input from receptors that sense both external (exteroception) and internal events (proprioception). Exteroception that the somatosensory system receives is mediated by receptors in the skin that are sensitive to touch, vibration, and warm and cool temperatures.

The different types of receptors that provide the input to the somatosensory system respond to different forms of mechanical stimulation. Receptors in the skin respond to touch, vibration, and temperature (warmth and cold), and nociceptors respond to painful stimuli including hot and cold. Receptors in muscles provide unconscious proprioception and respond to the length of the muscles. Receptors in tendons measure the stretch of tendons, and receptors in joints are sensitive to pressure. Receptors in internal organs, such as the intestines, are sensitive to stretching and chemicals such as those associated with ischemia.

The particular aspects of the receptors that provide the input to the somatosensory system are of minor importance for intraoperative monitoring where electrical stimulation of sensory nerves is the common way of stimulation. For a detailed description of sensory receptors, see for example Møller 2003, (*1*).

Ascending Somatosensory Pathways

The peripheral nerve fibers that receive input from sensory receptors of the body enter the dorsal horn of the spinal cord as dorsal roots (**Fig. 5.1**) and ascend in the dorsal column of the spinal cord on the ipsilateral side to terminate in cells in the dorsal column nuclei

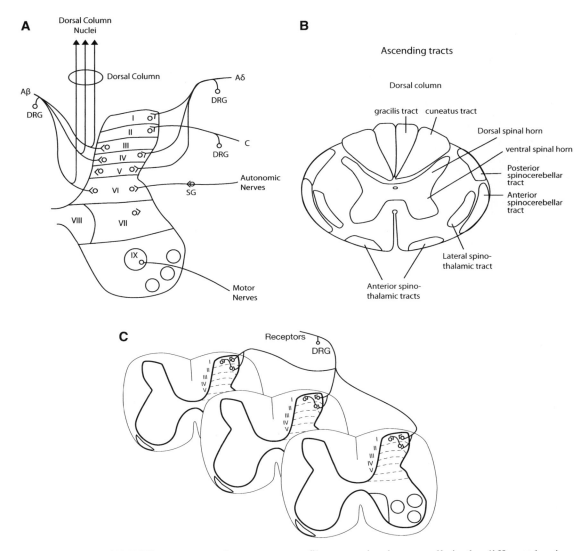

Figure 5.1: (**A**) Different types of sensory nerve fibers terminating on cells in the different lamina of the horn of the spinal cord (Rexed's classification (*2*)). (**B**) Anatomical localization of ascending tracts in the spinal cord. Based on Brodal 2004 (*74*). (**C**) Illustration of how dorsal root sensory fibers send ascending and descending branches to two adjacent segments of the spinal cord.

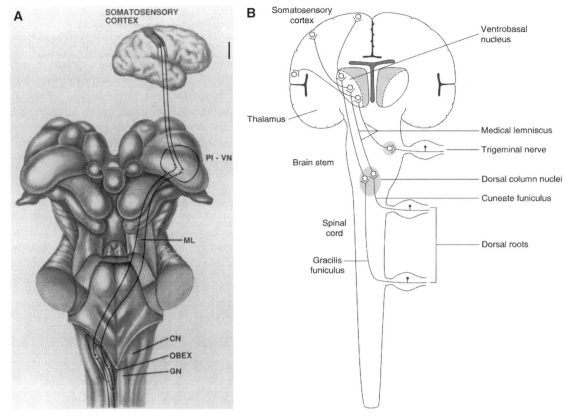

Figure 5.2: (**A**) Schematic diagram showing the neural pathway of the portion of the somatosensory system that travels in the dorsal column. *GN* gracilis nucleus, *CN* cuneate nucleus, *Pl-VN* Posteriolateral ventral nucleus of the thalamus, *ML* middle lemniscus. (Reprinted from (*75*)). (**B**) Schematic diagram showing the anatomical locations of the main components of the ascending somatosensory pathways (Reprinted from (*1*) with permission from Elsevier).

(**Fig. 5.2**). The cell bodies of these fibers are located in the dorsal root ganglia (DRG). (Sensory receptors of the head are innervated by cranial nerves.)

Several types of nerve fibers mediate sensory information to the spinal cord. Low threshold cutaneous receptors are innervated by Aβ fibers (6–12 μm diameter) with conduction velocities between 30 and 70 m/s. Proprioceptive fibers from muscle spindles, tendon organs, and receptors monitoring joint movements are large (Aα) fibers, but pain fibers are the smallest myelinated fibers (Aδ). Unmyelinated fibers (C fibers) also mediate pain.

The spinal horn has been divided into laminae (*2*). The dorsal roots of sensory nerve fibers enter the spinal cord, and some make synaptic contact with cells in different laminae of the dorsal horn of the spinal cord (**Fig. 5.2A**), whereas other fibers that travel in the dorsal column reach the dorsal column nuclei located in the lower medulla. The dorsal roots that enter the spinal cord branch several times, and the different branches make synaptic contact with cells in different parts of the dorsal horn of the segment on which they enter as well as on several adjacent segments. Some branches ascend uninterrupted on the same side of the spinal cord as they entered to form the dorsal column, and these axons make synaptic contact with cells in the dorsal column nuclei (**Fig. 5.1**). Some small, myelinated fibers that mediate pain (Aδ fibers) terminate on cells in lamina I and IV of the dorsal horn, and the axons of these cells cross the midline and ascend on the opposite side of the spinal cord as the spinotha- lamic tracts to reach the thalamus (**Fig. 5.1B**).

Dorsal Root Fiber Collaterals. The sensory nerve fibers that enter a segment of the spinal cord send collateral fibers to several adjacent segments (**Fig. 5.1C**), where they can activate cells in the dorsal horns of these segments. **Fig. 5.1C** only shows three adjacent segments of the spinal cord, one above and one below the segment, where the dorsal root enters, but there is anatomical evidence that these branches continue up and down the spinal cord to several more segments (*3*).

The efficacy of the synapses that connect these fibers to cells decreases with the distance from the segment where the nerve fibers enter the spinal cord, but the efficacy can change as a result of the activation of neural plasticity. The branches that terminate on cells in the first few of the neighboring segments can normally activate cells in the dorsal horn, while the branches that terminate on cells in segments that are more distant cannot normally activate cells because of insufficient synaptic efficacy. The efficacy of the synapses that connect these collaterals to cells in the dorsal horns gradually decreases with the distance from the segment where the dorsal root enters.

The synapses that normally are "dormant" can be "unmasked" when neural plasticity is activated. This may occur when the dorsal root that enters a segment is severed or when the input is otherwise reduced. Such increased syn- aptic efficacy caused by injury and subsequent lack of input to the segment to which the dorsal root was damaged occurs as a result of the acti- vation of neural plasticity (*4*).

This means that injury to a sensory nerve can have widespread effect on the excitability of dorsal horn neurons and cause an abnormal spread of sensory activity to more segments of the spinal cord than what normally occurs. This is one reason for the complex reactions that often occur from damage of a single dorsal root or a peripheral nerve.

Dorsal Column System. The dorsal column is entirely an anatomical structure with many kinds of nerve fibers, not a single tract. The majority of fibers are primary afferents and collaterals of primary afferents from sensory receptors. These first-order nerve fibers that receive input from receptors in the skin and muscles enter the dorsal horn of the spinal cord and ascend in the dorsal column (posterior funiculus consisting of the cuneate and gracilis funiculi) of the spinal cord on the ipsilateral side to terminate in cells in the dorsal column nuclei (**Fig. 5.3**).

The dorsal column has two parts, the funicu- lus cuneatus and the funiculus gracilis. The fibers of these two parts terminate on cells in the cuneate and gracilis nuclei, respectively. In addition, the dorsal column contains ascending fibers that originate in cell bodies of the dorsal horn of the spinal cord. These constitute what is known as the second order dorsal column pathway.

The fibers of the dorsal column that origi- nate in the upper portion of the body (thoracic and cervical segments) terminate in the neu- rons of the cuneate nucleus, while some of the nerve fibers that innervate receptors of the lower body terminate in the gracilis nucleus of the dorsal column nuclei.

The fibers of the second order dorsal column pathway mainly originate from cells in lamina IV of the spinal horn in the cervical enlargement of the spinal cord and from cells in lamina V and VI in the lumbosacral cord. Many of the fibers in the second order pathways are activated by receptors in joint and muscle receptors (*5*).

The primary afferents of the dorsal column system mediate fine touch (from skin recep- tors) and unconscious proprioception (from muscle spindles and tendon organs) from the upper and lower limbs, respectively. The cuneate nucleus also relays impulses from

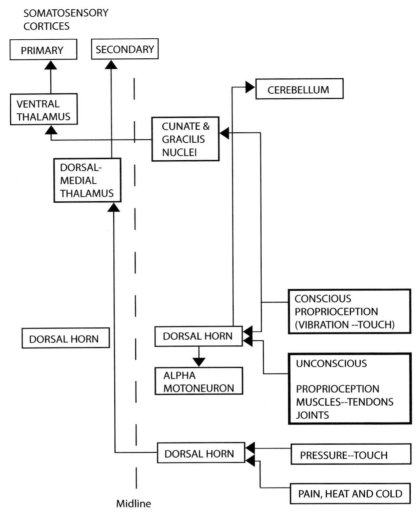

Figure 5.3: Simplified diagram of the most important ascending pathways of the somatosensory system.

slowly adapting receptors in muscles also from the lower body, and there are indications that damage to the dorsal column system may impair movement control.

The nucleus cuneatus and the nucleus gracilis, together known as the dorsal column nuclei, are located in the caudal portion of the medulla. The nucleus Z is located slightly rostral and medial to the dorsal column nuclei. Nucleus Z receives proprioceptive fibers from the lower body and low threshold skin receptors (6). It is

assumed to be mainly involved in unconscious proprioception.

Fibers that leave the dorsal column nuclei and the nucleus Z cross over to the other side of the medulla and ascend to form the medial lemniscus. The medial lemniscus ascends in the brainstem, first near the midline and later, more laterally, to terminate in the somatosensory nuclei (the ventral posterior lateral (VPL) nucleus, also known as the ventrobasal (VB) thalamus comprising the VPL and ventral posterior medial (VPM) nuclei, **Fig. 5.2**) of the thalamus, which is the second main relay nucleus of the somatosensory system. It is mainly the dorsal column that is monitored when using SSEP; (see Chap. 6).

This difference between the ascending pathways of the somatosensory system of the lower and upper body has important implications for the interpretation of the SSEP recorded in response to electrical stimulation of peripheral nerves of the lower limbs (peroneal or posterior tibial nerves) as well as when dermatomal stimulation is used, as we shall discuss later in this chapter. (When dermatomes of the lower body are stimulated electrically to elicit SSEP, it is probably mainly skin receptors that are activated, and such neural activity probably mainly travels in the dorsal column system; (see Chap. 6)).

Some of the fibers of the second order pathway terminate in the dorsal column nuclei and some terminate in nucleus Z in the cat and the external cuneate nucleus of the monkey. These fibers mediate proprioception that does not cause awareness such as information from muscle spindles and joint receptors (proprioception) in the lower body. These fibers travel ipsilaterally in the lateral fasciculi of the spinal cord and terminate in the nucleus Z, which is located more medially and rostral to the nucleus gracilis (6). Fibers that leave nucleus Z cross the midline and join the medial lemniscus. Nucleus Z of the cat medulla has been shown to act as a relay between the spinal cord and the ventral lateral (VL) nucleus of the motor thalamus (6). In one study, the authors presented evidence that group I muscle afferents from the hind limbs in the cat enter the dorsal lateral fasciculi at the L_3 level and terminate in nucleus Z (7). Tracey (1982) (5) showed that in the cat and the monkey, the fast-conducting group I muscle afferents from the lower limbs are likely to transverse the posterolateral funiculus.

Organization of the Somatosensory Cortex. The primary somatosensory cortex receives its input from the VPL nuclei of the thalamus as third-order neurons. These neurons travel in the posterior limb of the internal capsule and disburse over the somatosensory cortex (postcentral gyrus of the parietal cortex) in a somatotopic fashion, with the legs represented closest to the midline, followed in the lateral direction by the representation of the trunk, forearm, and hand (**Fig. 5.4**). Neurons in the primary cortex send axons to the secondary somatosensory cortex and to association cortices. Secondary somatosensory cortices occupy large parts of the somatosensory cortical areas (for details see (*1*)).

The primary somatosensory cortex also receives unconscious proprioceptive input, and evoked potentials have been recorded in response to electrical stimulation of deep tissue such as joints. Single cell recordings have confirmed that tracts that carry unconscious proprioception indeed project to cells in areas of the primary somatosensory cortex that are different from

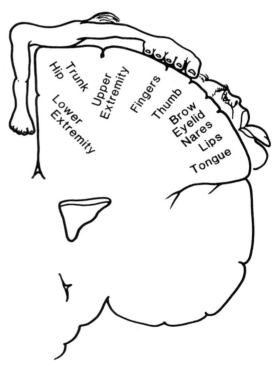

Figure 5.4: Somatotopic organization (homunculus) of the body surface on the somatosensory cortex by Penfield and coworkers (Reprinted from (*76*)).

those that receive conscious somatosensory input, such as from cutaneous receptors (*8*). In primates, it is area 2 (Brodmann's area, see Appendix A) of the primary somatosensory cortex that receives proprioceptive input (*9*). Humans may be assumed to have a similar organization.

The secondary cortex has been the target of attempts to modulate pain and tinnitus, and its connections may, therefore, become directly important for intraoperative monitoring where proper localization of the placement of recording electrodes may be facilitated by intraoperative recordings. Neurons in the S2 cortical region receive input from S1 and bilateral input from the thalamus. S2 neurons are topographically organized with the homunculus of the body surface similar to S1. These neurons also receive input from cells in the VB nuclei of the thalamus. There are also connections from S1 and S2 to the insular cortex.

Neurons in area 5, located in proximity to area 2, receive input from proprioceptors, such as muscle spindles and joint receptors, through input from the lateral posterior nucleus and the anterior nucleus of the pulvinar of the thalamus and corticocortical input from area 3a (*5*). Neurons in S2 also receive input from the anterior lateral system (thus pain information, see below) (**Fig. 5.5**).

Anterior Lateral System. Temperature and pain information travel in the anterior lateral system consisting of the spinothalamic tract, the spinomesencephalic tract, and the spinoreticular tract. The spinothalamic tract is the largest and probably the most important of these tracts. The anterior lateral system is concerned with less localized and more general tactile sensation in contrast to the dorsal column system, which communicates fine touch and has an almost 1:1 synaptic ratio, which provides for much more precise localization and discrimination.

The lateral and anterior spinothalamic tracts terminate on cells in the dorsal and medial thalamic (VPL) nuclei. The axons of these cells terminate in the secondary somatosensory cortex and association cortices (*1*). The anterior lateral system has great clinical importance, but intraoperative monitoring of this system has not been described (**Fig. 5.6**).

Anterior and Posterior Spinocerebellar System. The third ascending system consists of the anterior and the posterior spinocerebellar tracts (**Figs. 5.2** and **5.3**). This system furnishes unconscious proprioception and provides important feedback to the motor system, but it is not monitored intraoperatively either. The spinocerebellar tract may be regarded as belonging more to the motor system than to

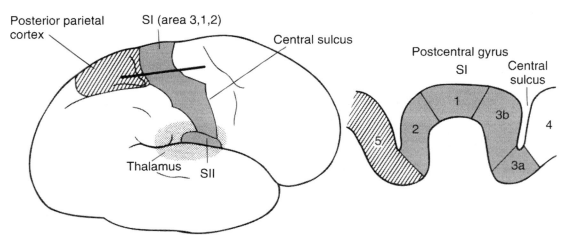

Figure 5.5: Somatosensory cortices, SI and SII (Reprinted from (*74*) with permission from Oxford University Press).

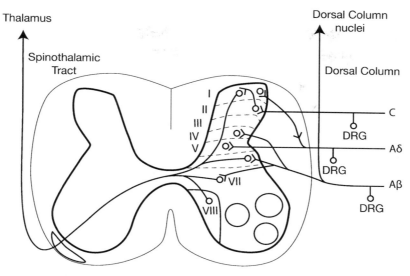

Figure 5.6: Illustration of the termination of the Aβ, Aδ fibers, and C fibers in the dorsal horn and their ascending connections that carry innocuous information to the dorsal column nuclei and pain pathways (spinothalamic tract). *DRG* Dorsal root ganglion. Lamina II is also known as substantia gelantinosa.

sensory systems. Both the anterior and posterior spinoreticular tracts receive their input not only from receptors in muscles (muscle spindles), tendons, and joints, but also from skin receptors. The fibers travel in peripheral nerves and enter the spinal cord as dorsal root fibers that terminate on cells in the central part of the spinal horn. The axons of these cells travel on both sides of the spinal cord and reach cells in the cerebellum without interruption. Collateral from the fibers in this tract reach nucleus Z of Brodal and Pompeiano (7) and terminate on its cells. These cells send axons to the thalamus where they terminate in the VPL.

The Trigeminal System. Tactile information from the face is mediated by the trigeminal system. The cell bodies of the trigeminal nerve (fifth cranial nerve) are located in the trigeminal ganglion (ganglion of Gasser or semilunar ganglion) where the trigeminal nerve central branches enter the sensory trigeminal nucleus that extends from the midbrain to the upper part of the spinal cord (**Fig. 5.7**). The ascending fibers from that nucleus join the medial lemniscus

on the contralateral side and extend to the thalamic nucleus (medial portion of the ventral posterior nucleus, VPN). The fibers from the VPN project to the somatosensory cortex (postcentral gyrus) lateral to the homunculus projection of the hand (**Fig. 5.4**). The rostral portion of the trigeminal nucleus is concerned with touch, warmth, and cool sensations, while the most caudal portion, the spinal nucleus of the trigeminal nerve, is mainly concerned with pain and cold and hot sensations. This part of the nucleus is involved in the generation of pain in patients with trigeminal neuralgia. Treatment may involve operations that involve microvascular decompression of the trigeminal nerve or operations where a small cut is made in the nerve. In such operations, it may be useful to map the trigeminal nerve using intraoperative neurophysiology (see Chap. 14).

Electrical Potentials Generated by the Somatosensory Nervous System

Recordings of evoked potentials from the somatosensory system play an important role in intraoperative monitoring of the spinal cord

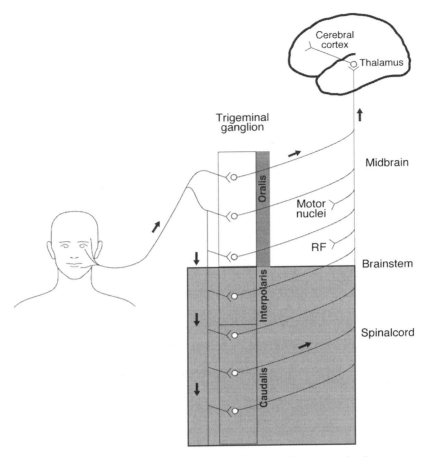

Figure 5.7: Schematic drawings of the pathways through the trigeminal sensory nucleus. The *upper part* is the sensory part and the *lower (shaded) part* is mainly involved in processing noxious stimuli (pain processing). *RF* Reticular formation. (Adapted from (*77*)).

and the brain, and both near-field and far-field potentials are used in various kinds of monitoring of SSEP.

In somatosensory system monitoring, peripheral nerves are often stimulated electrically while evoked potentials are recorded from electrodes placed on the scalp. There is a distinction between upper limb SSEP recorded in response to stimulation of the nerves at the wrist and lower limb SSEP stimulation performed at the knee or the foot. Responses from electrodes placed on the skin (dermatomes) are also used in intraoperative monitoring. Practical aspects regarding the monitoring of SSEP are detailed in Chap. 6.

Near-Field Evoked Potentials. Typical recordings made directly from the surface of the dorsal column nuclei in response to stimulation of the median nerve at the wrist are shown in **Fig. 5.8** compared with far-field SSEP recorded from electrodes placed on the vertex and the upper neck in a patient undergoing an operation where the dorsal column nuclei were exposed. It is seen that electrical stimulation of the median nerve gives a large response from the dorsal column nuclei (the cuneate nucleus) with a waveform that is typical for responses from a nucleus with an initial positive–negative potential followed by a broad negative potential (see Chap. 3).

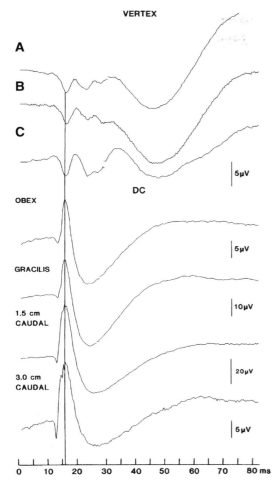

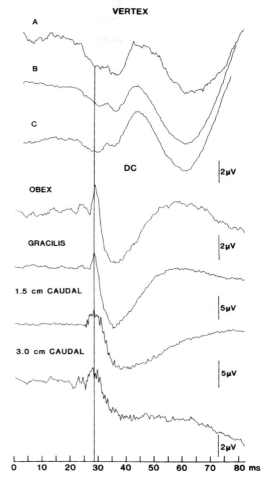

Figure 5.8: Responses to electrical stimulation by an electrode placed over the median nerve at the wrist. *Upper curves*: Far-field recordings (vertex-inion) obtained after the patient was anesthetized, but before the operation began (**A**), during direct recording (**B**), and during closure (**C**). *Middle curves*: Recordings from the surface of the cuneate nucleus using the opposite earlobe as a reference (DC). (Reprinted from (*20*) with permission from Wolters Kluwer Lippincott Williams & Wilkins).

Figure 5.9: Recordings are similar to those in **Fig. 5.8**, but were obtained from the gracilis nucleus in response to electrical stimulation of the peroneal nerve at the knee. As in **Fig. 5.8**, the *top tracings* were obtained by recording from electrodes placed on the scalp (vertex-inion) before the operation began. (Reprinted from (*20*) with permission from Wolters Kluwer Lippincott Williams & Wilkins).

The response from the gracilis nucleus to stimulation of the peroneal nerve has a similar waveform, but with longer latencies containing a series of wavelets (**Fig. 5.9**) that indicate that the neural pathway that is activated is longer than that involved in the response from

stimulation of the median nerve, and that there is a larger variation in fiber diameter. Therefore, the neural activity that arrives at the level of the upper spinal cord is dispersed in time.

The stimuli used to evoke the responses shown in **Fig. 5.8** and **5.9** were presented at a rate of 20 pps and the recording filters were set at 3–3,000 Hz. Sampling intervals were 160 μs, and each recording had 512 data points. Negativity is shown as an upward deflection. The results were obtained in a patient undergoing microvascular decompression to relieve spasmodic torticollis.

Far-Field Evoked Potentials. When peripheral nerves, such as the median nerve of the upper limb or the posterior tibial nerves and peroneal nerves of the lower limb, are electrically stimulated for the purpose of recording SSEP, both the dorsal column system and the anterior lateral system are most likely activated, but it is generally assumed that the anterior lateral system is not represented to any noticeable degree in the responses that are recorded, nor is the spinocerebellar tract contributing noticeably to the far-field potentials.

Upper Limb SSEP. SSEP recorded from electrodes placed on the scalp in response to

electrical stimulation of the median nerve at the wrist have a series of peaks and troughs. In recordings of such responses, the negative peaks are labeled with an "N" followed by the normal latency in milliseconds. The positive peaks (or valleys) of the SSEP are usually labeled with a "P" followed by a number that is the normal latency of that peak.

The SSEP recorded from electrodes placed on the scalp on the side contralateral to the stimulation, in an awake or lightly anesthetized person, are dominated by potentials that originate in the primary somatosensory cortex. These potentials are communicated through the dorsal column system and have a latency of ~20 ms (N_{20}), but potentials with shorter latencies can also be identified (**Fig. 5.10**). The waveform as well as the amplitude of the recorded potentials depends on the placement of the recording electrodes. A negative peak with latency of 18 ms

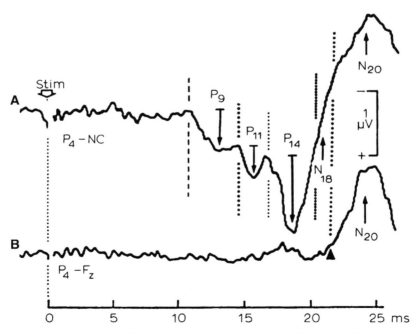

Figure 5.10: SSEP recorded in response to stimulation of the median nerve at the wrist. (**A**) Noncephalic reference. (**B**) Frontal references. *NC* Noncephalic; P4 and Fz (see 10–20 system, **Fig. 6.1**). (Reprinted from (*12*) with the permission from Elsevier).

(N_{18}) can be recorded from large areas of the scalp on both sides. These negative peaks are preceded by a series of positive peaks (P_9, P_{11}, P_{14}, P_{16}) which are best recorded from electrodes that are placed on the neck with a noncephalic reference (for instance, placed on the shoulder), but they can also be recorded from electrodes placed over the parietal region of the scalp and the upper neck (**Fig. 5.10**). Such electrode placement (contralateral–parietal to the upper dorsal neck) is practical for intraoperative monitoring and yields a clear representation of the P_{13-16} peaks as well as the N_{18} and N_{20} peaks (see also Chaps. 6 and 17 for discussions of various recording techniques).

The two main negative peaks – N_{18} and N_{20} – are followed by a positive deflection (P_{22}), a large negative peak (N_{30}), and another positive deflection (P_{45}) that is broader than the P_{22} peak (not seen in **Fig. 5.10**). The N_{20}, P_{22}, and P_{45} peaks are localized to the contralateral parietal region (3 cm behind C_3 or C_4), while the N_{18} and P_{14-16} components can be recorded from large regions of the scalp, including that of the contralateral side (**Fig. 5.10**). Subtracting the recordings from the ipsilateral and the contralateral sides yields more clearly identifiable N_{20}, P_{22}, and P_{45} peaks.

Evoked potentials that are generated by the brachial plexus in response to electrical stimulation of the median nerve may be recorded by placing an electrode at Erb's point (Erb's point is found just above the mid-portion of clavicle). These potentials are indicators of the degree of activation of the brachial plexus and are valuable in intraoperative monitoring of SSEP because their presence confirms that the electrical stimulation excites the median nerve.

Measuring the difference between the latencies of the different peaks in the SSEP and those of the potentials recorded from Erb's point eliminates the effect of changes in the conduction time of the median nerve in the arm (due, e.g., to changes in temperature). If the absolute value of the latencies of the various peaks in the SSEP is used, a prolongation in the conduction time of the central portion of the somatosensory pathway cannot be distinguished from a prolongation in the conduction time of the median nerve. Another

measure that eliminates the influence of neural conduction in the peripheral (median) nerve, as well as that in the dorsal column, is the frequently used central conduction time (CCT), which is the interval between the P_{14-16} and the N_{20} peaks (*10*) (**Fig. 5.11**). (Further details on this subject are discussed in Chap. 6).

Lower Limb SSEP. The latencies of the individual components of the lower limb SSEP depend on the height of the individual in whom they are recorded to a much greater extent than what is the case for upper limb SSEP. Large differences in these latencies are seen in children (*11*).

The SSEP elicited by stimulation of the posterior tibial or the peroneal nerves at the knee do not exhibit SSEP peaks as distinct and early as those elicited by median nerve stimulation. Because the nerve tracts involved in lower limb stimulation are much longer than those involved in median nerve stimulation, the latencies of the peaks in the lower limb SSEP are much longer than those of the peaks in the upper limb SSEP. The individual variability of these responses is much greater than the upper limb SSEP, and they are more affected by peripheral nerve neuropathy such as seen with age and diseases such as diabetes.

Recording of cortical responses elicited by lower limb stimulation may be performed using electrodes placed on the midline scalp (at C_z) level, or better yet, 3–4 cm posterior to C_z using F_{pz} or the ipsilateral mastoid as reference (**Fig. 5.12**). An electrode location 3–4 cm posterior to C_z with a noncephalic reference placed on the upper neck is also often used.

When recording potentials that are generated in the upper spinal cord and lower medulla, it may be advantageous to place the reference electrode on the upper neck, similar to that described for recording upper limb SSEP. However, the amplitudes of such early components are small and individually variable. From experience it is known that the earliest peaks in the lower limb SSEP (P_{17} and P_{24}) can only be recorded reliably from an electrode placed on the lower portion of the body, over the T_{12}

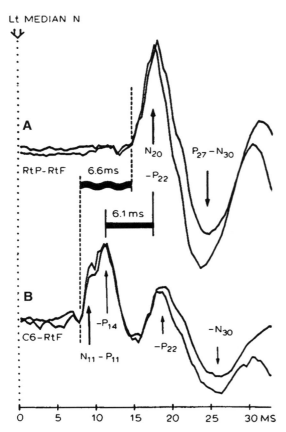

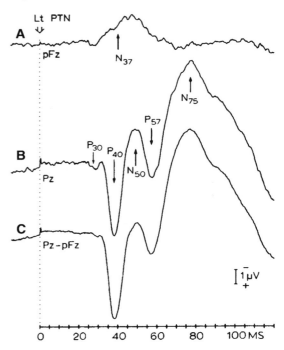

Figure 5.11: Illustration of how the CCT is determined based on recordings of the SSEP with two different electrode placements. The onset of the CCT is defined as the time of the earliest response from the spinal entry of the neural activity; the end is the beginning of the N_{20} component. (**A**) Recordings from a contralateral parietal location (behind C_3 or C_4) using a frontal reference. (**B**) Recording from a noncephalic (spinal C_6) location using the same frontal reference as in (**A**). (Modified from (*22*) with permission from Elsevier).

Figure 5.12: SSEP in response to stimulation of the left posterior tibial nerve using various locations for the recording electrodes (**A**) Recordings from a frontal location, F_{pz}. (**B**) Recording from a midline position, P_z. A noncephalic reference (on *left shoulder*) was used in both recordings. (**C**) The difference between the recording in (**A**) and the one in (**B**), mimicking a differential recording between F_{pz} and P_z. (Reprinted from (*22*) with the permission from Elsevier).

vertebra or below the hip (e.g., on a lower limb). Such an arrangement may be difficult to use for intraoperative monitoring because it often results in noisy recordings from electrical interference (*11*).

The response from the popliteal fossa (at the knee) to stimulation of the posterior tibial

nerve shows the activation of the peripheral nerve that is being stimulated, similar to that which is noted in recordings from Erb's point in upper limb SSEP. These responses indicate that proper stimulation has been applied to the respective (posterior tibial) nerve.

Neural Generators of the SSEP

The SSEP elicited by stimulation of the median nerve (upper limbs) and the peroneal or posterior tibial nerves (lower limbs) are fundamentally different, and the neural generators of these two types of SSEP are discussed separately.

Upper Limb SSEP. Studies of the neural generators of the SSEP confirm that the major contributions to the SSEP recorded from electrodes placed on the scalp originate in the dorsal column system.

The short latency evoked potentials, in response to electrical stimulation of the median nerve, are generated by the peripheral nerves, the spinal cord (the dorsal column fibers) and possibly by the medial lemniscus (*12–15*) while the dorsal column nuclei seems to produce very small far-field potentials (*16*).

Recordings from different locations along the spine have shown that the P_9 peak dominates at the spinal C_7 level, and it has been concluded that P_9 of the scalp-recorded SSEP represents the neural volley that enters the spinal cord from the brachial plexus. Evidence has been presented that the P_{11} peak is generated in the dorsal horn by neural structures that are not parts of the ascending somatosensory pathway. This is important to consider when the recordings of SSEP are used in intraoperative monitoring; it means that the P_{11} peak may be preserved, despite the compromise of ascending somatosensory tracts at the level of the foramen magnum.

The introduction of the use of a noncephalic reference for recording upper limb SSEP (13, 17) was a major breakthrough in studies of the neural generators of the SSEP studies because it made it possible to identify the early components of the SSEP and enabled investigators to study the origin of these potentials in more detail (12, 13). Some of these studies compared recordings from the scalp with recordings from the ventral side of the spinal cord using a recording electrode that was placed in the esophagus.

The origin of the P_{14-16} peaks is not entirely clear. Some investigators (18) assumed that P_{14} was generated in the medial lemniscus. These results are supported by work by other investigators, such as Allison and coworkers (19), while yet other investigators have arrived at different interpretations of the origins of these early components. These authors described the peaks as P_{13-16} peaks, thus assuming that the first of these occurred 1 ms earlier than other investigators. Some investigators (14) found evidence that P_{13} was generated more peripherally, namely, where the dorsal column passes through the foramen magnum and that P_{11} was generated by the dorsal root at the spinal C_2 level. It has been suggested that what these investigators Lueders et al. (14) identified as P_{13} was, in fact, the same peak as identified by the other investigators (the Desmedt group) and labeled P_{14}. The confusion between which peaks were P_{13} and which were P_{14} could have been a result of slightly different electrode placements and a small difference in the ways in which recordings were filtered by these two separate groups of investigators.

Studies comparing the responses from the exposed surface of the dorsal column nuclei evoked by electrical stimulation of the median nerve in patients undergoing neurosurgical operations, with those recorded from the scalp (SSEP) (20) (Fig. 5.8) recorded simultaneously with the intracranial recordings, indicate that P_{14} is most likely generated by the fiber tract that terminates in the cuneate nucleus.

Studies in the monkey (16) where the dorsal column nuclei were stimulated electrically and the elicited antidromic activity in the median nerve was recorded have provided accurate determinations of the neural conduction time in the median nerve. These studies indicated that the initial components of the potentials that are recorded from the surface of the dorsal column nuclei reflect ascending activity in the dorsal column (16) and support the assumption that the P_{14} peak in humans is generated by the termination of the dorsal column fibers on the cells of the cuneate nucleus.

Most studies, however, agree that the dorsal column nuclei themselves contribute little to the far-field potentials possibly because the organization of these nuclei is such that they produce a closed, or nearly closed, electrical field (*21*) (see Chap. 3). This is similar to the conclusions regarding the neural generators of the auditory brainstem responses (ABR), where the nucleus of the inferior colliculus was found to produce only a weak far-field response (see page 84).

The N_{18} peak that can be recorded over large regions of the scalp has a different origin than the N_{20} peak. The N_{18} is generated by bilateral brainstem structures while the somatosensory cortex generates N_{20}, which is specifically localized contralaterally to the side that is stimulated. The N_{18} peak is assumed to be the result of excitatory postsynaptic potentials in several nuclei that receive input from the medial lemniscus, such as the superior colliculus (22, 23). (It is important to keep in mind that fibers that constitute tracts such as the fibers of the medial lemniscus have many collaterals that connect to neurons in different parts of the CNS).

The N_{20} peak can only be recorded from a small area of the contralateral parietal scalp, and it is assumed to be generated by the primary somatosensory cortex, where it represents the early response of the input from the thalamus (22). The generators of the components (positive and negative peaks) that follow N_{20} (P_{22}, N_{30}, and P_{45}) are not known in detail, but the generators of these components are assumed to be higher brain structures that receive input from the primary somatosensory cortex, such as the secondary cortices and perhaps association cortices. There is considerable neural processing in the primary somatosensory cortex, and the result of that processing may contribute to some of the components in the SSEP that have latencies longer than 20 ms. These peaks are more individually variable, and they are more sensitive to anesthesia than earlier peaks, a sign that more synapses are involved.

Lower Limb SSEP. The generators of the lower limb SSEP (elicited by stimulation of the posterior tibial or the common peroneal nerves) have been studied much less comprehensively than the upper limb SSEP (elicited by stimulation of the median nerve). Likewise, the origins of the components of the lower limb SSEP are incompletely known. The N_{17} peak that can be seen in some recordings is assumed to be generated near the hip joint, and the P_{24} peak is assumed to be generated at the level of the twelfth thoracic vertebra. The P_{31} peak is probably generated where the spinal cord passes through the foramen magnum, and together with the P_{34} peak, these potentials may correspond to the P_{14-16} complex of the upper limb SSEP. The P_{34} peak is thus, assumed to be generated by structures in the brainstem (medial lemniscus), but this peak could also be analogous to the N_{18} peak of the upper limb SSEP (24) (see **Figs. 5.12** and **5.13**). The negative deflection (N_{34}) following these positive peaks may be generated in brainstem structures or in the thalamus. The lower limb response elicited by electrical stimulation of the posterior tibial nerve has a main positive peak with a latency of ~40 ms (P_{40}) followed by a large negative peak at a latency of 45 ms (N_{45}). (The exact latency of these peaks depends on the height of the person in question, but there are other causes for the considerable variations seen in lower limb SSEP.) This negative peak is generally assumed to be generated by cortical structures, and it is best recorded with an active electrode at the midline, 3–4 cm behind the C_z (22). A frontal reference is usually used for such recordings. However, as discussed in Chap. 6, this is not an optimal electrode placement for intraoperative monitoring.

One reason that interpretation of the neural generators of the different components of the lower limb SSEP is less certain than for those of the upper limb SSEP is that anatomical structures of the ascending somatosensory pathway from the lower portion of the body are more complex and diverse compared to structures in the upper portion of the body (page 69). The early peaks in the SSEP evoked by lower limb stimulation are less distinct than those evoked by upper limb stimulation because of the greater temporal dispersion of the neural activity that arrives at the brain from the lower portion of the body due to the longer pathway than those of the upper limb SSEP. When nerve fibers have different conduction velocities, the temporal coherence of neural activity decreases along such nerves. Long nerves, therefore, tend to deliver less temporally coherent neural activity to central neural structures than shorter pathways. Since the amplitudes of the various peaks in the far-field response depend on the degree of temporal coherence of the neural activity, such temporal dispersion results in the

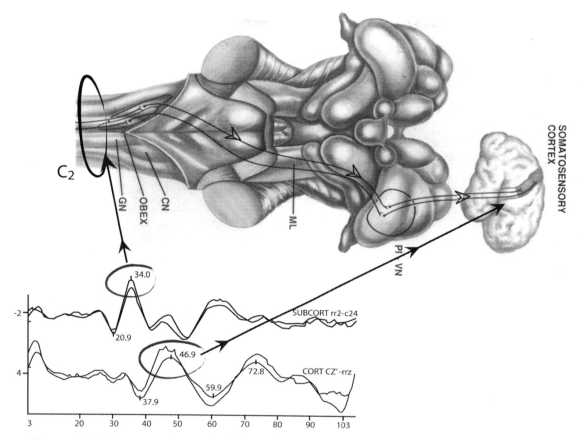

Figure 5.13: Response from stimulation of the posterior tibial nerve. *Upper trace*: Subcortical recording, Fpz-C$_2$S. *Lower trace*: Cortical response, recorded from Cz-Fpz.

peaks becoming broader and of smaller amplitudes compared to similar peaks in systems that have shorter pathways – such as the upper limb SSEP (see also discussion about the effect of temporal dispersion in Chap. 6, **Fig. 6.4**).

THE AUDITORY SYSTEM

Knowledge about the anatomy and physiology of the auditory system is a prerequisite for understanding not only the normal function of the auditory system, but also for understanding that changes in function may result from surgical manipulations of the auditory nerve and other, more central, structures of the auditory nervous system.

This section of this chapter describes the anatomy and physiology of the auditory system as applicable to intraoperative monitoring of different kinds of auditory evoked potentials (AEP). Generation of far-field auditory evoked potentials, auditory brainstem responses (ABR), near-field AEP, and compound action potentials (CAP) from the auditory nerve and cochlear nucleus are discussed. The practical aspects of hearing preservation in various types of operations and far-field/near-field recordings of ABR are discussed in detail in Chap. 7.

The Ear

The ear consists of the outer ear, the middle ear, and the inner ear (cochlea) where the first processing of sounds occurs and where the sensory receptors are located (**Fig. 5.14**).

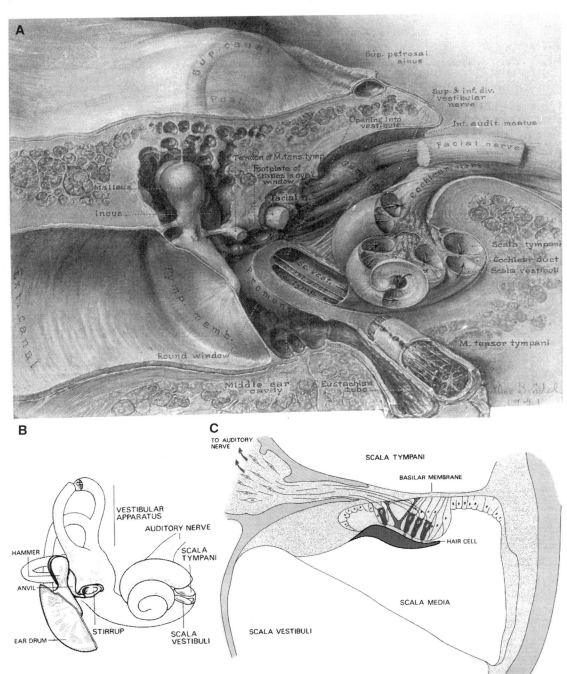

Figure 5.14: Anatomy of the ear. (**A**) Cross-section of the human ear. (Reprinted from (*78*)). (**B**) Schematic drawing of the ear. (Reprinted from (*79*)). (**C**) Cross-sectional drawing of the cochlea illustrating the fluid-filled canals and the basilar membrane with hair cells. (Reprinted from (*79*) with the permission from the Royal Swedish Academy of Science).

Sound Conduction to the Cochlea. The middle ear functions as an impedance transformer that facilitates transmission of airborne sound into vibrations of the fluid in the cochlea. This transformer action is the result of a difference between the area of the tympanic membrane and the area of the stapes footplate. The stapes footplate, which is located in the oval window, performs a piston-like, in–out motion that sets the fluid in the cochlea into motion. The middle ear cavity is filled with air and acts as a cushion behind the tympanic membrane. The proper function of the middle ear depends on the air pressure in the middle ear cavity being equal to the ambient pressure (*25*). This pressure equalization is normally maintained by the opening and closing of the Eustachian tube (**Fig. 5.14A**), which occurs naturally by the swallowing action. Since anesthetized individuals do not swallow, a negative pressure may build up in the middle ear cavity during anesthesia and that can cause a reduction in sound transmission for low-frequency sounds. Although the effect of such a reduction on the results of intraoperative monitoring of auditory evoked potentials has been discussed, there is no substantial evidence of any noticeable effect on the results of monitoring click-evoked auditory potentials. The reason is likely that negative pressure in the middle ear cavity mainly affects the transmission of low frequencies, and AEP elicited by click sounds mainly depend on the high frequency components of the sounds.

The acoustic middle ear reflex that normally reduces the transmission of mainly low frequency sounds through the middle ear is inactivated by the commonly used anesthetics. (For more details about the anatomy and physiology of the middle ear and the acoustic middle ear reflex, refer to books on the physiology of the ear, for instance, (*25, 26*).)

The Cochlea

The cochlea is shaped like a snail shell and has three fluid-filled compartments (scalae), which are separated by the cochlear partition (or basilar membrane) and the Reissner's membrane (**Fig. 5.14c**). The cochlea separates sounds according to their spectra, and it transforms each sound into a neural code in the individual fibers of the auditory portion of CN VIII. Another important function of the cochlea is that it compresses the amplitude range of sounds.

Frequency Analysis in the Cochlea. The special micromechanical properties of the basilar membrane are the basis for the frequency analysis that takes place in the cochlea. The basilar membrane is set into vibration by the fluid in the cochlea, which in turn is set into motion by the in-and-out motion of the stapes footplate. The particular properties of the basilar membrane and its surrounding fluid create a motion of the basilar membrane like that of a traveling wave. This traveling wave starts at the base of the cochlea and progresses relatively slowly toward the apex of the cochlea, and at a certain point along the basilar membrane, its amplitude decreases abruptly. The distance that this wave travels before its amplitude decreases is a direct function of the frequency of the sound. A low-frequency sound travels a long distance before being extinguished, while a high-frequency sound gives rise to a wave that only travels a short distance before its amplitude decreases abruptly. Thus, a frequency scale can be topographically mapped along the basilar membrane, with low frequencies at the apex and high frequencies at the base of the cochlea.

Each point on the basilar membrane may be regarded as being "tuned" to a specific frequency (**Fig. 5.15**). The region of the basilar membrane nearest the base is tuned to the highest frequencies, and the frequency to which the membrane is tuned decreases toward the top (apex) of the cochlea. The highest audible frequencies produce maximal vibration amplitude of the basilar membrane near the base of the cochlea.

The frequency tuning of the basilar membrane depends on the intensity of the sounds that reach the ear (*27, 28*). The basilar membrane is more frequency-selective for low intensity sounds than high intensity sounds as revealed by measuring the vibration amplitude

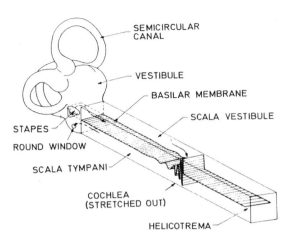

Figure 5.15: Schematic drawing of an ear with the cochlea uncoiled and shown as a straight tube to illustrate the traveling wave. (Reprinted from (*80*) with the permission of the American Institute of Physics).

of a single point of the basilar membrane when tones of different frequencies and different intensities are applied to the ear of an animal (guinea pig) (**Fig. 5.16**).

Sensory   Transduction   in   the Cochlea. Sensory cells, known as hair cells (because of their hair-like stereocilia), are arranged in rows located along the basilar membrane. There are two types of hair cells – outer and inner – and they are arranged along the basilar membrane as one row of inner hair cells and three to five rows of outer hair cells (**Fig. 5.17**). The human cochlea has ~30,000 hair cells. The axons of the cochlear portion of CN VIII connect to the two types of hair cells in distinctly different ways: each inner hair cell connects with several axons, while several outer hair cells connect with one nerve fiber (*29*) (**Fig. 5.18**) (for details see (*25*)). About 95% of the nerve fibers of the cochlear nerve connect to inner hair cells, while about 5% of the nerve fibers connect to outer hair cells.

The motion of the basilar membrane deflects the hairs on the hair cells – deflection in one direction causes the intracellular potentials of the hair cells to become less negative (depolari-

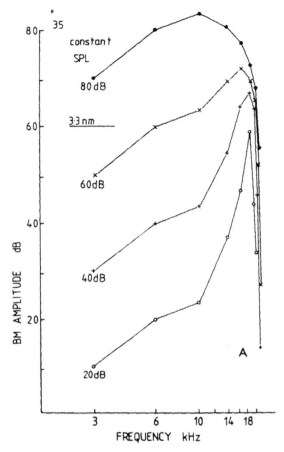

Figure 5.16: Frequency tuning of a point on the basilar membrane; the vibration amplitude of a point on the basilar membrane in a guinea pig is shown as a function of frequency. (Modified from (*81*), which was based on (*28*) with the permission of the American Institute of Physics).

zation), while a deflection in the opposite direction causes hyperpolarization (more positive).

The function of inner hair cells and that of outer hair cells is fundamentally different. Thus, while the inner hair cells function as transducers, which allow the motion of the basilar membrane to control the discharges of the individual auditory nerve fibers that connect to these hair cells, the outer hair cells function as "motors" that amplify the motion of the basilar membrane. Unlike the inner hair cells, outer hair

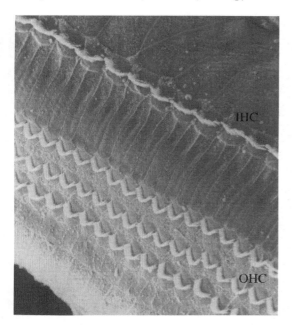

Figure 5.17: Scanning electron micrograph of hair cells along a small segment of the basilar membrane. *IH* inner hair cells, *OH* outer hair cells. (Courtesy of Dr. David Lim).

cells, as far as we know, do not participate in communicating information about the motion of the basilar membrane to higher auditory nervous centers. The active motion of the outer hair cells injects energy into the motion of the basilar membrane, and this injected energy compensates for the frictional losses in the basilar membrane that would have dampened the motion of the basilar membrane. Amplification by outer hair cells improves the sensitivity of the ear by about 50 dB, and it increases the frequency selectivity of the basilar membrane considerably, more so for weak sounds than for more intense sounds (see (25)).

Since low-frequency sounds give rise to the largest vibration amplitude of the apical portion of the basilar membrane, a low-frequency sound stimulates hair cells located in that region more than it stimulates hair cells in other regions. In a similar way, high-frequency sounds produce the largest vibration amplitude of more basal portions of the basilar membrane,

thereby exciting the hair cells in that region to a greater extent than they do hair cells in other regions of the basilar membrane.

An otoacoustic emission is a sound generated by the cochlea as a result of the active function of the outer hair cells, and it can be measured in the ear canal. The otoacoustic emission is increasingly becoming a valuable clinical test, but it has not yet been found to be of specific use in intraoperative monitoring.

Electrical Potentials Generated in the Cochlea. Several different types of electrical potentials can be recorded from the cochlea or in its vicinity as a result of excitation of the hair cells. The cochlear microphonics (CM) potential follows the waveform of a sound closely (hence, its name), and the summating potential (SP) follows the envelope of a sound. Excitation of the auditory nerve is the source of the action potentials (AP), which can best be elicited in response to click sounds or the sharp onset of a tone burst. Although all of these potentials can be evoked by the same sounds, each type responds best to specific types of sounds. Thus, the AP is most prominent in response to transient sounds, while the CM is most prominent in response to a pure tone of low-to-medium high frequency. The SP is most prominent when elicited in response to high-frequency tone bursts. **Fig. 5.19** shows how the sharp onset of the tone burst elicits a prominent AP, and the CM from the sinusoidal wave of the tone is seen over the entire duration of the tone. The baseline shift seen during the tone burst is the SP (see (25)). Clinically, these potentials are recorded from the cochlear capsule or the ear canal near the tympanic membrane, and in the clinic they are known as electrocochleographic (ECoG) potentials (for details see (30, 31)). These evoked potentials have gained little use in intraoperative monitoring. Some investigators have suggested that recording ECoG potentials can monitor the function of the auditory nerve, but the most common source of intraoperative damage to the auditory nerve is found in its intracranial

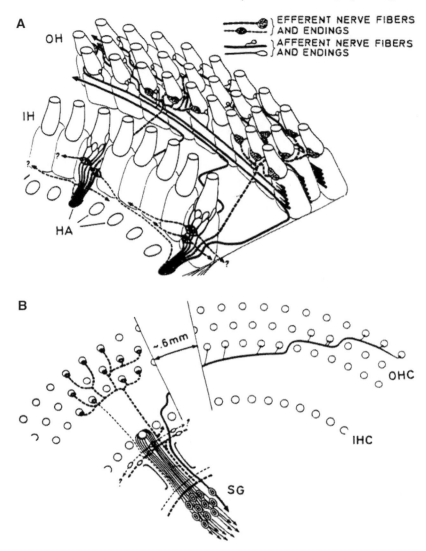

Figure 5.18: Schematic drawing of hair cells located along the basilar membrane with their connections to the ascending fibers of the auditory nerve (*solid lines*). Also shown are the efferent fibers (*dashed lines*). *OH* outer hair cells, *IH* inner hair cells, *HA* habenula perforate, *SG* spinal ganglion. (Reprinted from (*29*)).

course proximal to the generation of the ECoG (see Chap. 7).

Auditory Nervous System

The auditory nerve is longer in humans than in the small animals used for auditory research, which has had implications for the interpretation of human ABR (see page 79). The anatomy of the ascending auditory pathway is more complex than that of other sensory systems, such as the visual and somatosensory systems. There are two main, mostly parallel, ascending auditory pathways: the classical (or lemniscal pathways) and the nonclassical (or extralemniscal pathways). These two pathways are also known as the specific and the nonspecific or

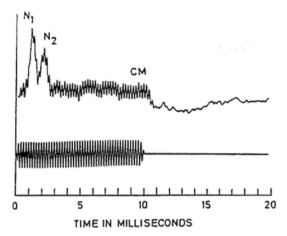

Figure 5.19: Different sound-elicited potentials that can be recorded from the round window of the cochlea. The recordings were obtained in a rat. The stimulus was a 5-kHz tone burst (10 ms). The cochlear microphonics appears as an oscillation with the frequency of the stimulus, the nerve action potentials appear as two upward peaks (N_1 and N_2), and the summating potential appears as the shift (*upward*) in the baseline recording that is seen during the time the stimulus was on. (From (*82*) with the permission from Elsevier).

polysensory pathways (*1, 25*). Much less is known about the anatomy and physiology of the nonclassical pathways than the classical pathways. In parallel to the ascending pathways are descending pathways.

Although the descending pathways are more abundant than the ascending pathways, much less is known about the descending pathways than the ascending pathways (*1, 25, 32*). The descending pathways may be regarded as reciprocal to the ascending pathways, and these two parts of the auditory pathways form loops in which information can circulate.

Anatomy

CLASSICAL (LEMNISCAL) PATHWAYS. The most important nuclei of the ascending auditory pathway and their connections are shown in **Fig. 5.20**. The first relay nucleus of the ascending auditory pathway is the cochlear

nucleus. All fibers of the auditory nerve (AN) are interrupted in this nucleus, which has three main divisions: the dorsal cochlear nucleus (DCN), the posterior ventral cochlear nucleus (PVCN), and the anterior ventral cochlear nucleus (AVCN). Each fiber of the cochlear nerve bifurcates to terminate in the PVCN and the AVCN. The fibers that reach the PVCN send collateral fibers to the DCN. In that way, all auditory nerve fibers reach cells in all three divisions of cochlear nucleus.

Recordings from the surface of the cochlear nucleus are used for monitoring the function of the auditory nerve in operations where the nerve is at risk of being injured. Implantation of stimulating electrodes on the surface of the cochlear nucleus is used as auditory prostheses in individuals who have congenital malformations that make the auditory nerve nonfunctional and in individuals with damage to the auditory nerve bilaterally from, for example, the removal of bilateral vestibular schwannoma.

The neurons of cochlear nucleus connect to the central nucleus (ICC) of the IC via several fiber tracts that cross the midline: the dorsal acoustic stria (DAS), the ventral acoustic stria (VAS), and the trapezoidal body (TB). There are also connections from cochlear nucleus to the IC that do not cross the midline. Some of the crossed fibers that originate in the cochlear nucleus reach the ICC without any synaptic interruption while other connections from the cochlear nucleus are interrupted in the nuclei of the superior olivary complex (SOC) (medial superior olivary nucleus, or MSO, lateral olivary nucleus, or LSO) or the TB. The fibers from these nuclei as well as those from cochlear nucleus proceed to the ICC as the fiber tract of the lateral lemniscus (LL). Some of the fibers of the LL reach the dorsal or ventral nuclei of the LL. All fibers that reach the ICC are interrupted in the ICC. The output fibers of the ICC form the brachia of the ICC and connect to the thalamic auditory relay nucleus, namely, the medial geniculate body (MGB). The MGB furnishes auditory information to the primary auditory cortex (A1) (**Fig. 5.20A**). (For details, see (*1, 25, 32*).)

The lengths of the different tracts of the ascending auditory pathways in humans

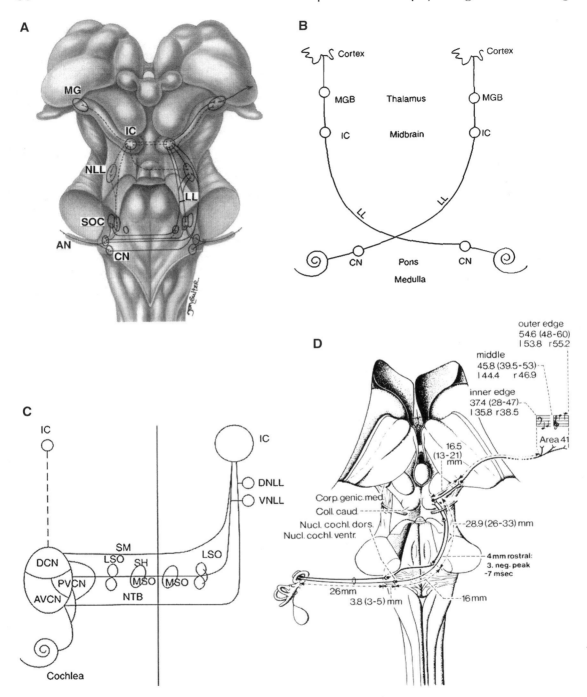

(**Fig. 5.20D**) are longer than those in the animals that are commonly used for the studies of the auditory system. This means that the travel time throughout the ascending auditory pathways is longer in humans than in animals and results in longer latencies of the different components of the ABR in humans compared with that in animals.

AUDITORY CORTEX. The auditory cortex in humans is located deep in Hechel's gyrus in the lateral fissure of the temporal lobe (Brodmann's area 41). The different areas of the auditory cortex are labeled primary cortex (A1), secondary cortex (A2), anterior auditory field (AAF), and posterior auditory field (PAF). The A1 area receives input from the ventral part of the auditory nucleus (MGB) of the thalamus and sends a large fiber tract back to the MGB (*33*). These descending connections from the cerebral cortex to the MGB are important in connection with recent developments where the auditory cortex is stimulated electrically to treat hyperactive auditory disorders, such as tinnitus and hyperacusis (*34*). The electrical stimulation that is applied to the cerebral cortex may have its effect by activating cells in the MGB via these descending pathways.

The connections from the MGB to the cortex and back again form a loop, the cortico-thalamic loop that may play an important role in creation of some forms of tinnitus (*35*).

Nonclassical   (Extralemniscal) Pathways. Nonclassical pathways project to the secondary and association cortices, thus bypassing the primary auditory cortex. These pathways use the dorsal thalamus whereas the classical pathways use the ventral thalamic nuclei.

Many of the neurons in the nonclassical pathways respond to other sensory modalities, and other sensory modalities can modulate the response to sound. Intraoperative neurophysiological monitoring does not involve nonclassical pathways as far as is known (for details about the nonclassical pathways, (*1, 25, 36*)).

Physiology. The physiology of the auditory system is covered only briefly here; more detailed descriptions can be found in Møller 2006 (*25*) and Møller 2003 (*1*).

FREQUENCY TUNING. Frequency or spectral selectivity is a prominent feature of the response from single auditory nerve fibers. Since each nerve fiber is tuned to a specific frequency, nerve cells in the nuclei of the ascending auditory pathway are tuned to a specific frequency as well. Complex processing of information takes place in the various nuclei of the ascending auditory pathway; the nature of the processing is not completely understood, but for the most part, processing seems to enhance changes in amplitude and frequency of sounds.

Figure 5.20: Anatomy of the ascending auditory pathway. (**A**) Illustration of how the main nuclei and fiber tracts are located in the brain. *AN* auditory nerve, *CN* cochlear nucleus, *SOC* superior olivary complex, *LL* lateral lemniscus, *IC* inferior colliculus, *MG* medial geniculate body. (From (*75*)). (**B**) Schematic drawing of the ascending auditory pathway. The crossed pathways are shown. *VCN* ventral cochlear nucleus, *DCN* dorsal cochlear nucleus, *IC* inferior colliculus, *MGB* medial geniculate body. (**C**) Schematic drawing of the pathways from the cochlear nucleus to the inferior colliculus. *DCN* Dorsal cochlear nucleus, *PVCN* Posterior ventral cochlear nucleus, *AVCN* Anterior ventral cochlear nucleus, *LSO* lateral superior olive, *NTB* nucleus of the trapezoidal body (NTB), *MSO* medial superior olive, *SH* stria of Held (intermediate stria), *SM* stria of Monakow (dorsal stria), *LL* lateral lemniscus, *DNLL* dorsal nucleus of the lateral lemniscus, *VNLL* ventral nucleus of the lateral lemniscus, *IC* inferior colliculus (Reprinted from (*25*) with permission from Elsevier). (**D**) Schematic drawing of the ascending auditory pathway showing the length of the auditory nerve and the various fiber tracts. Results from 30 specimens (Modified from (*55*) with the permission from Elsevier).

The temporal pattern of a sound is coded in the timing of the discharges of single auditory nerve fibers. Temporal coding of sounds provides information about the spectrum of a sound, as does the place code that is represented by the tuning of various neural elements. Both place and temporal coding of auditory information are important for the discrimination of complex sounds, such as speech and music, but either one alone can provide speech discrimination. It is evidenced from the efficacy of cochlear implants that place coding alone is sufficient for speech discrimination (37, 38), but temporal coding alone has been shown to suffice for speech discrimination also (37). Under normal circumstances, both temporal and place coding is used, and the fact that either one is sufficient for speech discrimination is an indication of redundancy in the auditory system.

TONOTOPIC ORGANIZATION. Nerve fibers of the auditory nerve as well as those of nerve cells of the nuclei of the ascending auditory pathway are arranged anatomically in accordance with the frequency at which their threshold is lowest (tonotopic organization). Thus, all neural structures of the classical ascending auditory pathway can be mapped to the frequency to which the neurons of these neural structures respond best (for details see (25)).

Descending Auditory Nervous System

Descending auditory pathways are abundant, and while the anatomy is relatively well understood, the function of these systems is not understood to any great detail (32, 39). As mentioned above, the descending pathways may be regarded as reciprocal to the ascending pathways, and together these two pathways form loops where information may circulate.

Anatomy. Efferent pathways extend from the auditory cerebral cortex to the hair cells in the cochlea (32). These pathways have been regarded as several separate systems, but it may be more appropriate to regard the descending systems as reciprocal to the ascending pathways. The best-known parts of these descending

pathways are the peripheral parts. Thus, the auditory nerve contains efferent nerve fibers that originate in the SOC and terminate mainly at the outer hair cells. These efferent fibers, also known as the olivocochlear bundle, consist of both crossed and uncrossed fibers. The efferent nerve fibers travel in the vestibular portion of the eighth cranial nerve (CN VIII) from the brainstem to Ort's anastomosis located deep in the internal auditory meatus, where they shift over to the cochlear portion of the CN VIII (for more details see (1, 25)).

Physiology. The function of the descending pathways is poorly understood. The abundant descending system from the primary auditory cortex to the thalamus may function to change the way the thalamus processes sounds. Electrical stimulation of the primary auditory cortex may therefore affect the thalamus, which is important to consider when such stimulation is used to control tinnitus (40). The olivocochlear bundles seem to influence outer hair cells, which are involved in "otoacoustic" emission. Therefore, measurements of otoacoustic emission can be used to investigate the function of this part of the efferent system.

Electrical Potentials from the Auditory Nervous System

For intraoperative monitoring, it is most important to know how the various nuclei of the ascending auditory pathways are connected, and how these nuclei, together with the fiber tracts that connect them, produce electrical activity when the ear is stimulated with transient sounds.

Factors that are important for interpreting the responses used in intraoperative monitoring include the design of the auditory nervous system in parallel pathways and the architecture of various auditory nuclei that contribute to farfield potentials, which are recorded from electrodes placed on the scalp.

The function of the descending system, as well as matters regarding coding of complex sounds in the nuclei of the ascending auditory nervous system, are described in textbooks on hearing (*25*) but are probably of relatively little importance to the understanding of how neural activity in these structures contributes to the electrical activity that is recorded from electrodes placed on the scalp (ABR). The sounds commonly used to elicit such responses are simple sounds, such as tone bursts and click sounds, and the complex processing that occurs in the auditory system of sounds, such as speech and music, probably does not affect the response to such simple sounds to any noticeable degree.

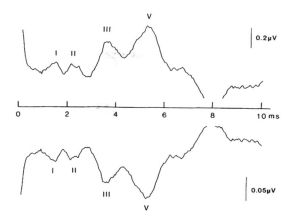

Figure 5.21: Typical recording of ABR obtained in a person with normal hearing. The recording is the summation of 4,096 responses to rarefaction clicks recorded differentially between the forehead and the ipsilateral mastoid with a band-pass of 10–3,000 Hz. The top recording is shown with vertex-positivity as an upward deflection, and the bottom curve is the same recording, but with vertex-positivity shown as a downward deflection. Reprinted from (*75*).

Auditory Brainstem Responses. ABR (also known as brainstem auditory evoked potentials, BAEP) are generated by the activity in structures of the ascending auditory pathways that occurs during the first 8–10 ms after a transient sound, such as a click sound, has been applied to the ear.

Traditionally, the ABR are recorded between electrodes placed at the vertex. When the ABR is recorded in the traditional way with one electrode placed on the vertex and another one placed on the earlobe or mastoid and each connected to the input of a differential amplifier, both of these electrodes are active (record sound-evoked potentials). The potentials that are recorded by each one of these two electrodes contribute to the recorded ABR. The standard way of displaying evoked potentials is to show negativity at the active electrode as an upward deflection. Since both electrodes are active, the ABR can be displayed in two different ways. A negative potential at the vertex electrode produces an upward deflection (as shown in the bottom tracing in **Fig. 5.21**) if the vertex electrode is connected to the inverting input (G_2) of the amplifier (see Chap. 18). If the vertex electrode is connected to the noninverting input (G_1), then a positive potential at the electrode placed at the vertex results in an upward deflection (**Fig. 5.21**, top tracing).

Obtained that way, in a person with normal hearing, the waveform is characterized by five or six (vertex-positive) peaks. These peaks are traditionally numbered consecutively using Roman numerals from I to VI (*41*) (**Fig. 5.21**).

The earlobe electrode contributes mainly to the first two (or three) peaks of the ABR while the vertex electrode makes the greatest contribution to peak V.

The waveform of the ABR depends on three key factors: the electrode placement used for recording ABR (the much used vertex-earlobe, or mastoid placement is not ideal), the stimuli used to elicit the responses, and how the recorded potentials are processed (filtered). (Discussed in Chaps. 7 and 18).

There is a certain distinct individual variation in the wave shape of the ABR – even in individuals with normal hearing. Pathologies that affect the auditory system (*42*) may result in abnormalities in the ABR that are specific for different pathologies. Hearing loss of various kinds may affect ABR in a complex way.

The fact that only the vertex-positive peaks in ABR are labeled (with Roman numerals) could imply that only vertex-positive peaks are important. This choice of labeling was, however, not based on any experimental evidence showing that the vertex-positive peaks of ABR are more important in diagnostics than the negative valleys, nor was this choice in labeling related to the neural generators of these peaks. This arbitrary choice of labeling only the vertex-positive peaks of ABR is unfortunate because it focuses only on vertex-positive peaks while the vertex negative peaks may be just as important for detecting functional abnormalities of the auditory system both in the clinic and in the operating room. (Studies of the neural generators of ABR have supported the assumption that vertex-negative peaks (or valleys) are indeed important (42)).

Only a few studies have made use of the traditional way of labeling the different components of the ABR using "N" for negative peaks, followed by the normal value of the latency of the peak; conversely, positive peaks are labeled with a "P" followed by a number that is the peak's normal latency.

Since the convention of labeling the vertex-positive peaks of the ABR with Roman numerals has been in use for a long time, this book uses this method for labeling ABR peaks.

Neural Generators of the ABR. Because of the (mainly) sequential activation of neural structures of the auditory pathways, ABR consist of a series of components that are separated in time. The peaks and valleys that form the ABR generally appear with different latencies in accordance with the anatomical location of their respective neural generators. **Fig. 5.22** shows a schematic and simplified picture of the present concept of the neural generators of the human ABR. This depiction is a simplified description of the relationship between the different components of the ABR and the anatomy of the ascending auditory pathway. It can only serve as a first approximation because of the complexity of the ascending auditory pathway with its extensive parallel systems of neural pathways. Neural activation of some nuclei may, therefore occur simultaneously, and the electrical activity of different nuclei and fiber tracts that is

elicited by a transient sound may, therefore overlap in time.

Comparisons between ABR made directly from the capsule of the cochlea in humans (ECoG) have shown evidence that peak I in the ABR is generated by the auditory nerve (distal portion). The finding that the negative peak of the CAP recorded from the exposed intracranial portion of the auditory nerve in humans has a latency close to that of peak II in the ABR (43–45) indicates that wave II is generated by the proximal portion of the auditory nerve, and this finding has been supported by later studies (46–48). This means that the auditory nerve in humans is the generator of both peaks I and II of the ABR and that no other neural structure contributes to either of these two peaks. These are the only components of the ABR that are generated from a single anatomical structure.

Peak II may be generated because neural activity propagates in the auditory nerve, where the electrical conductivity of the surrounding medium changes (14, 49) or when the propagation of neural activity stops (as it does when it reaches the cochlear nucleus). The importance of the electrical conductivity of the medium that surrounds the auditory nerve intracranially has been shown in studies of patients undergoing operations in the cerebella pontine angle (CPA) (50).

> The auditory nerve in animals commonly used in experimental research only generates one peak in the ABR (peak I). Peak II in such animals is generated by the cochlear nucleus (see, e.g. (51–54)). This difference between humans and animals commonly used in auditory research is due to the fact that the auditory nerve is much longer in humans (~26 mm (55, 56); Fig. 5.20D) than it is in many research animals, 8 mm in the cat (57), and similarly in monkeys (54).

The average diameter of axons in the auditory nerve in children is 2.5 μm with a narrow distribution in young individuals. With increasing age, the diameter increases and the variation becomes larger – 0.5–7 μm by the age of 40–50 years ((58) **Fig. 5.23**). Because the diameters of the fibers of the auditory nerve are relatively small, the conduction velocity in the

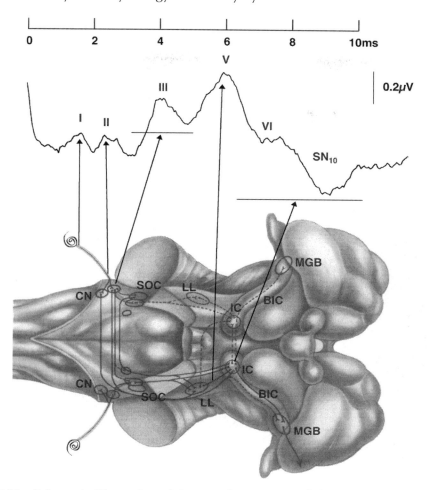

Figure 5.22: Schematic illustration of the neural generators of the ABR recorded in the traditional way and displayed with vertex positive potentials as an upward deflection. Reprinted from (*25*), by permission from Elsevier.

auditory nerve is only about 20 m/s (*59*). The time it takes for neural activity in the human auditory nerve to travel a distance of 2.6 cm from the ear to the brainstem is, therefore a little more than 1 ms. The fact that the amplitude of ABR decreases with age in humans may be explained by the greater variations in the diameter of the axons and thus, larger variations in conduction velocity and consequently, larger temporal dispersion of the nerve impulses that arrive at the cochlear nucleus.

The generators of the vertex positive peaks of the ABR with latencies that are longer than that of peak II are more complex, and these peaks most likely have multiple sources. The high degree of parallel processing in the auditory nervous system may result in different structures being activated simultaneously, and this may cause an individual component of the ABR, for example, peak IV, to receive contributions from fundamentally different structures of the ascending auditory pathway.

Intracranial recordings in patients undergoing neurosurgical operations have shown evidence that the earliest component in the ABR that originates in brainstem nuclei is peak III (*25*).

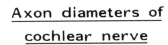

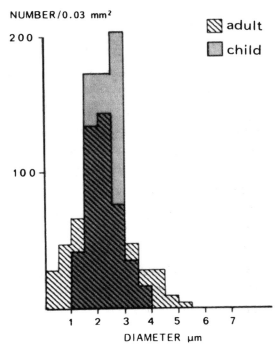

Figure 5.23: Distribution of the diameters of the axons of auditory nerve fibers for a child and an adult. (Reprinted from (*58*) by permission from Elsevier).

While the cochlear nucleus is most likely the main generator of that peak (*60*), there is evidence that the vertex-negative component between peaks III and IV also receive contributions from the cochlear nucleus (*42, 60*). Peak IV is not always visible, and the vertex negative component between peak III and peal IV is not always a prominent valley. The contralateral cochlear nucleus may contribute to the ABR (*42, 61*) through connections between the cochlear nuclei on the two sides.

Less is known about the source of peak IV than the sources of peaks I–III and peak V of the ABR. Peaks I, II, and III receive input from only the ipsilateral side (see **Fig. 5.23**) (*42*), while peak IV is likely to be the earliest positive peak of the ABR that receives contribu-

tions from contralateral structures of the ascending auditory pathway (see also (*25*)). Thus, peak IV may thus receive contributions from both sides of the brainstem. There is evidence that the anatomical location of the source of peak IV is deep in the brainstem (near the midline), maybe in the pons (the SOC) (*42, 62*). Most likely, other structures contribute to peak IV, such as the cochlear nucleus and the distal parts of the lateral lemniscus.

Comparisons between the latencies of the different components of responses recorded intracranially and the vertex-positive and vertex-negative peaks of the ABR (*42, 63*) also emphasize that it is not only the vertex-positive peaks of the ABR that have anatomically distinct neural generators, but also the vertex-negative valleys in the ABR recorded in the conventional way. In fact, the vertex-negative components may be just as important as indicators of pathologies.

Some studies (*42*) show that the response recorded from the dorsal acoustic stria, on the floor of the fourth ventricle, generates a peak that is slightly shorter than that of peak V. This indicates that if the lateral lemniscus is interrupted along its more rostral course (by surgically induced injury or by disease processes), the lateral lemniscus, and maybe even the DAS itself, may generate a peak in the ABR that is indistinguishable from the normal peak V of the ABR (except for a slightly shorter latency than the normal peak V).

Peak V of the ABR in humans has a complex origin. There is evidence that the sharp tip of peak V is generated by the lateral lemniscus, where it terminates in the inferior colliculus (*64*). There is also evidence from animal experiments that the inferior colliculus itself generates only a very small far-field response, even though a large evoked potential can be recorded from its surface (*54*). The reason for this phenomenon may be found in the anatomical organization of the inferior colliculus, where its dendrites may point in many directions so that the nucleus generates a "closed field" (*21*). The slow negative potential in the ABR in humans that occurs with a latency of ~10 ms (SN_{10}) (*65*) most likely represents postsynaptic potentials generated by the dendrites of the cells of the inferior colliculus. The amplitude of this component varies widely from individual-to-individual, but the filters used in the recordings of ABR often attenuate it.

Studies in patients undergoing neurosurgical operations that included comparisons among the ABR and intracranial potentials recorded from different locations along the lateral side of the brainstem have confirmed that peaks I–III receive contributions mainly from ipsilateral structures of the ascending auditory pathway, while peak V receives its major contributions from contralateral structures (42).

Little is known about the generators of peaks VI and VII, but these components of the ABR may be generated by neural firing in cells of the inferior colliculus (somaspikes) (48, 64, 66).

THE VISUAL SYSTEM

Visual evoked potentials (VEP) have been used in connection with intraoperative monitoring during operations in which the optic nerve or optic tract is involved, such as those to remove pituitary tumors, tumors of the cavernous sinus, and aneurysms in this area (67). However, intraoperative monitoring of the visual system plays a much smaller role than monitoring of the auditory and somatosensory systems because of technical difficulties in presenting adequate stimuli to the eye of anesthetized individuals (68, 69). The adequate stimulus for the visual system is a pattern that changes in contrast (for details see (1)), such as a reversing checkerboard pattern. The use of such a stimulus requires that the pattern be focused on the retina, which is not possible in an anesthetized patient. Therefore, flash stimulation is the only form of stimulation that can be used in an anesthetized patient, and that is not an appropriate stimulus for evoking VEP for the purpose of detecting changes in the function of the visual nervous system (see Chap. 8).

The Eye

Before it reaches the retina, light passes through the conductive apparatus of the eye consisting of the cornea, the lens, and the pupil. The optic apparatus of the eye projects a sharp image on the retina, where the light-sensitive receptors are located together with a complex neural network that enhances the contrast between areas with different degrees of illumination. Much of the neural processing of visual stimuli takes place in the neural network in the retina of the eye itself. This processing is also the basis for the representation of differences in illumination over the visual field, and there are optic nerve fibers that have small excitatory fields that are surrounded by inhibitory areas, while others have inhibitory center areas that are surrounded by excitatory areas. The position of the eye is controlled by six extraocular eye muscles that are innervated by three cranial nerves (CN III, CN IV, and CN VI) (see Chap. 11 and Appendix B).

Receptors. There are two kinds of sensory cells, cones and rods, in the human retina. The outer segments of cones and rods contain light sensitive substances (photo pigment) (1). The three different kinds of photo pigment in the cones, one for each of the three principal colors, blue, green, and red, provide the eye's color sensitivity (photopic vision). Rods are more sensitive than cones and provide vision in low light (scotopic vision).

Adaptation of the photoreceptors plays an important role for the processing of information in the visual system, as it does in other sensory organs. Adaptation of the eye is a form of automatic gain control that adapts the sensitivity of the eye to the ambient illumination. The adaptation of photoreceptors provides most of the eye's automatic gain control. The pupil also provides some automatic gain control, the range of which varies among species.

Adaptation of the eye is often referred to as dark adaptation, which refers to the recovery of sensitivity that occurs after the exposure to bright light. The first part of the dark-adaptation curve is steeper than the following segment and represents the dark-adaptation of cones; the second segment is related to the function of rods. Light adaptation (the opposite of dark adaptation) is caused by the exposure to bright light causing reduced sensitivity of the eye.

Ascending Visual Pathways

Two different afferent pathways have been identified, the classical and the nonclassical pathways, which are similar to that of the auditory and the somatic sensory systems (*1*). In this book, only the classical pathway, known as the retino-geniculo-cortical pathway, is described. This pathway involves the lateral geniculate nucleus (LGN) of the thalamus and the primary visual cortex (striate cortex, V1) (**Fig. 5.24**).

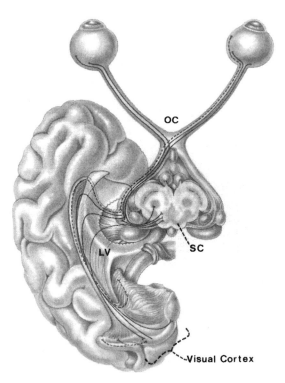

Figure 5.24: Schematic drawing of the major visual pathways. OC, optic chiasm; SC, superior colliculus; LV, lateral ventricle. (Reprinted from (*75*)).

After processing in the neural network in the retina, all visual information travels in the optic nerve (CN II) that enters the optic chiasm, where the fibers of the optic nerve reorganize. From the optic chiasm, the information travels in the optic tracts to the LGN in the thalamus, from which there are connections to the visual cortex (V1), which is located in the posterior portion of the brain.

The organization of the part of the optic nerve that belongs to the classical visual pathways is best illustrated by the effect on vision from visual defects that are caused by lesions of the optic nerve and the optic tract at different locations. If the optic nerve from one eye is severed, no visual information from that eye will reach the LGN. If the optic tract is severed on one side between the optic chiasm and the LGN in animals with forward pointed eyes, the result is homonymous hemianopsia. Visual information from the nasal field on the same side and the temporal field of the opposite eye does not reach the LGN, but visual information from the temporal field on the same side and the nasal field of the opposite eye is unaffected. Midline sectioning of the optic chiasm causes loss of vision in the temporal field in both eyes (the crossed pathways) causing "tunnel vision."

Lesions at more central locations of the visual pathways, such as the LGN or the visual cortex, can cause complex visual defects such as scotoma that manifest by blind (black) spots in the visual fields.

Visual Evoked Potentials

VEP show large individual variations and depend on the stimuli used to elicit the responses and the placement of recording electrodes. A positive peak with a latency of 75–100 ms (P100) usually dominates the VEP recorded from electrodes placed on the scalp (*70*), and sometimes a small peak with a latency of 45–50 ms and a negative peak with a latency of ~70 ms (N70) can be recognized (**Fig. 5.25**).

Neural Generators of the VEP. Years of intensive research on coding in the visual system have resulted in the accumulation of wealth of

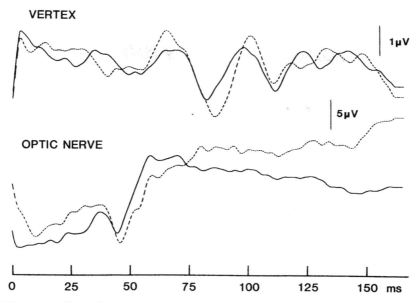

Figure 5.25: Recordings from an electrode placed directly on the optic nerve and from an electrode placed on the scalp at a location approximately overlying the visual cortex in response to stimulation with flashes of light delivered by light-emitting diodes (LED) attached to a contact lens (Reprinted from (*72*) with the permission from Futura Publishing Co.).

knowledge about the responses from single nerve cells in the visual cortex and the LGN as well as from the neural network in the retina. Unfortunately, the information about the generators of the evoked response from the optic nerve and LGN is sparse, and the relationship between the different components of the VEP and the potentials that can be recorded directly from the different parts of the visual system (near-field potentials) is poorly understood.

It is assumed that the N70 and P100 peaks are somehow generated in the visual cortex (striate cortex, Broadman's area 17, see Appendix A) (*1, 71*), but little is known about how these potentials relate to the normal functioning of the visual system. The exact anatomical location of the generators of early components of the VEP is poorly understood. Intraoperative recordings from the optic nerve show an early positive deflection with a latency of 75 ms followed by a broad negative potential with a latency of ~55 ms, in response to short light flashes (*72*) (**Fig. 5.25**). These poten-

tials do not seem to have any corresponding components in the scalp recorded far-field potentials.

The reason that the optic nerve produces such a small far-field potential may be that the medium surrounding the optic nerve and the optic tract is relatively homogeneous with regard to electrical conductivity. The abrupt change in conductivity of the medium around the nerve, which is regarded to be a prerequisite for a nerve to generate stationary far-field peaks (*14, 49, 73*), does not seem to exist for the optic nerve.

REFERENCES

1. Møller AR (2003) *Sensory Systems: Anatomy and Physiology.* Amsterdam: Academic Press.
2. Rexed BA (1954) Cytoarchitectonic atlas of the spinal cord. J. Comp. Neurol. 100:297–379.
3. Brown AG (1981) *Organization in the Spinal Cord: The Anatomy and Phsysiology of Identified Neurons.* New York: Springer.

4. Møller AR (2006) *Neural Plasticity and Disorders of the Nervous System*. Cambridge: Cambridge University Press

5. Tracey DJ (1982) Pathways in proprioception. In: G Garlick, (Ed.) *Proprioception, Posture, and Emotion*. Kensington, N.S.W: University of New South Wales Press, 23–56.

6. Landgren S and H Silfvenius (1971) Nucleus Z, the medullary relay in the projection path to the cerebral cortex of group i muscle afferents from the cat's hind limb. J. Physiol. (Lond.) 218:551–71.

7. Brodal A and O Pompeiano (1957) The vestibular nuclei in cat. J. Anat. 91:438–54.

8. Mountcastle VB (1957) Modality and topographic properties of single neurons of cat's somatic cortex. J. Neurophysiol. 20:408–34.

9. Powell TPS and VB Mountcastle (1959) Some aspects on the functional organization of the cortex of the postcentral gyrus obtained in a single unit analysis with cytoarchitecture. Bull. Johns Hopkins Hosp. 105:133–62.

10. Hume AL and BR Cant (1978) Conduction time in central somatosensory pathways in man. Electroencephalogr. Clin. Neurophysiol. 45:361–75.

11. Gilmore R (1992) Somatosensory evoked potential testing in infants and children. J. Clin. Neurophysiol. 9:324–41.

12. Desmedt JE and G Cheron (1980) Central somatosensory conduction in man: Neural generators and interpeak latencies of the far-field components recorded from neck and right or left scalp and earlobes. Electroencephalogr. Clin. Neurophysiol. 50:382–403.

13. Desmedt JE and G Cheron (1981) Non-cephalic reference recording of early somatosensory potentials to finger stimulation in adult or aging normal man: Differentiation of widespread N18 and contra-lateral N20 from the prerolandic P22 and N30 components. Electroencephalogr. Clin. Neurophysiol. 52:553–70.

14. Lueders H, RP Lesser, JR Hahn et al (1983) Subcortical somatosensory evoked potentials to median nerve stimulation. Brain 106:341–72.

15. Mauguiere F, JE Desmedt and J Courjon (1983) Neural generators of N18 and P14 far-field somatosensory evoked potentials studied in patients with lesion of thalamus or thalamo-cortical radia-tions. Electroencephalogr. Clin. Neurophysiol. 56:283–92.

16. Møller A, R, PJ Jannetta and JE Burgess (1986) Neural generators of the somatosensory evoked potentials: Recording from the cuneate nucleus in man and monkeys. Electroencephalogr. Clin. Neurophysiol. 65:24 1–248.

17. Cracco RQ and JB Cracco (1976) Somatosensory evoked potentials in man: Farfield potentials. Electroencephalogr. Clin. Neurophysiol. 41:60–466.

18. Desmedt JE and G Cheron (1981) Prevertebral (oesophageal) record-ing of subcortical somatosensory evoked potentials in man: The spinal Pl3 component and the dual nature of the spinal gen-era-tors. Electroencephalogr. Clin. Neurophysiol. 52:257–75.

19. Allison T and L Hume (1981) A comparative analysis of short-latency somatosensory evoked potentials in man, monkey, cat, and rat. Exp. Neurol. 72:592–611.

20. Møller AR, PJ Jannetta and HD Jho (1990) Recordings from human dorsal column nuclei using stimulation of the lower limb. Neurosurgery 26:291–9.

21. Lorente de Nó R (1947) Action potentials of the motoneurons of the hypoglossus nucleus. J. Cell Comp. Physiol. 29:207–87.

22. Desmedt JE (1989) Somatosensory evoked potentials in neuromonitoring. In: JE Desmedt (Ed.) *Neuromonitoring in Surgery*. Amsterdam: Elsevier Science Publishers, 1–21.

23. Berkley KJ, RJ Budell, A Blomqvist et al (1986) Output systems of the dorsal column nuclei in the cat. Brain Res. Rev. 396:199–226.

24. Erwin CW and AC Erwin (1993) Up and down the spinal cord: Intraoperative monitoring of sensory and motor spinal cord pathways. J. Clin. Neurophysiol. 10:425–36.

25. Møller AR (2006) *Hearing: Anatomy, Physiology, and Disorders of the Auditory System*, 2nd edition. Amsterdam: Academic Press.

26. Pickles JO (1988) *An Introduction to the Physiology of Hearing*, 2nd edition. London: Academic Press.

27. Rhode WS (1971) Observations of the vibration of the basilar membrane in squirrel monkeys using the mossbauer technique. J. Acoust. Soc. Am. 49:1218–31.

28. Sellick PM, R Patuzzi and BM Johnstone (1982) Measurement of basilar membrane motion in the guinea pig using the Mossbauer technique. J. Acoust. Soc. Am. 72:131–41.

29. Spoendlin H (1970) Structural basis of periph-
    eral frequency analysis. In: R Plomp and GF
    Smoorenburg (Eds.) *Frequency Analysis and
    Periodicity Detection in Hearing*. Leiden: A. W.
    Sijthoff, 2–36.

30. Eggermont JJ, DW Odenthal, DH Schmidt et al
    (1974) Electrocochleography: Basic principles
    and clinical applications. Acta Otolaryngol.
    (Stockh.) Suppl. 316:1–84.

31. Eggermont JJ, A Spoor and DW Odenthal
    (1976) Frequency specificity of tone-bursts elec-
    trocochleography. In: RJ Ruben, C Elberling and
    G Salomon (Eds.) *Electrocochleography*,
    Baltimore, MD: University Park Press, 215–46.

32. Winer JA and CC Lee (2007) The distributed
    auditory cortex. Hear. Res. 229:3–13.

33. Andersen P, PL Knight and MM Merzenich
    (1980) The thalamocortical and corticothalamic
    connections of AI, AII, and the anterior field
    (AAF) in the cat: evidence for two largely seg-
    regated systems of connections. J. Comp.
    Neurol. 194:663–701.

34. Baguley DM (2003) Hyperacusis. J R Soc Med.
    96:582–5.

35. Llinas RR, U Ribary, D Jeanmonod et al (1999)
    Thalamocortical dysrhythmia: A neurological
    and neuropsychiatric syndrome characterized
    by magnetoencephalography. Proc. Natl. Acad.
    Sci. 96:15222–7.

36. Møller AR and P Rollins (2002) The non-clas-
    sical auditory system is active in children but
    not in adults. Neurosci. Lett. 319:41–4.

37. Shannon RV, F-G Zeng, V Kamath et al (1995)
    Speech recognition with primarily temporal
    cues. Science 270:303–4.

38. Loizou PC (2006) Speech processing in voco-
    der-centric cochlear implants. In: AR Møller
    (Ed.) *Cochlear and Brainstem Implants*. Basel:
    Karger, 109–43.

39. Winer JA, ML Chernock, DT Larue et al (2002)
    Descending projections to the inferior colliculus
    from the posterior thalamus and the auditory
    cortex in rat, cat, and monkey. Hear. Res.
    168:181–95.

40. De Ridder D, G De Mulder, V Walsh et al
    (2004) Magnetic and electrical stimulation of
    the auditory cortex for intractable tinnitus. J.
    Neurosurg. 100:560–4.

41. Jewett DL and JS Williston (1971) Auditory
    evoked far fields averaged from scalp of humans.
    Brain 94:681–96.

42. Møller AR, HD Jho, M Yokota et al (1995)
    Contribution from crossed and uncrossed brain-
    stem structures to the brainstem auditory evoked
    potentials (BAEP): A study in human.
    Laryngoscope 105:596–605.

43. Møller AR and PJ Jannetta (1981) Compound
    action potentials recorded intracranially from the
    auditory nerve in man. Exp. Neurol. 74:862–74.

44. Hashimoto I, Y Ishiyama, T Yoshimoto et al
    (1981) Brainstem auditory evoked potentials
    recorded directly from human brain stem and
    thalamus. Brain 104:841–59.

45. Spire JP, GJ Dohrmann and PS Prieto (1982)
    Correlation of brainstem evoked response with
    direct acoustic nerve potential. J Courjon, F
    Manguiere and M Reval (Ed.). Vol. 32. Raven
    Press: New York.

46. Scherg M and D von Cramon (1985) A new
    interpretation of the generators of BAEP waves
    I V: Results of a spatio temporal dipole.
    Electroencephalogr. Clin. Neurophysiol.
    62:290–9.

47. Møller AR, PJ Jannetta and LN Sekhar (1988)
    Contributions from the auditory nerve to the
    brainstem auditory evoked potentials (BAEPs):
    Results of intracranial recording in man.
    Electroencephalogr. Clin. Neurophysiol.
    71:198–211.

48. Møller AR, (1994) Neural generators of audi-
    tory evoked potentials. In: JT Jacobson (Ed.)
    *Principles and Applications in Auditory Evoked
    Potentials*. Boston: Allyn & Bacon. 23–46.

49. Kimura A, A Mitsudome, DO Beck et al (1983)
    Field distribution of antidromically activated
    digital nerve potentials: Models for far-field
    recordings. Neurology 33:1164–9.

50. Martin WH, H Pratt and JW Schwegler (1995)
    The origin of the human auditory brainstem
    response wave II. Electroencephalogr. Clin.
    Neurophysiol. 96:357–70.

51. Buchwald JS and CM Huang (1975) Far field
    acoustic response: Origins in the cat. Science
    189:382–4.

52. Achor L and A Starr (1980) Auditory brain stem
    responses in the cat: I. Intracranial and extracra-
    nial recordings. Electroencephalogr. Clin.
    Neurophysiol. 48:154–73.

53. Achor L and A Starr (1980) Auditory brain stem
    responses in the cat: II. Effects of lesions.
    Electroencephalogr. Clin. Neurophysiol.
    48:174–90.

54. Møller AR and JE Burgess (1986) Neural generators of the brain stem auditory evoked potentials (BAEPs) in the rhesus monkey. Electroencephalogr. Clin. Neurophysiol. 65:361–72.

55. Lang J (1985) Anatomy of the brainstem and the lower cranial nerves, vessels, and surrounding structures. Am. J. Otol. Suppl, Nov:1–19.

56. Lang J (1981) Facial and vestibulocochlear nerve, topographic anatomy and variations. In: M Samii and P Jannetta (Eds.) *The Cranial Nerves*. New York: Springer, 363–77.

57. Fullerton BC, RA Levine, HL Hosford Dunn et al (1987) Comparison of cat and human brain stem auditory evoked potentials. Hear. Res. 66:547–70.

58. Spoendlin H and A Schrott (1989) Analysis of the human auditory nerve. Hear. Res. 43: 25–38.

59. Møller AR, V Colletti and FG Fiorino (1994) Neural conduction velocity of the human auditory nerve: Bipolar recordings from the exposed intracranial portion of the eighth nerve during vestibular nerve section. Electroencephalogr. Clin. Neurophysiol. 92:316–20.

60. Møller AR and PJ Jannetta (1983) Auditory evoked potentials recorded from the cochlear nucleus and its vicinity in man. J. Neurosurg. 59:1013–8.

61. Møller AR and HD Jho (1988) Responses from the brainstem at the entrance of the eighth nerve in human to contralateral stimulation. Hear. Res. 37:47–52.

62. Møller AR and PJ Jannetta (1982) Auditory evoked potentials recorded intracranially from the brainstem in man. Exp. Neurol. 78:144–57.

63. Møller AR, PJ Jannetta and HD Jho (1994) Click-evoked responses from the cochlear nucleus: A study in human. Electroencephalogr. Clin. Neurophysiol. 92:215–24.

64. Møller AR and PJ Jannetta (1982) Evoked potentials from the inferior colliculus in man. Electroencephalogr. Clin. Neurophysiol. 53:612–20.

65. Davis H and SK Hirsh (1979) A slow brain stem response for low-frequency audiometry. Audiology 18:441–65.

66. Møller AR and PJ Jannetta (1983) Interpretation of brainstem auditory evoked potentials: Results from intracranial recordings in humans. Scand. Audiol. (Stockh.) 12:125–33.

67. Wilson WB, WM Kirsch, H Neville et al (1976) Monitoring of visual function during parasellar surger. Surg. Neurol. 5:323–9.

68. Cedzich C, J Schramm and R Fahlbusch (1987) Are flash-evoked visual potentials useful for intraoperative monitoring of visual pathway function? Neurosurgery 21:709–15.

69. Cedzich C, J Schramm, CF Mengedoht et al (1988) Factors that limit the use of flash visual evoked potentials for surgical monitoring. Electroencephalogr. Clin. Neurophysiol. 71: 142–5.

70. Chiappa K (1997) *Evoked Potentials in Clinical Medicine*, 3 rd edition. Philadelphia: Lippincott-Raven.

71. Kraut MA, JC Arezzo and HGJ Vaughan (1985) Intracortical generators of the flash VEP in monkeys. Electroencephalogr. Clin. Neurophysiol. 62:300–12.

72. Møller AR (1987) Electrophysiological monitoring of cranial nerves in operations in the skull base. In: LN Sekhar and VL Schramm Jr (Eds.) *Tumors of the Cranial Base: Diagnosis and Treatment*. Mt. Kisco, New York: Futura Publishing Co, 123–32.

73. Kimura J, A Mitsudome, T Yamada et al (1984) Stationary peaks from moving source in far-field recordings. Electroencephalogr. Clin. Neurophys. 58:351–61.

74. Brodal P (2004) *The Central Nervous System*, 3 rd edition. New York: Oxford University Press.

75. Møller AR (1988) *Evoked Potentials in Intraoperative Monitoring*. Baltimore: Williams and Wilkins.

76. Penfield W and T Rasmussen (1950) *The Cerebral Cortex of Man: A Clinical Study of Localization of Function*. New York: Macmillan.

77. Sessle BJ (1986) Recent development in pain research: Central mechanism of orofacial pain and its control. J. Endod. 12:435–44.

78. Brodel M (1946) *Three Unpublished Drawings of the Anatomy of the Human Ear*. Philadelphia: W.B. Saunders.

79. Møller AR (1975) Noise as a health hazard. Ambio 4:6–13,.

80. Zweig G, R Lipes and JR Pierce (1976) The cochlear compromise. J. Acoust. Soc. Am. 59:975–82.

81. Johnstone BM, R Patuzzi and GK Yates (1986) Basilar membrane measurements and the traveling wave. Hear. Res. 22:147–53.

82. Møller AR (1983) On the origin of the compound action potentials (N_1N_2) of the cochlea of the rat. Exp. Neurol. 80: 633–44. $1C_z$, C_3, C_4, F_{pz}, F_z, and O_z refer to the international 10-20 system for placement of EEG electrodes (105) (see **Fig. 6.1**).

6

Monitoring Somatosensory Evoked Potentials

From: *Intraoperative Neurophysiological Monitoring: Third Edition*,
By A.R. Møller, DOI 10.1007/978-1-4419-7436-5_6,
© Springer Science+Business Media, LLC 2011

INTRODUCTION

Intraoperative recordings of somatosensory evoked potentials (SSEP) were recorded among the earliest used electrophysiological methods for monitoring function of the spinal cord, and for that matter, of any neurological system. Orthopedics was the first specialty of surgery where this method was used, beginning in the 1970s in operations for scoliosis (1–3).

When SSEP are monitored during operations involving the spinal cord, the responses are usually elicited by electrical stimulation of a peripheral nerve and recorded from electrodes placed on the scalp. The SSEP obtained in that way are generated by successive excitation of neural structures of the ascending somatosensory pathway. These potentials, thus, consist of different components that appear with different latencies (see the description of the neural generators of the SSEP in Chap. 5).

SSEP elicited by electrical stimulation of areas of the skin (dermatomes) that are innervated by part of peripheral nerves that originate in specific dorsal roots of the spinal cord were later introduced for more specific monitoring of the spinal cord segments and spinal nerve roots.

Intraoperative recordings of SSEP are also used for monitoring peripheral nerves (see Chap. 13). When used for monitoring of the function of the spinal cord, it must be considered that SSEP only represent the dorsal (sensory) portion of the spinal cord. When suitable methods developed for monitoring the ventral (motor) portion of the spinal cord, such monitoring became an important part of intraoperative monitoring in operations where the spinal cord is at risk of being injured. The value of SSEP monitoring should not be ignored, however, because changes in the recorded SSEP indicate that somatosensory functions have been affected by surgical manipulations or by changes in blood supply to parts of the spinal cord or the brain. More specifically, when used in operations on the spine or in operations on the spinal cord, the SSEP mainly represent the integrity of the dorsal horn of the spinal cord

and the ascending somatosensory tracts in the spinal cord. It is assumed that SSEP represent activity in the dorsal column system and the primary somatosensory cortex. However, it is known that at least one component of the SSEP is generated by other structures, namely, the rostral brainstem (Peak N_{18} – see Chap. 10).

Damage to dorsal column structures is primarily associated with the loss of sensation of touch, vibration, heat, cold, and pain. It should not, however, be ignored that the same areas also serve unconscious proprioception. Unconscious proprioception provides feedback to the spinal cord and the brain of body movements (muscle contraction, tendon stretch, and joint pressure), but does not produce any conscious awareness. This kind of proprioception is absolutely essential for motor control and loss or impairment causes serious movement deficits. This is just another example of overlap between sensory and motor functions. This also means that monitoring the ventral spinal cord that is usually associated with motor functions is not sufficient to reduce the risk of postoperative motor deficits – damage to the dorsal spinal cord causes severe motor deficits if structures that are involved in proprioception are injured. No intraoperative monitoring has been described that specifically is directed to monitor proprioception, but monitoring SSEP is assumed to also cover proprioception at least partly when the SSEP are elicited from peripheral nerves, though the details about what structures contribute to the SSEP as it is commonly recorded are unknown.

Monitoring of SSEP is also used for detecting brain ischemia (4), and changes in the recorded SSEP have been used to estimate cerebral blood flow in areas of the brain that generate the SSEP (5). The use of intraoperative monitoring of SSEP as an indicator of brain ischemia is valuable during operations on aneurysms in which the anterior circulation of the brain may be affected (6). In such operations, upper limb SSEP, elicited from the median nerve of the wrist, are used. The component of the recorded SSEP that is generated by the primary somatosensory cortex (N_{20}) is used as an indicator of ischemia.

In some operations, SSEP have also been used to monitor brainstem function, although auditory brainstem responses (ABR) are usually found to be superior to SSEP for this purpose (see Chap. 7) or may provide additional information. The ascending auditory pathway has several nuclei located in the brainstem, which can explain why ABR seem to be more sensitive for detecting the effect of ischemia and surgical manipulations of the brainstem than SSEP; the somatosensory system has basically only a fiber tract (the medial lemniscus) passing through the brainstem.

Recording of SSEP is used intraoperatively for mapping of the cerebral cortex to confirm the location of the central sulcus before resection is attempted, such as in operations for intractable epilepsy and pain (7).

SSEP IN MONITORING OF THE SPINAL CORD

Intraoperative monitoring of spinal cord function is indicated in operations in which the blood supply to the spinal cord may be compromised as well as in surgical procedures in which the spinal cord may be manipulated. Manipulations of the spinal cord and ischemia may occur in operations on the spine, such as corrective surgery for scoliosis, operations for spinal stenosis, disc removal, in trauma surgery, operations on the spinal cord to remove spinal cord tumors, tethered cord, and syringomyelia are the most frequently performed operations.

> Beginning in the 1970s, orthopedic surgery was the first surgical specialty to introduce intraoperative monitoring of the spinal cord using the recordings of SSEP (1–3). This was the only technique available at that time for monitoring spinal cord function; motor systems could not be monitored because it was not possible to activate descending motor

pathways in anesthetized individuals. Intraoperative monitoring of SSEP only monitors the sensory pathways of the spinal cord and thus, theoretically, the nonsensory pathways, such as the descending motor pathways, may be injured without any noticeable change occurring in the recorded SSEP. This has been regarded to be a serious problem, especially because the blood supply to the part of the spinal cord where the ascending sensory pathways travel (the dorsal portion of the spinal cord) differs from the blood supply of the anterior (ventral) portion of the spinal cord where the descending motor pathways are located, and there are large individual variations. Thus, a deficiency of blood supply causing ischemia or injury to the ventral portion of the spinal cord may cause impairment of motor function (such as paraplegia) without any noticeable changes in the recorded SSEP. This matter has been discussed in much detail, and many efforts were made to remedy this problem by developing methods for monitoring of the motor system. It is now possible to monitor the descending motor pathway intraoperatively due to the development of practical ways to activate the descending spinal motor pathways (8) (see Chap. 10).

There are three limitations in this theoretical argument regarding the separation of the motor and sensory parts of the spinal cord that are important to understand. First, ischemic injury does not always exactly respect the division between the ventral and dorsal spinal cord so that vascular injuries to the ventral portion of the spinal cord can be reflected in changes in the SSEP (9). There are considerable individual variations in the blood supply to the spinal cord that contribute to the uncertainty regarding the blood supply to the spinal cord. Second, in surgery on the spinal cord, mechanical injury to the cord outside of the anatomical location of intramedullary surgery often affects both the ventral and dorsal portions of the spinal cord. Third, insults to the ventral portion of the spinal cord may cause a "spinal shock," and thereby, affect the SSEP transiently because of the abundant connections in the spinal cord that connect different parts of the spinal cord.

Finally, the pathways contributing to the SSEP are not purely limited to the dorsal column system (*10*), and pathways in the lateral cord, such as the dorsal spinocerebellar tract that involves proprioception, but does not produce awareness, may contribute to the SSEP.

Areas 1 and 2 of the somatosensory cortex receive input from deep pressure, limb position, and joint movement receptors, and areas 3 and 4 receive input from active and passive movement of forelimbs (in monkeys) probably from group I muscle afferents (muscle spindles) (for a review see York 1985 (*10*)). This would mean that SSEP evoked by stimulation of peripheral nerves (but probably not from stimulation of dermatomes) and recordings from the scalp include proprioception that travels in ascending fiber tracts that are located in the lateral spinal cord, which is a different location than tactile sensation and vibration that travels in the dorsal column (see Chap. 5).

Many studies have shown evidence that intraoperative monitoring of SSEP reduces the risk of postoperative deficits in many different operations on the spine, most prominently, in corrective operations not only for scoliosis and other deformities of the spine, but also for other spine operations and in operations on the spinal cord such as those for tumors, syringomyelia, and adhesion (tethered cord) (*11–15*). Only a few studies have concerned the use of SSEP in vascular and cardiac operations (*16*).

Combining monitoring of motor evoked potentials (MEP) and SSEP is now common in corrective spine operations (*17, 18*) and in operations on the spinal cord (*19*) (Chap. 10). SSEP and MEP monitoring in vascular operations, such as thoracic aneurysm repair, is controversial (*20*).

Practical experience, obtained from thousands of spine operations in which SSEP were monitored intraoperatively, has shown that monitoring of the SSEP reduces the risk of paralysis and pareses in operations on the spine (21). Of the 184 patients who suffered postoperative deficits in 51,263 operations, injuries in 150 of these 184 patients were predicted on the basis of the results obtained in intraoperative SSEP monitoring.

SSEP failed to detect abnormalities in 34 patients (false negatives). While that represents a very small incidence of false negative results of monitoring (34 of 51,263 operations, or 0.063%), the false negative responses in the 184 who suffered postoperative deficits was high (34 in 184, 18.5%).

Recordings of SSEP are sensitive methods to detect changes in neural conduction, and small changes in the function of the dorsal column pathway in the spinal cord can be easily detected. However, changes in the waveform of such recordings may not only occur as a result of manipulations of the spinal cord that imply a risk of postoperative neurological deficits, but also harmless events such as changes in body temperature or changes in the anesthetic level may cause changes in the recorded potentials.

Stimulation

Electrical stimulation of peripheral nerves on the limbs is used almost exclusively to elicit the SSEP for intraoperative monitoring, but SSEP elicited by electrical stimulation of specific areas of the skin (dermatomes) offers advantages in some operations. Monitoring the sensory part of the upper cervical portion of the spinal cord or the somatosensory pathways in the brainstem can be performed by observing SSEP elicited by electrical stimulation of the median nerve at the wrist. The median nerve contributes to dorsal roots of C_{6-8} and T_1. The potentials that are evoked by stimulation of the ulnar nerve may be used as well. The ulnar nerve contributes to the dorsal roots of C_8 and T_1, whereas the radial nerve, which is rarely stimulated for evoking SSEP, contributes to C_{5-8}, and somewhat to T_1.

Since the median nerve at the wrist contributes to C_8 (and T_1) dorsal roots, the SSEP that are elicited by stimulation of the median nerve should be sensitive to injury of the spinal cord at and above the C_8 level. If the spinal cord below C_8 is at risk, the SSEP must be elicited by stimulation of a peripheral nerve on a lower limb (or an appropriate dermatome).

It has also been shown that mechanical stimulation of the skin to activate receptors can be used to elicit SSEP responses (22), but this way of eliciting SSEP is not in general use in the operating room at present – mainly because the responses are of lower amplitude and have higher variability than those produced by electrical stimulation of a peripheral nerve.

Upper Limb SSEP

When SSEP are recorded in a clinical setting, several recording channels are used to differentiate between the different components of the response (23); similar recordings can be made in the operating room because most of the equipment used in the operating room has 16 amplifiers and can, thus, record in up to 16 channels simultaneously. However, for monitoring purposes, it suffices to record SSEP in a few channels only.

The cortical (N_{20}) and midbrain (N_{18}) potentials evoked by stimulation of the upper limb SSEP may be recorded with the active electrode placed over the contralateral parietal cortex; 2 cm behind C_3 or C_4 called C_3' or C_4' (10–20 system (24), **Fig. 6.1**). The reference electrodes for such recordings are often placed on the forehead. A derivation involving an active electrode on the scalp and a noncephalic reference electrode placed on the shoulder or sternum (25, 26) provides a better identification of early subcortical components of the SSEP in response to median nerve stimulation (P_9, P_{11}, P_{14-16}). SSEP have been effectively recorded with the reference electrode placed on the upper neck in the midline (**Fig. 6.2**) and the active electrode placed on the contralateral parietal scalp about 7 cm lateral to the midline and 2–3 cm behind the plane of the C_z level (corresponding to C_3' or C_4') (25).

The P_9, P_{11}, and P_{14-16} and the N_{18} are also of value for monitoring the cervical spinal cord. The P_9 is generated where the nerves from the brachial plexus enter the spinal cord; P_{11} is generated internally in the dorsal horn of the spinal cord. P_{14-16} are generated close to the termination of the dorsal column or in the dorsal column nuclei (27). Although the P_{14} is classically thought of as generated at the cervico-medullary junction, there is evidence that it has generators

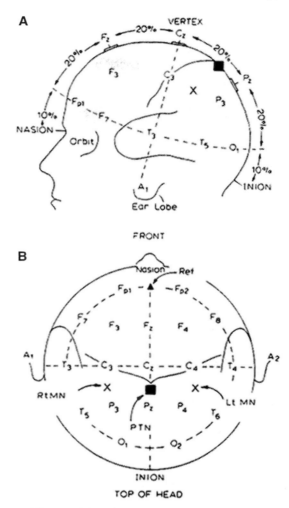

Figure 6.1: The 10–20 electrode system as described by the International Federation of Clinical Neurophysiology. Reprinted from (24) with permission from Elsevier.

in many locations in the cord, and hence, this component of the SSEP may not always change dramatically with injury to the cord (28). The N_{18} of the upper limb SSEP that is generated by structures of the rostral brainstem can be recorded over a large part of the scalp. The N_{20} of the SSEP that is generated in the primary somatosensory cortex can only be recorded on the side of the scalp that is contralateral to the stimulus site (median nerve at the wrist). Recordings from Erb's point reflect activity in

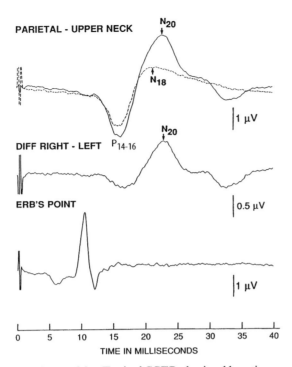

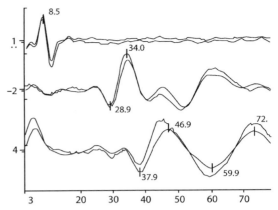

Figure 6.3: Recordings in response to stimulation of the posterior tibial nerve. *Top traces*: Recordings from the common peroneal nerve in the popilitery fossa. *Middle traces*: Recordings of subcortical components of the SSEP from Fpz-C2S. *Lower trace*: Recordings of cortical components of the SSEP from Cz-Fpz. Positive potentials in the recordings (with one replication) are shown with positive potentials at the active electrode on the upper neck (C2S) and Cz as an upward deflection. The reference electrodes were placed at a frontal midline position (Fpz).

Figure 6.2: Typical SSEP obtained by stimulating the median nerve at the wrist while recording on two channels from the two parietal positions 3 cm behind C_3 and C_4 (X in **Fig. 6.1A**), with the reference electrode placed on the upper back, in a patient undergoing microvascular decompression to relieve spasmodic torticollis. The *middle curve* is the difference between the two recordings. The curve is, thus, similar to recording differentially between the two parietal locations, and it shows mainly peak N_{20}. Also shown is the response from Erb's point (response from the brachial plexus).

the brachial plexus and thus, are of value for ensuring effective stimulation of the median nerve (**Fig. 6.2**).

Lower Limb SSEP

Recordings of lower limb SSEP are usually performed with the active electrode placed on C_z (or 2 cm behind) and the reference electrode either at a frontal scalp position or at a noncephalic location (shoulder or upper neck).

There are cortical components (P_{40} or P_{37}) and subcortical components (N_{34}, N_{21}) of the lower limb SSEP that can have value for intraoperative monitoring (see **Fig. 6.3**). The waveform of the recorded potentials depends on the placements of the recording electrodes (see also Chap. 5, **Fig. 5.12**).

Recordings of the cortical components of the lower limb SSEP are usually made with the active electrode placed 2 cm posterior to the vertex (C_z') and the reference electrode placed at the forehead.

The N_{34} component of the subcortical component of the SSEP originates in the brainstem. It is typically recorded using electrodes placed at Fpz and the upper neck. It is readily recorded in most patients, but can be of low amplitude. The advantage of monitoring this component during spine surgery is that it is much less sensitive to anesthetic effects than the components that originate from the cortex. The subcortical N_{21} component of the SSEP is elicited by lower limb stimulation and recorded from an electrode placed at T_{12} vertebra with the reference electrode on the iliac crest. This early component has, however, not found wide use in intraoperative monitoring, and the electrode placement for recording this potential usually causes unacceptable levels of electrical interference.

Recordings from peripheral nerves in the popliteal fossa can be used to record the action potential volley traveling cranially in the nerve that is being stimulated at more distal locations, such as the posterior tibial nerve. This is of value for demonstrating that the stimulation produced an effective activation of the peripheral nerve.

Which Nerves Should Be Stimulated?. For lower limb SSEP, it is common praxis to stimulate the posterior tibial nerve at the ankle as recommended by the American Clinical Neurophysiology Society (2006) Guideline 9D: guidelines on short-latency SSEP (*29*) and in the report of an IFCN committee, 1994 (*30*) and by a position statement by the American Society of Neurophysiological Monitoring (ASNM) (*31*).

One would think that it would be better to stimulate the common peroneal nerve at the knee because the length of the peripheral nerve that the nerve impulses have to travel before reaching the spinal cord is shorter than when the posterior tibial nerve is used. Using a shorter path to the spinal cord by stimulating at a more proximal location makes the dispersion of the neural activity that arrives at the spinal cord less than when elicited by stimulation of a more distal location, such as the posterior tibial nerve, which is the traditional location for stimulation. It would, therefore, seem to be better to stimulate the peroneal nerve at the knee (the popliteal fossa). However, the common praxis of stimulating the posterior tibial nerve is based on laboratory studies that show that scalp SSEP have larger amplitudes when elicited from the posterior tibial nerve compared with SSEP elicited by stimulating the common peroneal nerve (*32*).

Another advantage of stimulating the posterior tibial nerve is that recording the response from the popliteal fossa at the knee provides a convenient check that the stimulation is adequate; it can detect conduction blocks such as from ischemia of the leg, which would cause deterioration of the SSEP response. One other reason for stimulating the posterior tibial nerve instead of the common peroneal nerve is that it is often easier to access the ankle than the knee in a person placed on the operating table.

Therefore, based on laboratory studies in participants without neurological disorders (such as peripheral nerve disorders), stimulation of the posterior tibial nerve is the best choice in most patients. Verification of these results by studies in the operating room has not been published.

Stimulation of the common peroneal nerve should be reserved for use in patients with peripheral nerve neuropathy, where it may be better to stimulate the common peroneal nerve at the knee because of the shorter peripheral nerve path that would be involved and would be less effected from the neuropathy. It is also important to consider that conduction deficits from neuropathy are the greatest in the distal portions of a nerve, and neuropathy's effect on the dispersion of neural activity at the target neuron increases with the length of the nerve that is involved causing temporal dispersion of the neural activity that arrives at cells in the spinal cord.

There is little doubt that the volleys of nerve impulses elicited from stimulation of a nerve on the foot arrive at the brainstem level more dispersed in time (lower degree of temporal coherence) than activity that is elicited from sites on nerves that are closer to the spinal cord, such as the common peroneal nerve, because of the longer nerves involved. It is generally assumed that temporally dispersed neural activity is less effective in activating the target neuron because it causes an excitatory post synaptic potential (EPSP) with a lower amplitude than neural activity that is less temporally dispersed (Fig. 6.4). Experimental studies of SSEP elicited from the

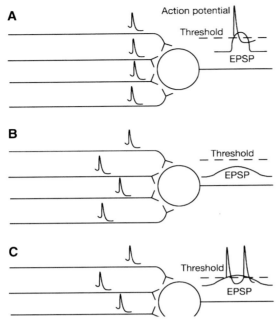

Figure 6.4: Hypothetical illustration of the effect of spatial integration by a cell on which many axons converge. (**A**) Little spatial dispersion, one stimulus impulse elicits one impulse in the target neuron's axon. (**B**) Increased spatial dispersion causing broadening of the EPSP and lower amplitude. The high threshold of the target neuron prevents it from firing. (**C**) The same degree of spatial dispersion as in (**B**), but threshold of the target neuron is lower. The prolonged EPSP makes the neuron fire twice. Reprinted from (*33*) with the permission of Cambridge University Press.

posterior tibial nerve compared with SSEP elicited from stimulation of the common peroneal nerve, however, show that stimulation of the posterior tibial nerve is more effective in eliciting SSEP responses by Pelosi et al. (32). There seems to be little doubt that the neural activity that reaches the first neuron (in the dorsal column nuclei) is more dispersed when elicited from the posterior tibial nerve compared with the activity elicited from the common peroneal nerve (because of the longer distance). The study by Pelosi et al., thus, seems to show that increased temporal dispersion is advantageous and indicates that activity that is more dispersed

may cause greater activation of the somatosensory system. The reason could be that prolonged EPSPs at the target neuron can cause more than one nerve impulse in the axon of this neuron (see Fig. 6.4C) (33).

The increased temporal dispersion of the neural volley elicited by electrical stimulation of peripheral nerves on the lower limbs is greater in older individuals and is usually regarded as the cause of the difficulties experienced in eliciting SSEP in older individuals. The effect is amplified by different kinds of neuropathies, such as those seen in diabetic patients or in postpoliomyelitis patients. This would indicate that a broadening of the elicited EPSP and subsequent lower amplitude would be the cause of the reduced activation of the somatosensory system, thus in accordance with the hypothetical situation illustrated in **Fig. 6.4B**.

Recording SSEP in response to upper limb (median nerve) stimulation usually can be recorded without difficulty in patients, where recordings of lower limb SSEP fail because of such neuropathies. In situations where neuropathy makes it difficult to obtain satisfactory SSEP responses, it might be worth trying double impulses or short pulse trains for the stimulation.

It is evident from the hypothetical situations displayed in **Fig. 6.4** that both the intensity and the duration of the stimulation are important for synaptic activation. There are two ways of increasing neural excitation, increasing the stimulus intensity, thus increasing the number of nerve fibers being activated, or increasing the number of nerve impulses in individual nerve fibers. This means that not only the intensity of electrical stimulation of a peripheral nerve to elicit SSEP is important, but also the duration of the activation of nerve fibers is important.

Thus, if electrical stimulation with a single impulse causes nerve fibers to fire more than one nerve impulse, it may increase the activation of the target neuron in the spinal cord. While it is well known that stimulation with a train of impulses is more effective for eliciting motor responses than single impulses (Chap. 10), increasing the duration of the activation of a peripheral nerve by using trains of impulses instead of a single impulse has not been described for SSEP.

Dermatomal Evoked SSEP

Monitoring of the spinal cord by SSEP recordings that are elicited by stimulation of peripheral nerves as described above represents the sum of the neural conduction in many spinal nerve roots. Peripheral nerves receive input from large areas of the body, and electrical stimulation of peripheral nerves, therefore, simulates the normal activation of sensory receptors (muscle receptors, joint receptors, and skin receptors) located in many different parts of the body. Such stimulation activates the spinal cord in a spatially unspecific manner because the peripheral nerve that is stimulated provides input to many segments of the spinal cord. Injury to a specific dorsal root or segment of the spinal cord may not affect the recorded SSEP to a great extent because the contributions from intact dorsal roots mask the deficit in a single dorsal root or a single segment of the spinal cord.

The neural conduction in one or a few dorsal roots or spinal cord segments can be monitored by applying the stimulation to a well-defined small part (skin) of the body. Individual dorsal roots of the spinal cord carry the sensory nerve supply to patches of the skin, known as dermatomes, as illustrated in **Fig. 6.5**. SSEP obtained in response to electrical stimulation of individual dermatomes provide a way to monitor the function of specific dorsal roots and specific parts of the spinal cord (**Fig. 6.6**).

Stimulation of dermatomes provides a more specific form of monitoring of spinal nerves and their roots than that which can be obtained by stimulation of peripheral nerves that activate many roots. If one root is injured, the SSEP will only decrease by a small amount, whereas such an injury has a large effect on the SSEP when elicited from the dermatome that is innervated by nerve fibers from the root that is damaged.

Dermatomal SSEP are much more sensitive to localized changes in neural conduction in dorsal roots and injury to a single spinal cord segment than the SSEP that are elicited by stimulation of peripheral nerves, although dermatomes overlap to some extent, and more than one dorsal root may be activated when a dermatome is stimulated. However, the amplitude of dermatomal SSEP tend to be lower, and the response exhibits a greater degree of variability than those obtained in response to stimulation of peripheral nerves (**Fig. 6.6**).

RECORDING SSEP FOR MONITORING PERIPHERAL NERVES

If an operation is performed distally on the arm or the leg, it is possible to record from the respective nerve proximal to the location of the operation while stimulating the nerve electrically at a location that is distal to the site of the operation. This method is described in detail in Chap. 13.

However, it is often more practical to monitor SSEP elicited by electrical stimulation of the nerve in question at a location distal to that where the nerve is being operated upon. In that way, the recorded SSEP can serve to monitor neural conduction in peripheral sensory nerves. Vrahas et al. (*34*) described the technique of monitoring the sciatic nerve during operations for pelvic and acetabular fractures, during which surgical manipulations may injure the sciatic nerve. Any component of the SSEP can be used to detect changes in neural conduction in a peripheral nerve. The signs of injuries to a peripheral nerve, like the sciatic nerve, are prolonged latencies and the reduction of the evoked potentials' amplitudes. Prolongation of neural conduction in the peripheral nerve from which the SSEP are elicited affects the latencies of all peaks equally. The amplitude of the response (CAP) recorded directly from a nerve in response to electrical stimulation decreases in direct proportion to the relative

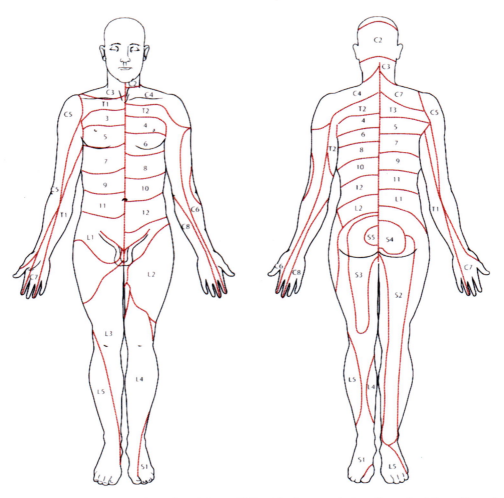

Figure 6.5: Dermatomes. (Reprinted from (*80*) with the permission from the Mayo Foundation: Rochester, Minnesota).

number of nerve fibers in which neural conduction is blocked, but the amplitude of the different components of the SSEP decreases to a lesser degree. The amplitude of the components of the SSEP that are of cortical origin is likely to decrease less than those of earlier components. It is, therefore, appropriate to use components of the SSEP that are generated by more peripheral structures than the cortex for monitoring.

The response recorded from the T_{12} location is an example of a peripherally generated evoked potential that is assumed to originate in the dorsal column and thus, represents neural activity that has not undergone any neural transformation in a nucleus. The amplitude of this response, therefore, accurately reflects the number of fibers of a nerve that is conducting, providing that supramaximal stimulation is used. A reduction in the amplitude of the T_{12} response by, for instance, 30% can be assumed to indicate that 30% of the nerve fibers are no longer active. Since the variation in conduction velocity of the different nerve fibers that make up the nerve in question is likely to increase, the CAP recorded from the nerve broadens.

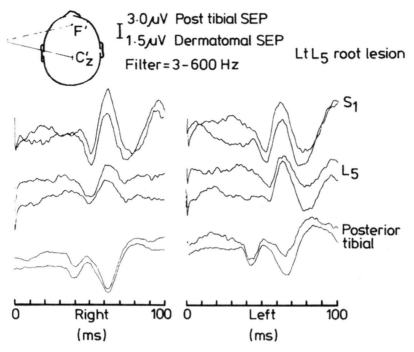

Figure 6.6: Comparison between responses elicited by stimulation of the S_1 and L_5 dermatome and the posterior tibial nerve. (Reprinted from (*81*) with permission from the British Medical Journal Publishing Group).

The amplitude of the CAP is, therefore, not an accurate measure of the number of active nerve fibers, but the area of the CAP is a better measure.

Other factors than injury may affect the CAP recorded from a nerve. Thus, the CAP, as well as the far-field evoked potentials (SSEP), may be affected by changes in the course of the peripheral nerve that is being tested or by changes in the geometry of the nerve, which, for example, may occur if the leg is abducted. Such manipulations may cause changes in the amplitude of the response (*35*) that should not be mistaken for signs of injuries to nervous tissue.

It may be practical to use sequential stimulation of the sciatic nerve on both sides so that the SSEP that are elicited by stimulation of the sciatic nerve on the operated side can be compared with that from the (assumed) unaffected side. Using the difference in the SSEP that are recorded from the two sides eliminates any influence caused from changes in the temperature of the limbs and other general changes, such as in the level of anesthesia or blood pressure. Such changes would affect both sides equally.

Neural conduction in peripheral nerves of the arm and in the brachial plexus can be monitored by recording SSEP and using methods similar to those described above for the lower limb. In such cases, it is practical to use the P_{14-16} complex of the SSEP elicited by stimulation of the median nerve or the ulnar nerve, depending on which of these two nerves is at risk of being affected by the operation.

Injuries to the brachial plexus may occur from positioning of the patient on the operating table. Such injuries may occur even in operations that are not affecting peripheral nerves on the arm or the brachial plexus at all. Injuries to the brachial plexus from positioning of the patient are rather common, and it is justified to record SSEP in response to median nerve stimulation during the positioning of patients where the arm and shoulder are involved.

Recording from Erb's point may also be useful because such recordings yield responses from the brachial plexus and thus, reflect changes in neural conduction of a peripheral nerve on the area that is proximal to the site of stimulation (**Fig. 6.2**).

Peripheral nerves of the arm and leg are mixed nerves in which the same nerve carries both sensory and motor fibers. When SSEP are used to monitor neural conduction in such nerves, it is the sensory fibers that are tested. When direct recordings from nerves are used for monitoring, then it is neural conduction in both sensory and motor fibers that is tested, and when muscle responses are recorded in response to electrical stimulation of a mixed nerve, then it is the motor portion of the nerve that is tested. It is useful to record responses from muscles that are innervated by nerves that are at risk of being injured during an operation; this may serve to monitor neural conduction in peripheral nerves as a supplement or replacement for recording of SSEP.

The amplitudes of the responses that are obtained at the end of an operation may serve as a prognostic measure of the extent of an injury to a peripheral nerve; although such information should be treated cautiously because the responses obtained at the end of the operation cannot distinguish a temporary injury from a permanent injury.

For stimulation and recording, needle electrodes or wire hook electrodes should be used; they should be placed percutaneously to reach the nerves in question, or within their close proximity. In operations to repair brachial plexus injuries, it may be of value to stimulate spinal roots electrically in the surgical field while observing the cortical component of the SSEP for the purpose of discriminating a root avulsion.

Pedicle Screws

Pedicle screws are used to hold spinal instrumentation in place, and when inserted, there is a risk that these screws injure spinal nerve roots. Recording of SSEP has been used for monitoring sensory nerve roots of the spinal cord during the placement of pedicle screws.

However, as discussed above, SSEP elicited by electrical stimulation of a peripheral nerve activate several nerve roots that enter the spinal cord; if one is damaged (for example by the pedicle screw), the input to the spinal cord will only decrease marginally and may not cause a sufficient change in the SSEP to be detected. The specificity of such monitoring can be improved by using stimulation of dermatomes instead of peripheral nerves (see page 101). Both forms of monitoring of SSEP have shortcomings for monitoring insertion of pedicle screws, and these two methods of recording SSEP are now largely replaced by recording of motor (muscle) potentials (electromyographic potentials (EMG), either stimulated or free-running) (*36, 37*) as discussed in Chap. 10.

STIMULATION TECHNIQUE AND PARAMETERS FOR SSEP MONITORING

SSEP are commonly elicited by electrical stimulation of peripheral nerves on the limbs or by stimulation of dermatomes.

Peripheral Nerves

Electrical stimulation of peripheral nerves can be accomplished using surface electrodes, subdermal needle electrodes or wire hook electrodes. The electrodes should be placed close to the nerves that are to be stimulated. The distance between the two stimulating electrodes should be 1–2 cm. The negative electrode should be placed closest to the trunk (most proximal). For stimulation of specific dermatomes, surface electrodes (such as EKG pads) should be placed on the skin within the dermatome that is to be stimulated, 5–10 cm apart on one side of the body. A constant-current stimulator is the best choice for stimulation of peripheral nerves and dermatomes because changes in the electrode impedance do not affect the current that is delivered to the nerve.

When stimulating a peripheral and mixed nerve in an anesthetized patient who is not paralyzed, the stimulus current should be increased to a level where a noticeable muscle twitch can be seen (a twitch of the thumb when stimulating the median nerve, a twitch of the muscles on the leg when stimulating the peroneal nerve at the knee, or a twitch of the big toe when stimulating the posterior tibial nerves). If the anesthesia regime includes a muscle relaxant, a muscle response will not be detectable, and the stimulus current level should be set to three to four times the threshold for a preoperative twitch. (Muscle relaxants do not influence the effectiveness of stimulation since muscle relaxants do not affect neural conduction in peripheral nerves.) If the optimal stimulus intensity cannot be determined in an individual patient, a setting of 20 mA has been recommended (*38*), although others use current levels as high as 100 mA.

The number of nerve fibers that are activated by electrical stimulation increases with increasing stimulus strength up to the level at which the stimulation depolarizes all nerve fibers in the nerve that contribute to the SSEP. A strong stimulus, therefore, produces a response with the highest possible amplitude. The optimal level of stimulation cannot be used in patients who are conscious because it causes intolerable pain, but in anesthetized patients it is possible to use optimal stimulus strength.

Optimal Stimulus Rate. The stimulus rate should be set so that an interpretable record can be obtained in as short a time as possible. The number of responses that can be collected in a certain time increases with increasing stimulus rate (**Fig. 6.7**). A high stimulus rate, therefore, allows faster collection of an interpretable response. However, when the stimulus rate is increased above a certain value, the amplitude of each individual response decreases. There is, therefore, an optimal choice of the stimulus rate at which an interpretable record can be obtained within the shortest amount of time, namely, the rate at which the product of the

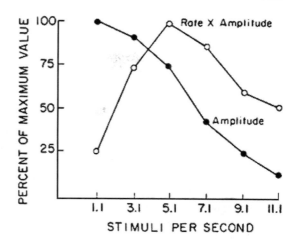

Figure 6.7: Effect of increasing the rate of the stimulus presentation (*filled circles*) on the amplitude of the SSEP in response to electrical stimulation of the posterior tibial nerve. *Open circles* show the product of the amplitude of the SSEP and the stimulus rate. (Reprinted from (*39*) with permission from Elsevier).

amplitude of the response and the stimulus rate has its maximal value (*38, 39*).

The stimulus rate affects various components of the SSEP differently, and the optimal rates are, therefore, different for the different components. The optimal rate is lower when the evoked responses are elicited from the lower limbs than it is when elicited from the upper limbs. In most patients, the optimal stimulus rate for observing the primary cortical components (N_{20} peak for upper limb SSEP and N_{45} peak for lower limb) in the SSEP is ~10 pulses per second (pps) when elicited by stimulation of a nerve on the upper limbs (medial nerve) and approximately 5 pps when elicited by stimulation of the lower limbs (posterior tibial nerve) (**Fig. 6.7**).

There is, however, considerable individual variation in the optimal stimulus rate. In patients with peripheral neuropathy, such as may be caused by diabetes mellitus, a lower stimulus rate yields a better response. In all situations, avoid selecting rates that are multiples of 60 Hz in North America and 50 Hz in Europe in order to reduce contamination of the recordings with power line frequency signals (see Chap. 18).

If nerves on both extremities are to be stimulated, the nerve on each extremity should be stimulated, one at a time, or the stimulation of the two extremities should be alternated and the responses displayed separately. Although some investigators have described the use of bilateral stimulation, this is not recommended because injury to one side only causes a small change in such bilaterally elicited potentials because the response from the intact side dominates, and it may be impossible to detect even severe changes in the response from one side if the response from the other side were unchanged.

Dermatomes

The stimulus strength used for stimulation of dermatomes should be adjusted so that it does not stimulate underlying structures (muscles) in patients who are not paralyzed. Stimulation of dermatomes may produce smaller response amplitudes, and thus, more responses may need to be collected and averaged to obtain an interpretable record (**Fig. 6.6**). It may be practical to alternate between stimulating dermatomes that correspond to the level of the spinal cord that is being operated upon and stimulating a peripheral nerve that includes that same area of the spinal cord.

Recording of SSEP

Recording SSEP from the scalp can be performed using needle or wire hook electrodes or surface electrodes. Needle or wire hook electrodes should be applied after the patient is anesthetized. Surface electrodes can be applied before the patient is anesthetized. Needle and wire hook electrodes can provide stable recordings over many hours.

The response to stimulation of the median nerve (upper limb SSEP) is best recorded from electrodes placed over the contralateral parietal region of the scalp, 3–4 cm behind the central plane through C_3 and C_4 and 7 cm lateral from the midline (C_3' and C_4') (10–20 system, see **Fig. 6.1**). It is helpful in distinguishing between

N_{18} and N_{20} to record two channels of SSEP, one channel differentially between an electrode on the right parietal scalp with a reference at the upper neck, and the other channel from the left parietal scalp with the same reference (**Fig. 6.1**). (Most modern equipment offer as many as 16 channels for recordings, see Chap. 18).

It is practical to record SSEP from both sides simultaneously, with a shared reference at the upper neck. This yields a clear N_{20} from the contralateral recording and a clear N_{18} on the recording from the side ipsilateral to the one where the stimulation is applied. If recorded with the active electrode placed at C_z, the N_{20} peak of the SSEP is much more attenuated, and the N_{18} peak may dominate that region of the recording. The N_{20} peak may not be noticeable at all if the active electrode is placed on the ipsilateral parietal region of the scalp. Thus, recording from different locations on the scalp makes it possible to differentiate between the N_{18} and the N_{20} peaks.

A clear representation of the potentials generated in the dorsal column nuclei (P_{14-16}) can be obtained by placing the reference electrode at the inion or the upper neck. If the reference electrode is placed at the frontal portion of the scalp (F_z) or the forehead, these potentials are not prominent at all, and the recorded potentials will be dominated by potentials of cortical origin (N_{20}) when the contralateral median nerve is stimulated. With the reference electrode placed at the neck the recordings also yield earlier peaks, such as P_9, which is generated by the activity entering the spinal cord, and P_{11}, which is generated internally in the spinal cord (see Chap. 5).

When recording the responses elicited by stimulation of the lower limbs, the active electrode should be placed in the midline, 3–4 cm posterior to the plane of the C_z and the reference electrode placed either at a frontal location in the midline (F_{pz}) or on the upper neck. Since the potentials are recorded from the midline, the same electrode position can be used regardless of which side is being stimulated. To visualize early components of the lower limb

SSEP, the reference electrode should be placed over the T_{12} vertebra. Recording differentially between C_z and T_{12} can be noisy due to the long distance between the two electrodes, and, therefore, more responses must be averaged to get an interpretable record than when recording between C_z and a frontal location. In many situations, it is not possible to obtain useable recordings from T_{12}.

Optimization of SSEP Recordings. Optimization of recording conditions can make it possible to record SSEP from lower limbs without the use of signal averaging (*40*) as illustrated in **Fig. 6.8**.

Optimization of recordings of SSEP is most important for lower limb SSEP, which show greater individual variations than upper limb SSEP. Optimization involves achieving the best signal-to-noise ratio (SNR) by reducing noise (see Chap. 18) and achieving the largest signal amplitude (*40, 41*). The amplitude of the recorded potentials depends on the placement of the recording electrodes, the anesthesia, and the stimulation.

Different kinds of anesthesia suppress the recorded potentials to different degrees; total intravenous anesthesia (TIVA) consisting of Propofol, benzodiazepines, Ketamine, Etomidate, and opioids as favorable agents that seem to suppress SSEP the least (*40*) (similar anesthesia regimen is favorable for use in connection with the monitoring of MEP (*42, 43*) as such monitoring is often performed together with SSEP monitoring, see Chap. 10).

The best SNR is achieved by reducing electrical noise from the environment, biological noise from the patient, and reducing the amount of noise picked up by the electrodes, which depends on their placement (distance between electrodes and electrode impedance) (see Chaps. 17 and 18).

The amplitude and the waveform of the recorded SSEP depend on the placement of the recording electrodes, and the electrical interference and the spontaneous EEG that are picked up by the recording electrodes also depend on the electrode placement (*41*), as seen in the

recordings in **Fig. 6.7**, where the amplitude of the P_{37} component had a maximum when the active electrode was placed at C_z for each nerve. This is the case where the pathways have a normal crossing of the midline (decussation) as confirmed by the presence of ipsilateral P_{37} fields and contralateral N_{37} potentials. **Fig. 6.7** also shows that bipolar recording from locations C_z–C_{p4} and C_z–C_{p3} was optimal regarding the amplitude of the recorded SSEP. The recordings in **Fig. 6.8** also reveal greater noise in -F_{pz} derivations resulting in less reproducibility of the recorded waveform.

This means that it is worth paying attention to the placement of recording electrodes. Optimal placement can decrease the number of responses that must be collected to obtain an interpretable response, and it can focus on the components of the SSEP that are most important for the actual monitoring. Using optimal stimulation is also important (see **Fig. 6.8**).

In some individuals, the somatosensory pathways are not crossed as they are normally, and that affects the recordings of SSEP. In a study of 206 consecutively monitored thoracolumbar spine surgeries involving 173 patients MacDonald et al. (*40*) found that sensorimotor pathways were not crossed in four patients with horizontal gaze palsy and progressive scoliosis (HGPPS) (six surgeries, one patient had three surgeries) as they are normally. SSEP monitoring in such patients must take that into account and use a different electrode placement.

The waveform of the SSEP is not only influenced by electrode positions, but it also depends on the recording parameters. The filter settings of the amplifiers affect the waveform of the recorded potentials considerably, and it affects the contamination of the recorded potentials from electrical interference and from biologic signals, such as spontaneous EEG and muscle activity. It is, therefore, important to use optimal filtering to minimize the number of responses that must be averaged in order to obtain an interpretable record. As is described in detail in the chapter on monitoring of auditory brainstem responses (ABR) (Chap. 7), zero phase finite impulse response digital filters have advantages

A

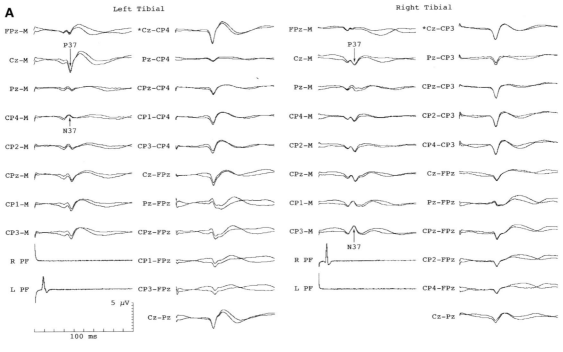

B

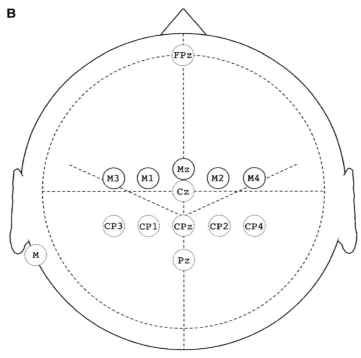

over the traditionally used analog filters, including the digital filters that emulate such analog filters (see Chap. 18). Similar filters as those described in the chapter on ABR may be used for filtering SSEP. If only analog filters are used, the low cutoff should be set at between 1 and 5 Hz (high-pass filter) and for the high cutoff (low-pass filter), a setting of between 125 and 250 Hz will reproduce cortical responses clearly. These filter settings may cause smoothing and attenuation of early components, such as the P_{14-16} peak of the SSEP elicited by stimulation of the median nerve. If these components are important for the interpretation of the SSEP, a higher low-pass cutoff setting should be chosen, for instance, between 500 and 1,000 Hz.

Responses elicited by median nerve stimulation should be viewed in a 40 or 50-ms wide time window, while potentials that are elicited by lower limb stimulation should be viewed in an 80- to 100-ms wide time window. The sampling rate for the analog-to-digital conversion should be at least 2,000 Hz (0.5 ms sampling time) when a low-pass filter setting of 500 Hz is used, but it is more appropriate to use a 5–10 kHz sampling rate (see Chap. 10). Most modern equipment uses a sampling rate that is assumed to be adequate and which the user cannot normally alter (and it may not even be known to the user).

All modern equipment has the possibility for artifact rejection, which is based on the amplitude of the response. If the response includes an initial artifact from electrical stimulation, the first part of the recording should not be used for determining whether a record should be rejected or not (see Chap. 18).

It is imperative to be able to display the output of the amplifiers directly so that the source of interference that may occur suddenly during

an operation can be identified. A prerequisite for being able to eliminate such intermittent interferences is that its source is identified. The waveform of the averaged response cannot be used for this purpose; only the directly recorded waveform can reveal the source of the interference. If the interference is so strong that it activates the artifact rejection all the time, there is no way to characterize the nature of the interference. Only examination of the waveform of the raw output from the amplifiers can lead to the identification of the interference.

For the detection of changes that may occur during an operation, it is important to be able to compare every recording made during an operation with a baseline. The continuous comparison between the baseline and the actual recordings is the most effective way of detecting changes in the SSEP. The popular "waterfall" (or "stack") display is useful for documentation, but not for the detection of changes during an operation. Rather, such a display may miss slow changes and distract from observing changes that occur during an operation.

Baseline recordings should be made for the individual patient preferably after the patient has been anesthetized, but before the operation is begun. The recordings made during the operation should be compared to that of the baseline. The display of the baseline recording should be superimposed on the current recordings.

INTERPRETATION OF SSEP

In some operations, monitoring of the amplitude of any component is sufficient; whereas in other operations, it is of importance to be able to identify the structures that are affected. Knowledge about the neural generators of the

---

Figure 6.8: (A) Illustration of the waveform and amplitude of cortical SSEP elicited by electrical stimulation of the tibial nerve and recorded from the scalp using surface electrodes (impedance <2 kΩ), placed as indicated using the scheme shown in (B). No signal averaging was used. M Mastoid, PF Popliteal fossa. (B) Electrode placement for the recordings in (A). Reproduced from (*40*) with the permission Lippincott Williams & Wilkins.

SSEP is essential in order to make correct interpretation of changes in the SSEP with regard to the anatomical location of the injury that has caused the observed changes in the SSEP. For example, if peak N_{18} is mistaken for peak N_{20}, an error in interpretation of the anatomical location of the injury will occur because the neural generators of these two peaks are anatomically different (upper brainstem versus sensory cortex) (see page 72).

What Kinds of Changes Are Important?

Changes in the amplitude of specific components (peaks) in the SSEP are important indicators of surgically induced injuries, but prolonged latencies are also important to consider (44, 45). Some studies seem to indicate that changes (decreases) in the amplitude of the SSEP are more indicative of injury than are changes in the latencies (44). The Jones (44) study showed that if the amplitude of either the earliest or the second component of the lower limb SSEP decreased more than 40%, injuries that could cause permanent postoperative deficits were likely to have occurred. A 60% decrease was associated with a 50% risk of postoperative complications. Nuwer et al. (45) generally agreed with this evaluation. Studies have shown that the duration over which such changes occur is important, and if the duration of the disappearance of the recorded potentials is short, even a total disappearance of recordable potentials does not mean that (measurable) postoperative neurological deficits will occur (45). What constitutes "a short time" is debated, and it has been indicated that even a 30-min disappearance of evoked potentials may not indicate that postoperative sensory deficits are likely to occur. In addition, it is important to be aware of the large individual variations in the tolerance for changes in function that may occur during an operation. Older people can be regarded as having lower tolerance than younger and healthy individuals.

Large, but transient, changes in the SSEP may be indications of spinal shock that could be caused by injury or ischemia of the ventral part of the spinal cord, and the fact that the changes are usually only transient should not be interpreted to indicate that the function has recovered. However, transient changes in the SSEP should be considered a serious warning that requires immediate attention. Brown and Nash have emphasized the need to perform a wake-up test if changes occur in the SSEP that cannot be regarded as being minimal (46) because such changes in the SSEP may indicate that descending motor pathways have become injured.

Effect of Temperature and Other Nonpathological Factors

Lowering the temperature of the limb on which a peripheral nerve is being stimulated electrically below that of normal body temperature causes a decrease in the neural conduction velocity of peripheral nerves and thus, an increase in the latency of the SSEP. Less is known about the effect of abnormally high temperature (fewer). The latency of SSEP elicited by stimulation of the median nerve often increases during an operation because the temperature of the limb that is stimulated decreases. Often an arm or a leg is located outside the drape and thus, exposed to the cold air of the operating room (47). Lower limb SSEP can usually be recorded at body temperatures as low as 25°C, and SSEP elicited by stimulation of the median nerve may be recorded in patients with body temperatures as low as 20°C, but the latency of the different component is prolonged.

A decrease in the core temperature of the patient causes decreased conduction velocity of the somatosensory pathway in the spinal cord and the brain. For SSEP elicited by stimulation of the posterior tibial nerve, the prolongation of the latency has been estimated to be 1.15 ms/°C for the P_{40} peak (48).

Amplitudes of the different components of evoked potentials are more susceptible to random changes than are the latencies of specific components. Better control of stimulation and recording has reduced nonsurgically induced variations in the amplitude of the SSEP and thus, made it possible to interpret changes in the SSEP with a higher degree of certainty.

EVOKED POTENTIALS FROM THE SPINAL CORD

Techniques have been described to record evoked potentials from electrodes placed close to the spinal cord (*49–54*), and methods for direct electrical stimulation of the spinal cord have also been developed for intraoperative monitoring of the spinal cord (*15, 55–59*).

Spinal Evoked Potentials Elicited by Stimulation of Peripheral Nerves

Evoked potentials, recorded directly from the exposed spinal cord or from locations close to the spinal cord in response to electrical stimulation of peripheral nerves, have been utilized for many years to monitor the integrity of the spinal cord (*51, 58–61*). Such recordings are invasive, and the electrodes are located closer to the neural generators, and therefore, the recorded evoked potentials have much larger amplitudes than those recorded from the scalp.

Recording directly from the spinal cord while stimulating a peripheral nerve yields evoked potentials (**Fig. 6.9**) that are generated in different parts of the spinal cord. The recorded potentials are largely unaffected by anesthesia, which is not the case for the potentials that are generated in the cortex and recorded from the surface of the scalp. Since the recorded potentials have larger amplitudes than those recorded from the scalp, an interpretable record can be obtained much faster than when recording from scalp electrodes. The potentials that are recorded directly from the spinal cord have sharper peaks than the SSEP (**Fig. 6.9**), and therefore, it is easier to detect smaller changes in the latencies of the potentials recorded from the spinal cord than it is for potentials recorded from the scalp.

Two specific disadvantages of recording directly from the spinal cord exist; recording electrodes require placement on the surface of the spinal cord or near the spinal cord (*50*), and it is necessary to obtain a specific electrode position and maintain that position throughout the operation. Considerable changes may occur in the evoked potentials if the recording electrodes move only slightly during the operation.

Neurogenic Evoked Potentials. The responses that can be recorded at one location on the spinal cord to stimulation at another location of the spinal cord have been interpreted as being neurogenic motor evoked potentials (NMEP). The NMEP recordings were assumed to represent the motor (ventral) portion of the spinal cord, and as such, they were regarded to be a valuable substitution for recording MEP (*59*). However, later studies seem to show that the NMEP (mainly) reflect activity in the sensory pathways of the dorsal column (*62*), but a small motor component can be detected (*63*). These results were based on collision studies, where stimulation of the spinal cord and that of a peripheral nerve are applied with appropriate time differences to determine which pathways (sensory or motor) such general electrical stimulation of the spinal cord activates (see Chap. 14).

Stimulation Technique and Parameters

The same stimulus parameters that are used when stimulating a peripheral nerve to elicit cortical SSEP can be used to elicit spinal cord potentials, but it is possible to use a more rapid stimulus rate when recording spinal cord potentials. This may not be so important because of the large amplitudes of the responses that are recorded directly from the spinal cord that make it possible to obtain an interpretable record in a short time. The electrodes used for stimulation and recording from the spinal cord are introduced using small catheters.

Limited experience of recordings of sensory evoked potentials from the spinal cord prevents assessment of the value of such recordings as indicative of spinal cord injuries. The technique of direct stimulation and recording from the spinal cord is more popular outside the USA (such as in Japan) than in the USA.

Combination of SSEP and MEP Monitoring

Monitoring of SSEP and MEP are often combined in operations that affect the spinal cord. A technique for combining recordings from sensory

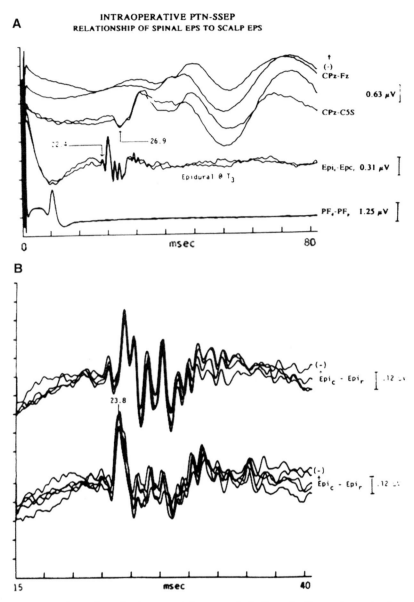

Figure 6.9: Examples of evoked potentials recorded directly from the spinal cord in response to stimulation of the posterior tibial nerve. (Reprinted from (*82*) with the permission Lippincott Williams & Wilkins).

and MEP taken from the surgical field have been described for use in connection with mapping of spinal roots in operations on conus medullaris and cauda equina of the spinal cord (*53*) (**Fig. 6.10**). In such operations, it is useful to monitor the bulbocavernosus reflex response, which can be recorded from the sphincter ani externus after stimulation of the pudendal nerve with a train stimulus paradigm. Usually, recordings were made from the sphincter, the tibialis anterior and the abductor hallucis. The quadriceps, gastrocnemius, and virtually any other lower extremity

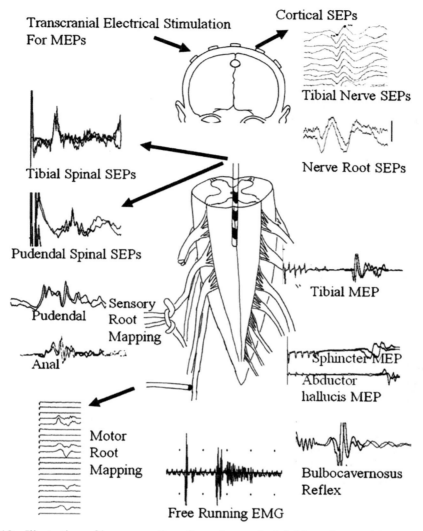

Transcranial Electrical Stimulation
For MEPs

Cortical SEPs

Tibial Nerve SEPs

Tibial Spinal SEPs

Nerve Root SEPs

Pudendal Spinal SEPs

Pudendal Sensory
Root
Mapping

Anal

Tibial MEP

Sphincter MEP

Abductor
hallucis MEP

Motor
Root
Mapping

Bulbocavernosus
Reflex

Free Running EMG

Figure 6.10: Illustration of how recordings from the surgical field can be combined with recordings from the body surface. Recordings of motor evoked potentials from a variety of muscles are shown together with epidural spinal recordings of potentials elicited by stimulation of the tibial nerve and the pudendal nerve. Recordings for identification of individual dorsal roots of pudendal or anal nerves using direct recording from the dorsal roots using hook electrodes are shown. Stimulation was cutaneous over the tibial nerve or over the penis/clitoris. (Reprinted from (53) with the permission from Springer).

muscle can be used for recording. Kothbauer also recorded cortical responses to tibial nerve stimulation or direct electrical stimulation of a nerve root (53).

Fig. 6.10 shows examples of how monitoring of many functions related to the spinal cord can be made together in a patient undergoing an operation affecting the lower spinal cord (conus medullaris and cauda equina).

EMG responses elicited by electric stimulation of motor nerve roots were used for identifying motor nerves in spinal ventral roots. Free running electromyographic recordings from the same muscles provide for the identification of surgery-induced sustained EMG activity from a variety of muscles (motor unit potentials and trains).

SSEP AS AN INDICATOR OF ISCHEMIA FROM REDUCED CEREBRAL BLOOD PERFUSION

Monitoring of SSEP is now in common use in operations where the frontal circulation may be compromised such as in aneurysm operations (6, 64). Monitoring of SSEP is superior to the monitoring of visual evoked potentials. The use of monitoring of MEP (see Chap. 10) is also valuable as an indicator of cerebral ischemia, and the use of that technique is increasing. The use of monitoring of VEP for the detection of ischemia has been suggested, but changes in the VEP do not correlate well with ischemia of the occipital cortex or with insults to the visual pathways (65) (see Chap. 8).

Basis for the Use of SSEP in Monitoring Cerebral Ischemia

The prolongation of the time interval between the P_{14} and the N_{20} peaks of the SSEP, known as the central conduction time (CCT) (see Chap. 5, **Fig. 5.12**) (66), is used as an indicator to detect changes in the function of the central somatosensory nervous system structures. A prolongation of the CCT is taken as an indication of the

beginning of ischemia and is a sign that the blood flow through the region of the brain that is involved in generating these potentials has decreased. (The conduction time of the median nerve often increases because the arm becomes cooler during long operations – but that does not affect the CCT).

Experiments in baboons showed that the SSEP disappear when cerebral blood flow falls below 15–18 ml/100 g/min, but a more severe decrease (to about 10 ml/100 g/min) in blood flow is necessary to disturb ionic homeostasis to an extent that there is risk of permanent damage (67). The animal experiments by Branston et al. (5) have shown that there is a direct relationship between the time it takes for the SSEP to disappear and the degree of ischemia. Studies in humans by Symon et al. (4, 64) have shown that there is a direct relationship between the time it takes for the N_{20} peak of the SSEP elicited by stimulation of the median nerve to disappear after the occlusion of an artery (a branch of middle cerebral artery; MCA, **Fig. 6.11**) in aneurysm surgery and the risk of occurrence of permanent neurological deficit. The time it takes for the SSEP to no longer be detectable following occlusion (clamping) of a branch of the MCA was found to be crucial to the outcome of the operation. The shorter the time it takes, the higher the risk of permanent postoperative deficits; if the time is <2 min, the risk is high for permanent deficits. Occlusion causes a lesser

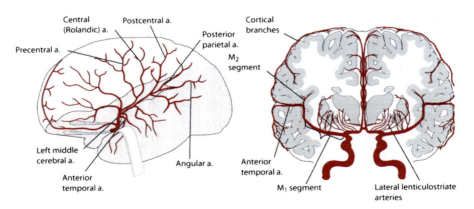

Figure 6.11: Blood supply by the middle and the anterior cerebral arteries. (Reprinted from (80) with the permission from the Mayo Foundation, Rochester, Minnesota).

degree of ischemia, and it takes a longer time for the SSEP to disappear. Patients in whom it took 4 min or more for the SSEP to disappear after the carotid artery or the MCA was occluded could tolerate 20 min of absence of the N_{20} peak of the SSEP. If the time it took for the N_{20} peak to disappear was <4 min, the estimated time of tolerance was reduced to 10 min (68). Studies in animals and in humans (69) have shown that the SSEP disappear more rapidly after repeated episodes of ischemia such as, for instance, from repeated temporary clipping of an artery, which is often performed in aneurism surgery.

The use of SSEP in intraoperative monitoring of operations on aneurysms is not as effective when the anterior cerebral artery is affected. Symon and Murota (64) suggested that the use of SSEP elicited from the lower limbs (posterior tibial nerve stimulation) may be more effective in detecting ischemia caused by the occlusion of the anterior cerebral artery than the use of SSEP elicited from the median nerve.

Symon and his group had also advocated the usefulness of SSEP monitoring as a predictor of outcome of basilar artery surgery, but Friedman et al. (70) pointed out that occlusion of the basilar artery may cause ischemia in areas of the brain other than those that affect the SSEP, and the occurrence of such ischemia may, therefore, escape detection when monitoring SSEP.

Monitoring of SSEP can provide prediction of the outcome of operations on patients in whom intraoperative complications occur, such as bleeding of an aneurysm. Prolonged CCT at 5 days postoperative was found to indicate poor outcome (64).

The same criteria for changes in CCT based on SSEP elicited from the median nerve have been used in other operations in which the blood flow may be altered intentionally to allow for surgical repair. Carotid endarterectomy, in which the carotid artery has to be clamped during the removal of the atherosclerotic plaque, is one example of an operation during which monitoring of SSEP is useful for evaluating whether the patient can tolerate an occlusion of the carotid artery (71). However, monitoring of EEG and cerebral oximetry are now used more often for that purpose (outside the scope of this book).

Practical Aspects of Recording SSEP for Detecting Ischemia

When SSEP monitoring is used for detecting cerebral ischemia in the brain, it is assumed that neural transmission in the spinal cord is not at risk. SSEP, elicited by stimulation of the median nerve, is, therefore, as useful as SSEP elicited by stimulation of a nerve on the lower limbs. Since the former method of SSEP elicitation is more reliable than the latter method, median nerve SSEP are usually chosen to detect cerebral ischemia. The median nerves at the wrists should be stimulated one at a time. Stimulation of both median nerves at the same time should not be used for the reasons described above (page 68).

Determination of the CCT that is used as a measure of ischemia requires that P_{14} and N_{20} be reproduced well in the recordings of the SSEP. The P_{14} component is best recorded from an electrode placed at the neck area, and the N_{20} peak is best recorded from an electrode placed over the contralateral parietal scalp (see **Fig. 6.3** and Chap. 5, **Fig. 5.12**). It is, therefore, appropriate to record differentially between electrodes placed on the contralateral scalp (3–4 cm behind C_3 or C_4) and the dorsal neck. It is practical to record from two channels, each one recording from either side of the scalp (3 and 4 cm behind C_3 and C_4, respectively) using the same reference at the neck for both channels. When operating on one side of the brain principally, the contralateral median nerve should be stimulated, and the recording should be obtained from the scalp on the side of the operations. Recording the SSEP from the opposite side in response to stimulation of the median nerve on the operated side to get the contralateral N_{20} may be useful, but it is important to make clear at all times which side is being stimulated and from which side the recordings are made.

When SSEP are used as an indicator of ischemia, it must be remembered that there are other factors that may affect the CCT such as the level of anesthesia, retraction of the brain, hypothermia, and hypotension. While brain retraction may only affect one hemisphere, and thus, SSEP recorded on one side only, general hypotension, hypothermia, and anesthesia affect both sides almost equally. That is one reason why it is valuable to record from both sides of the cortex by alternately stimulating the median nerves of both wrists. The anesthesia team often lowers the blood pressure in operations for aneurysms and other operations of the vascular system and that may affect the SSEP. The neurophysiology monitoring team should, therefore, watch the patient's blood pressure closely.

If the blood flow in the MCA is affected, it can be expected to only cause changes in the response on one side, in which case recordings from the other side may be used as a control to determine if changes are caused by general factors, such as hypotension or the effect of anesthesia. In cases where the basilar circulation is manipulated, such as it may be in operations on basilar aneurysms, the SSEP recorded from both sides may be affected by a reduction in blood flow due to clamping vessels in operations for aneurysms or other interference with the circulation in the basilar system.

Clamping the anterior communicating artery sometimes affects the blood supply to both hemispheres, thus affecting the SSEP in response to stimulation of median nerves on both sides. Alternately stimulating the two median nerves and displaying the recorded potentials as separate traces is ideal for monitoring SSEP for the purpose of detecting cerebral ischemia.

SSEP Compared with Direct Measurement of Blood Flow

Monitoring cerebral blood flow intraoperatively is valuable in some situations, but monitoring SSEP may be more suitable in many operations because it detects the effect of ischemia, while ischemia is indirectly only related to the amount of reduction in blood flow. Because SSEP measures changes in neuronal function (such as that caused by ischemia), it is probably a more reliable indicator of risk of permanent injury than measurements of blood flow, especially since ischemic

tolerances vary from patient to patient and may be different under different circumstances.

However, recordings of SSEP do not provide any information about how much oxygenation has decreased after it has reached the level at which the SSEP can no longer be recorded. After the loss of SSEP, there is, thus, a "blind area" where no information about the progression of ischemia can be obtained. The rate of change in the SSEP, as mentioned above, can be used as a guide by extrapolation for how fast that critical level is reached after the N_{20} has disappeared. This extrapolation is based on the assumption that ischemia progresses at the same rate after the SSEP no longer can be recorded as it did before SSEP loss. Direct measurement of blood flow would cover such a "blind area" and would provide information all the way down to zero flow. Therefore, both SSEP and blood flow should be monitored in operations where there is risk of ischemia in specific regions of the brain.

SSEP AS AN INDICATOR OF BRAINSTEM MANIPULATION

The benefit from intraoperative monitoring of SSEP in patients undergoing operations in which the brainstem may be manipulated is not as obvious as is the benefit from monitoring ABR (see Chap. 7) because there are no brainstem relay nuclei in the somatosensory system. The fiber tract of the medial lemniscus that passes through the brainstem may be affected by brainstem manipulation in a way that can be recorded as a change in the cortical SSEP, but presumably to a lesser degree than would nuclei in the brainstem ascending auditory pathways.

PRE- AND POSTOPERATIVE TESTS

Disorders that affect neural conduction in peripheral nerves may severely affect the outcome of intraoperative monitoring of SSEP, particularly, lower limb SSEP. If the patient has a moderate-to-severe neuropathy, from, for example, diabetes mellitus, it may not be possible to elicit an interpretable response by electrical stimulation of a peripheral nerve or a dermatome. Older people, even without definite symptoms, normally have lower amplitudes of their SSEP because of (normal) age-related reduction of the number of active nerve fibers in peripheral nerves and a larger variation of conduction velocities. These factors reduce the temporal coherence of the nerve activity that arrives at the dorsal column nuclei. These changes have greater effect on lower limb SSEP than upper limb SSEP because of the longer nerve paths in the spinal cord and the longer peripheral nerves and spinal ascending sensory nerve tracts. The decreased temporal coherence results in a distorted pattern of the recorded SSEP and lower amplitudes and longer latencies of all components. In mild cases of neuropathy, the amplitudes of the recorded SSEP may be lower than normal, and the latencies may differ only slightly from those of patients without such pathologies.

TRIGEMINAL EVOKED POTENTIALS

Although trigeminal evoked potentials (TEP) may be regarded as a "member" of the group of sensory evoked potentials known as SSEP, TEP are rarely used in intraoperative monitoring. When TEP are elicited by electrical stimulation of branches of the trigeminal nerve, a response can be recorded from electrodes placed on the scalp (C_z and O_z) (72, 73) as well as from the intracranial portion of the trigeminal nerve when exposed, such as in operations for microvascular decompression of the trigeminal nerve root, to treat trigeminal neuralgia (74). Short-latency, negative components elicited by electrical stimulation of branches of the trigeminal nerve have latencies of 0.9, 1.6, and 2.6 ms when recorded from the trigeminal nerve where it enters the brainstem (74). These potentials represent neural activity in the trigeminal nerve

– not in any other rostral structures – and such recordings can, thus, only be used to monitor the trigeminal (sensory) nerve (75). Recordings from electrodes on the scalp can be used for monitoring the ascending trigeminal sensory pathways when elicited by electrical stimulation of the peripheral trigeminal nerve. (In conscious individuals, TEP can also be elicited by tactile stimulation (air puffs) (76)). This method has not been described for use intraoperatively.

There are considerable differences in the results obtained in different laboratories regarding recording of TEP and by different investigators, in particular, with regard to long-latency (>5 ms) components of the TEP elicited by electrical stimulation of a peripheral branch of the trigeminal nerve (74). It has been shown that monitoring of TEP is useful in intraoperative monitoring of the medulla oblongata and in trigeminal rhizotomy in patients with trigeminal neuralgia in whom it may be of value to monitor neural conduction in the trigeminal nerve (74) (see Chap. 14).

ANESTHESIA REQUIREMENTS FOR MONITORING CORTICAL EVOKED POTENTIALS

The effect of anesthesia on SSEP is different for different components of the recorded SSEP. The subcortical components of the upper limb SSEP, P_{14-16}, are little affected by any commonly used anesthetics (43). However, most intraoperative monitoring of SSEP is based on recording cortical evoked potentials from electrodes placed on the scalp. Inhalation anesthetics that were in general use earlier are rarely used now in connection with the monitoring of SSEP. The ability to suppress SSEP is different for different kinds of inhalation anesthetics, and it is directly correlated to the concentration in which such agents are administrated[1] (77) (**Fig. 6.12**).

---

[1]The effect of different anesthetic agents is often described by their "mean alveolar concentration" (MAC), which is the concentration that induces anesthesia in an average person (50% of the recipients move, in response to incision).

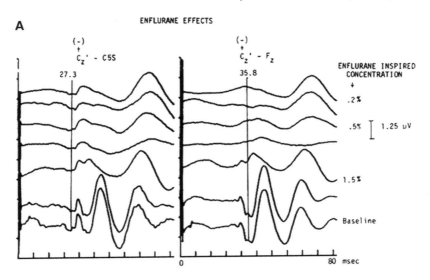

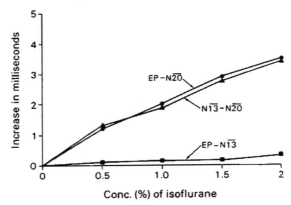

Figure 6.12: (**A**) Effect of anesthesia (enflurane) on the SSEP elicited by stimulating the posterior tibial nerve (Reprinted from Ref. (*83*)). (**B**) Effect of isoflurane on the neural conduction times that are represented by the difference in the latencies of the different peaks in the SSEP elicited by stimulating the median nerve at the wrist. No effect is seen in the conduction from the brachial plexus (Erb's point; EP) to the dorsal column nuclei (EP-N$_{13}$), but there is a gradual increase in the central conduction time (CCT, N$_{13}$–N$_{20}$) with increasing concentration of isoflurane. (Reprinted from (*83*) with the permission from Springer).

Instead of inhalation anesthetics, TIVA techniques are coming into more frequent use. TIVA can be designed so that it affects the SSEP much less than that of inhalation anesthetics. It is now common to use TIVA, composed of drugs such as Propofol, Ketamine, etomidate, and opioids as favorable agents that seem to suppress SSEP the least (*40*). Muscle relaxant drugs are often included for operations in which the motor systems are not monitored (see Chap. 16). Benzodiazepines such as Midazolam, are also often included, but probably with little effect on recordings of SSEP.

Some anesthetics, such as etomidate, seem to enhance the cortical components of the

SSEP rather than suppress them when administrated in low dosages. Etomidate causes an increase in the amplitude of SSEP of cortical origin (78).

Brown and Nash (46) noted that the administration of anesthetics by bolus injection has adverse effects on intraoperative monitoring, such as the recording of the SSEP. The adverse effect on the recordings of sensory evoked responses can be minimized by using drug infusion at a constant rate to avoid transient bolus effects. Anesthetic agents used to maintain anesthesia should, therefore, be administered by continuous infusion techniques. However, bolus administration is still used despite excellent equipment being available for programed infusion.

Agents such as opioids (narcotics) that are used to achieve freedom of pain, and beta-adrenergic blockers, nitroglycerine, and sodium nitroprusside, used to control blood pressure, have little effect on the monitoring of SSEP in normal dosages and neither do commonly used cardiovascular drugs. However, vasodilators may cause shunting of blood flow away from the spinal cord, and their use should be discouraged during procedures where there is a risk of reduced blood flow to the spinal cord.

ABNORMALITIES AND PATHOLOGIES THAT OCCUR BEFORE THE OPERATION THAT IS TO BE MONITORED

Trauma, previous operations, diseases, and congenital malformations that occur before an operation may affect the ability of recording SSEP or result in abnormal recording. Age-related changes in neural conduction of peripheral nerves are common and may make it difficult to elicit SSEP, especially from lower limbs. The presence of neuropathies, such as those resulting from diabetes, may make it impossible to elicit SSEP, and it is possible that the latencies are prolonged and amplitudes are lower than normal. Some individuals, especially those with scoliosis, may have certain

additional neural abnormalities, such as mainly uncrossed ascending somatosensory pathways (79), and this makes the monitoring of SSEP more difficult than the monitoring in individuals with normal anatomy.

REFERENCES

1. Brown RH and CL Nash (1979) Current status of spinal cord monitoring. Spine 4:466–78.
2. Nash CL, RA Lorig, LA Schatzinger et al (1977) Spinal cord monitoring during operative treatment of the spine. Clin Orthop 126:100–5.
3. Engler GL, NI Spielholtz, WN Bernard et al (1978) Somatosensory evoked potentials during Harrington instrumentation for scoliosis. J Bone Joint Surg 60A:528–32.
4. Symon L, J Hargadine, M Zawirski et al (1979) Central conduction time as an index of ischemia in subarachnoid haemorrhage. J Neurol Sci 44:95–103.
5. Branston NM, L Symon, HA Crockard et al (1974) Relationship between the cortical evoked potential and local cortical blood flow following acute middle cerebral artery occlusion in the baboon. Exp Neurol 45:195–208.
6. Neuloh G and J Schramm (2004) Monitoring of motor evoked potentials compared with somatosensory evoked potentials and microvascular Doppler ultrasonography in cerebral aneurysm surgery. J Neurosurg 100:389–99.
7. Pagni CA, M Naddeo and Mascari (1988) History of evoked potential recording in humans, in *Evoked potentials: Intraoperative and ICU Monitoring*, RL Grundy and RM Villani, Editors. Springer: Wien. 17–44.
8. Deletis V (2002) Intraoperative neurophysiology and methodologies used to monitor the functional integrity of the motor system, in *Neurophysiology in Neurosurgery*, V Deletis and JL Shils, Editors. Academic Press: Amsterdam. 25–51.
9. Robertazzi RR and JNJ Cunningham (1998) Monitoring of somatosensory evoked potentials: A primer on the intraoperative detection of spinal cord ischemia during aortic reconstructive surgery. Semin Thorac Cardiovasc Surg 10:11–7.
10. York DH (1985) Somatosensory evoked potentials in man: differentiation of spinal pathways

responsible for conduction from the forelimb vs hindlimb. Prog Neurobiol 25:1–25.

11. Khealani B and A Husain (2009) Neurophysiologic intraoperative monitoring during surgery for tethered cord syndrome. J Clin Neurophysiol 26:76–81.

12. Nuwer MR (1999) Spinal cord monitoring. Muscle Nerve 22:1620–30.

13. Slimp J (2004) Electrophysiologic intraoperative monitoring for spine procedures. Phys Med Rehabil Clin N Am 15:85–105.

14. Yamada T, M Yeh and J Kimura (2004) Fundamental principles of somatosensory evoked potentials. Phys Med Rehabil Clin N Am 15:19–42.

15. Møller A, S Ansari, L Osburn et al (2010) Techniques of intraoperative monitoring for spinal cord function: Their past, present and future directions. Neurol Res. In press

16. Stecker M (2004) Evoked potentials during cardiac and major vascular operations. Semin Cardiothorac Vasc Anesth 8:101–11.

17. Kelleher M, G Tan, R Sarjeant et al (2008) Predictive value of intraoperative neurophysiological monitoring during cervical spine surgery: a prospective analysis of 1055 consecutive patients. J Neurosurg Spine 8:215–21.

18. Quraishi N, S Lewis, M Kelleher et al (2009) Intraoperative multimodality monitoring in adult spinal deformity: Analysis of a prospective series of one hundred two cases with independent evaluation. Spine 34:1504–12.

19. Hyun S and S Rhim (2009) Combined motor and somatosensory evoked potential monitoring for intramedullary spinal cord tumor surgery: correlation of clinical and neurophysiological data in 17 consecutive procedures. Br J Neurosurg 23:393–400.

20. Keyhani K, CR Miller, A Estrera et al (2009) Analysis of motor and somatosensory evoked potentials during thoracic and thoracoabdominal aortic aneurysm repair. J Vasc Surg 49:36–41.

21. Nuwer MR, EG Dawson, LG Carlson et al (1995) Somatosensory evoked potential spinal cord monitoring reduces neurologic deficits after scoliosis surgery: Results of a large multicenter study. Electroencephalogr Clin Neurophysiol 96:6–11.

22. Pratt H and A Starr (1986) Somatosensory evoked potentials in natural forms of stimulation, in *Frontiers of Clinical Neuroscience*, RQ Cracco and I Bodis-Wollner, Editors. Alan R. Liss, Inc: New York. 28–34.

23. Chiappa K (1997) *Evoked Potentials in Clinical Medicine*, 3rd edn. Lippincott-Raven: Philadelphia.

24. Jasper HH (1958) The ten twenty electrode system of the International Federation. Electroencephalogr Clin Neurophysiol 10:371–5.

25. Desmedt JE and G Cheron (1981) Non-cephalic reference recording of early somatosensory potentials to finger stimulation in adult or aging normal man: Differentiation of widespread N18 and contra-lateral N20 from the prerolandic P22 and N30 components. Electroencephalogr Clin Neurophysiol 52:553–70.

26. Cracco RQ and JB Cracco (1976) Somatosensory evoked potentials in man: Farfield potentials. Electroencephalogr Clin Neurophysiol 41:60–466.

27. Møller AR, PJ Jannetta and HD Jho (1990) Recordings from human dorsal column nuclei using stimulation of the lower limb. Neurosurgery 26:291–9.

28. Mauguiere F (2000) Anatomic origin of the cervical N13 potential evoked by upper extremity stimulation. J Clin Neurophysiol 17:236–45.

29. American Clinical Neurophysiology Society (2006) Guideline 9D: Guidelines on short-latency somatosensory evoked potentials. Am J Electroneurodiagnostic Technol 46:287–300.

30. Nuwer MR, M Aminoff, J Desmedt et al (1994) IFCN recommended standards for short latency somatosensory evoked potentials. Report of an IFCN committee. Electroencephalogr Clin Neurophysiol 91:6–11.

31. Toleikis JR (2005) American Society of Neurophysiological Monitoring. Intraoperative monitoring using somatosensory evoked potentials. A position statement by the American Society of Neurophysiological Monitoring. J Clin Monit Comput 19:241–58.

32. Pelosi L, JB Cracco, RQ Cracco et al (1988) Comparison of scalp distribution of short latency somatosensory evoked potentials (SSEPs) to stimulation of different nerves in the lower extremity. Electroencephalogr Clin Neurophysiol 71:422–8.

33. Møller AR (2006) *Neural Plasticity and Disorders of the Nervous System*. Cambridge University Press: Cambridge.

34. Vrahas M, RG Gordon, DC Mears et al (1992) Intraoperative somatosensory evoked potential

monitoring of pelvic and acetabular fractures. J Orthoped Trauma 6:505–8.

35. Desmedt JE, TH Nguyen and J Carmeliet (1983) Unexpected latency shifts of the stationary P9 somatosensory evoked potential far field with changes in shoulder position. Electroencephalogr Clin Neurophysiol 56:628–34.

36. Maguire J, S Wallace, R Madiga et al (1995) Evaluation of intrapedicular screw position using intraoperative evoked electromyography. Spine 20:1068–74.

37. Toleikis JR (2002) Neurophysiological monitoring during pedicle screw placement, in *Neurophysiology in Neurosurgrey*, V Deletis and JL Shils, Editors. Elsevier: Amsterdam. 231–64.

38. Nuwer MR (1986) *Evoked Potential Monitoring in the Operating Room*. Raven Press: New York.

39. Nuwer MR and EC Dawson (1984) Intraoperative evoked potential monitoring of the spinal cord: Enhanced stability of cortical recordings. Electroencephalogr Clin Neurophysiol 59:318–27.

40. MacDonald D, Z Zayed and A Saddig (2007) Four-limb muscle motor evoked potential and optimized somatosensory evoked potential monitoring with decussation assessment: Results in 206 thoracolumbar spine surgeries. Eur Spine J 16:171–87.

41. MacDonald D (2001) Indiividually optimizing posterior tibial somatosensory evoked potential P37 scalp derivations for intraoperative monitoring. J Clin Neurophysiol 18:364–71.

42. Sloan T (2002) Anesthesia and motor evoked potential monitoring, in *Neurophysiology in Neurosurgery*, V Deletis and JL Shils, Editors. Elsevier Science: Amsterdam. 451–74.

43. Sloan TB and EJ Heyer (2002) Anesthesia for intraoperative neurophysiologic monitoring of the spinal cord. J Clin Neurophysiol 19:430–43.

44. Jones SJ, L Howard and F Shawkat (1988) Criteria for detection and pathological significance of response decrement during spinal cord monitoring, in *Neurophysiology and Standards of Spinal Cord Monitoring*, TB Ducker and RH Brown, Editors. Springer: New York. 201–6.

45. Nuwer MR, J Daube, C Fischer et al (1993) Neuromonitroing during surgery. Report of an IFCN committee. Electroencephalogr Clin Neurophysiol 87:263–76.

46. Brown RH and CLJ Nash (1988) Standardization of evoked potential recording, in *Neurophysiology and Standards of Spinal Cord Monitoring*, TB Ducker and RH Brown, Editors. Springer: New York. 1–10.

47. Coles JG, MJ Taylor, JM Pearce et al (1984) Cerebral monitoring of somatosensory evoked potentials during profoundly hypothermic circulatory arrest. Circulation 70:1096–102.

48. Rheineck Van Leyssius AT, CJ Kalkman and JG Bovill (1986) Influence of moderate hypothermia on posterior tibial nerve somatosensory evoked potentials. Anesth Analg 5:475–80.

49. Lueders H, RP Lesser, JR Hahn et al (1983) Subcortical somatosensory evoked potentials to median nerve stimulation. Brain 106:341–72.

50. Lueders H, A Gurd, J Hahn et al (1982) A new technique for intraoperative monitoring of spinal cord function: Multichannel recording of spinal cord and subcortical evoked potentials. Spine 7:110–5.

51. Maccabee PJ, DB Levine, EI Pinkhasov et al (1983) Evoked potentials recorded from scalp and spinous processes during spinal column surgery. Electroencephalogr Clin Neurophysiol 56:569–82.

52. Kothbauer KF (2007) Intraoperative neurophysiologic monitoring for intramedullary spinal-cord tumor surgery. Neurophysiol Clin 37: 407–14.

53. Kothbauer KF and V Deletis (2010) Intraoperative neurophysiology of the conus medullaris and cauda equina. Childs Nerv Syst 26:247–53.

54. Accadbled F, P Henry, JS de Gauzy et al (2006) Spinal cord monitoring in scoliosis surgery using an epidural electrode. Results of a prospective, consecutive series of 191 cases. Spine 31:2614–23.

55. Tamaki T, H Takano and K Takakuwa (1985) Spinal cord monitoring: Basic principles and experimental aspects. Cent Nerv Syst Trauma 2:137–49.

56. Tsuyama N, N Tsuzuki, T Kurokawa et al (1978) Clinical application of spinal cord action potential measurement. Int Orthop (SICOT) 2:39–46.

57. Tamaki T, H Tsuji, S Inoue et al (1981) The preven-tion of iatrogenic spinal cord injury utilizing the evoked potential. Int Orthop (SICOT) 4:313–17.

58. Owen JH (1993) Intraoperative stimulation of the spinal cord for prevention of spinal cord injury. Adv Neurol 63:271–88.

59. Owen JH, KH Bridwell, R Grubb et al (1991) The clinical application of neurogenic motor evoked potentials to monitor spinal cord function during surgery. Spine 16:S385–90.

60. Cohen AR, W Young and J Ransohoff (1981) Intraspinal localization of the somatosensory evoked potential. Neurosurgery 9:157–62.

61. Jones SJ, MA Edgar and AO Ransford (1982) Sensory nerve conduction in the human spinal cord: Epidural recordings made during scoliosis surgery. J Neurol Neurosurg Psychiatry 45:446–51.

62. Toleikis JR, JP Skelly, AO Carlvin et al (2000) Spinally elicited peripheral nerve responses are sensory rather than motor. Clin Neurophysiol 111:736–42.

63. Pereon Y, ST Nguyen, J Delecrin et al (2002) Combined spinal cord monitoring using mixed evoked potentials and collision techniques. Spine 27:1571–6.

64. Symon L and T Murota (1989) Intraoperative monitoring of somatosensory evoked potentials during intracranial vascular surgery, in Neuromonitoring in Surgery, JE Desmedt, Editor. Elsevier Science Publishers: Amsterdam. 263–74.

65. Cedzich C, J Schramm and R Fahlbusch (1987) Are flash-evoked visual potentials useful for intraoperative monitoring of visual pathway function? Neurosurgery 21:709–15.

66. Hume AL and BR Cant (1978) Conduction time in central somatosensory pathways in man. Electroencephalogr Clin Neurophysiol 45:361–75.

67. Astrup J, L Symon, NM Branston et al (1977) Cortical evoked potentials and extracellular K+ and H+ at critical levels of brain ischemia. Stroke 8:51–7.

68. Momma F, AD Wang and L Symon (1987) Effects of temporary arterial occlusion on somatosensory evoked responses in aneurysm surgery. Surg Neurol 27:343–52.

69. Spetzler R, W Selman, CJ Nash et al (1979) Transoral microsurgical odontoid resection and spinal cord monitoring. Spine 4:506–10.

70. Friedman WA, BJ Kaplan, AL Day et al (1987) Evoked potential monitoring during aneurysm operation: Observations after fifty cases. Neurosurgery 20:678–87.

71. Manninen P, R Sarjeant and M Joshi (2004) Posterior tibial nerve and median nerve somatosensory evoked potential monitoring during carotid endarterectomy. Can J Anaesth 51:937–41.

72. Bennett MH and PJ Jannetta (1980) Trigeminal evoked potentials in human. Electroencephalogr Clin Neurophysiol 48:517–26.

73. Landi A, SA Copeland, Wynn CB et al (1980) The role of somatosensory evoked potentials and nerve conduction studies in the surgical management of brachial plexus injuries. J Bone Joint Surg (Brit) 62B:492–6.

74. Stechison MT and FJ Kralick (1993) The trigeminal evoked potential: Part I. Long-latency responses in awake or anesthetized subjects. Neurosurgery 33:633–8.

75. Oikawa T, M Matsumoto, T Sasaki et al (2000) Experimental study of medullary trigeminal evoked potentials: development of a new method of intraoperative monitoring of the medulla oblongata. J Neurosurg 93:68–76.

76. Hashimoto I (1988) Trigeminal evoked potentials following brief air puff: Enhanced signal-to-noise ratio. Ann Neurol 23:332–8.

77. Wang AD, IE Costa e Silva, L Symon et al (1985) The effect of halothane on somatosensory and flash evoked potentials during operations. Neurol Res 7:58–62.

78. McPherson RW, S Bell and RJ Traystman (1986) Effects of thiopental, fentanyl, and etomidate on upper extremity somatosensory evoked potentials in humans. Anesthesiology 65:584–9.

79. MacDonald D, L Streletz, Z Al-Zayed et al (2004) Intraoperative neurophysiologic discovery of uncrossed sensory and motor pathways in a patient with horizontal gaze palsy and scoliosis. Clin Neurophysiol. 115.

80. Benarroch EE, JR Daube, KD Flemming et al (2008) Mayo Clinic Medical Neurosciences, 5th edn. Mayo Foundation: Rochester, Minnesota.

81. Katifi HA and EM Sedgwick (1987) Evaluation of the dermatomal somatosensory evoked potential in the diagnosis of lumbo-sacral root compression. J Neurol Neurosurg Psychiatry 50:1204–10.

82. Erwin CW and AC Erwin (1993) Up and down the spinal cord: Intraoperative monitoring of sensory and motor spinal cord pathways. J Clin Neurophysiol 10:425–36.

83. Samra SK (1988) Effect of isoflurane on human nerve evoked potentials, in Neurophysiology and Standards of Spinal Cord Monitoring, TB Ducker and RH Brown, Editors. Springer: New York. 147–56.

Monitoring Auditory Evoked Potentials

From: *Intraoperative Neurophysiological Monitoring: Third Edition*,
By A.R. Møller, DOI 10.1007/978-1-4419-7436-5_7,
© Springer Science+Business Media, LLC 2011

INTRODUCTION

Monitoring of the auditory system makes use of subcortical evoked potentials [Auditory Brainstem Responses (ABR) and CAP recorded from the exposed auditory nerve]. These modalities of evoked potentials are not affected by commonly used anesthetics.

One purpose of monitoring auditory evoked potentials is to reduce the risk of injury to the eighth cranial nerve (CN VIII), which is at risk of being injured by surgical manipulations in microvascular decompression (MVD) operations to relieve trigeminal neuralgia (TGN), hemifacial spasm (HFS), glossopharyngeal neuralgia (GPN) (1, 2), and in connection with MVD operations of the eighth nerve in patients with tinnitus and disabling positional vertigo (DPV) (3). Preservation of auditory function during the removal of small vestibular schwannoma has recently improved due to advancements in operative techniques and through the introduction of intraoperative neurophysiological monitoring of the auditory nerve (4–9).

ABR were some of the earliest sensory evoked potentials to be used intraoperatively for the purpose of reducing intraoperative injuries to the auditory nerve (1, 10). In operations to remove vestibular schwannoma, recordings of ABR have been supplemented by recording CAP from the exposed CN VIII (2, 4–7) and from recording evoked potentials from the vicinity of the cochlear nucleus (8, 11, 12) for monitoring of the integrity of the function of the auditory nerve.

Only the auditory part of CN VIII can be monitored, but it has been shown that the vestibular part of CN VIII can be injured in MVD operations and can produce symptoms and signs that indicate insult to the balance system (13). The advantages and disadvantages of different methods for monitoring the integrity of the auditory nerve are discussed, and different ways to optimize such recordings are described.

Recording from the vicinity of the cochlea (electrocochleography, ECoG) has been described as a technique for monitoring hearing in operations on vestibular schwannoma (14, 15). However, since the risk of damage to the auditory nerve in most operations affects its intracranial portion, and the ECoG potentials only reflect the CAP of the distal part of the nerve, the usefulness of monitoring ECoG is limited. Changes in the ECoG potentials, however, indicate impairment of blood supply to the ear. If that is caused by permanent damage to the labyrinthine artery, it is normally not reversible and monitoring cannot prevent permanent loss of hearing.

The choice of acoustic stimuli and how they are presented, as well as the hearing status of the patient, can influence the amplitude, latency and waveform of the recorded potentials (ABR or CAP). It is, therefore important to consider these factors in the interpretation of the results of intraoperative monitoring of auditory evoked potentials. Thus, all patients in whom intraoperative monitoring of auditory evoked potentials is to be performed should have hearing tests performed preoperatively. Included in such tests should, at the very least, include pure tone audiometry, determination of speech discrimination (using recorded speech material), and ABR. It is also preferable to include testing of the acoustic middle ear reflex.

Such preoperative tests are also a prerequisite in order to quantitatively evaluate a change in hearing status that may occur as a result of an intraoperative injury to the auditory nerve. These tests also assess the value of intraoperative monitoring of auditory evoked potentials and the value of any modification in the usual surgical methods that may be made in an attempt to improve hearing preservation (see Chap. 19).

This chapter discusses the practical aspects of hearing preservation in various types of operations using recordings of ABR or CAP directly from the auditory nerve or the vicinity of the cochlear nucleus. Recordings of ABR have been used to detect effects on the brainstem from surgical manipulations during operations on large vestibular schwannoma and on other types of masses that may occur in the cerebellopontine angle (CPA) (*6, 16, 17*), as well as on tumors or other space-occupying lesions in the region of the fourth ventricle.

AUDITORY BRAINSTEM RESPONSES

The ABR was described in Chap. 5. The technique used in recording ABR for intraoperative monitoring is similar to that used clinically to obtain ABR for diagnostic purposes. However, when recording ABR intraoperatively, several modifications in this technique are necessary because of the special environment of the operating room and because it is important to be able to obtain an interpretable record in as short a time as possible.

It is mainly changes in the latencies of specific components of the recorded evoked potentials (ABR or CAP from the auditory nerve or the cochlear nucleus) that are used as indications of injuries to the auditory nerve, but changes in amplitude of the recorded evoked potentials are also valuable signs of surgically induced injuries (*18*).

Changes in CAP recorded from the auditory nerve provide direct information about changes in the function of the auditory nerve, while interpretation of the intraoperatively recorded ABR is more complex.

Since the purpose of intraoperative monitoring of ABR is to detect changes that occur in the patient's auditory system during an operation, the recordings that are made during the operation must be compared with a baseline recording obtained in the same patient before the operation began rather than with a standard ABR recording as is made when ABR are used for clinical diagnostics.

How to Obtain an Interpretable Record in the Shortest Possible Time?

The ABR obtained during an operation must be interpreted immediately after they are completed so that changes in the ABR can be identified with the shortest possible delay, and the

information can be conveyed promptly to the surgeon. The criteria for obtaining a response as quickly as possible have similarities with those for SSEP, but the amplitudes of the ABR are much smaller than those of SSEP.

Because the ABR have much smaller amplitudes than the background of noise in the operating room (consisting of ongoing biological activity such as spontaneous activity from the brain, muscle activity, and electrical interference), many responses must be added (averaged) to obtain an interpretable record. The time it takes to obtain an interpretable record, therefore, depends on the amplitude of the ABR in relation to the background noise (the signal-to-noise ratio) and how many responses can be added per unit of time, based on the repetition rate of the stimuli. The most important factors for obtaining an interpretable record in the shortest possible time are:

1. Stimulus intensity
2. Stimulus repetition rate
3. Electrode placement
4. Electrical and other interferences
5. Filtering of recorded potentials
6. Quality control that does not add time to data collection.

Stimulus Intensity. The stimulus intensity should be adequately high, without imposing a risk of causing noise-induced hearing loss (NIHL) so that the amplitude of the recorded ABR is as high as possible. Clicks at an intensity of 105 dB peak equivalent sound pressure level (PeSPL) have been used for intraoperative monitoring for many years without problems. This intensity corresponds to ~65 dB hearing level (HL) (HL – dB above the average threshold of hearing in individuals with normal hearing, when click sounds are presented at a rate of 20/s).

Stimulus Repetition Rate. When the stimulus repetition rate is increased, the number of responses that can be collected within a certain period of time increases. If the amplitude of the responses were independent on the repetition

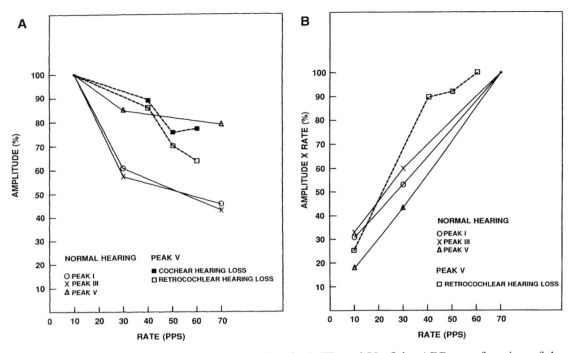

Figure 7.1: Decrease in the amplitude of peaks I, III, and V of the ABR as a function of the stimulus repetition rate (pulses per second, pps). (**A**) *Solid lines* are from patients with normal hearing (data from (*19*)), and *dashed lines* (only peak V) are from patients with hearing loss of both cochlear origin (*circles*) and retrocochlear origin (*crosses*) (data from (*20*)). Amplitude was normalized to 100% at 10 pps. (**B**) Same data as in (**A**), but the amplitudes of the peaks were multiplied by the repetition rate and normalized to 100% at 60 and 70 pps.

rate, then the time it would take to obtain an interpretable record would be inversely proportional to the repetition rate, thus a doubling of the repetition rate would shorten that time by a factor of two. However, this is only the case below a certain repetition rate because the amplitude of the peaks decreases with increasing repetition rate above a certain repetition rate and diminishes the gain of increasing the repetition rate. The decrease in amplitude that occurs when the repetition rate is increased is minimal at low repetition rates, but it accelerates with increasing repetition rate (**Fig. 7.1A**). There are only small changes in the ABR when stimulus repetition rates are increased from a few stimuli per second up to 20 stimuli per second. At a certain repetition rate, the reduction in amplitude of the recorded potentials becomes so great that it outweighs the gain from producing more responses per unit

time (**Fig. 7.1B**). This is the repetition rate that provides an interpretable record in the shortest possible time. If the repetition rate is increased beyond that rate, it will take a longer time to obtain an interpretable record. No data are available for the optimal stimulus repetition rate for ABR.

The relationship between the repetition rate of the stimulation and the amplitude of the individual peaks of the ABR depends on the individual's age and hearing loss, and increasing the stimulus repetition rate affects the different peaks differently. Peaks I–III are much more affected by an increased repetition rate than peak V, which is the most robust of the peaks of the ABR with regard to high repetition rate of the stimulus (*19*).

Hearing loss of cochlear origin does not seem to affect the way that the amplitude of the ABR peaks decrease with increasing repetition rate of click stimuli, but hearing loss of retro-cochlear origin, such as caused by an injury to the auditory nerve, affects how the amplitude of peak V decreases with increasing repetition rate of the stimulus. The product of the amplitude of peak V and the repetition rate of the click stimuli in individuals with hearing loss of retrocochlear origin (presumably from injury to the auditory nerve) nearly reaches a plateau somewhere above 40 pps (*20*) (**Fig. 7.1B**). Other investigators (*21*) obtained similar results. On the basis of these results, it seems advantageous to use repetition rates of at least 50 pps, and perhaps as high as 70 pps. That is much higher than the commonly used repetition rate (10–20 pps) (*20*) (**Fig. 7.1**). (Because the time required to obtain an interpretable record when recording ABR in the clinic is not important, most clinical recordings of ABR employ a low repetition rate of 10 to 20 pps).

Since it is not completely known how disease processes that affect the ear and the auditory nerve can affect the relationship between stimulus repetition rate and the amplitudes of the various peaks, it may not be advisable to use repetition rates higher than 50 pps. When the repetition rate is increased, caution should be exercised because the risk of (noise-induced) hearing loss from the sound increases accordingly, and it may not be advisable to use repetition rates higher than 40 pps if an intensity of 105 dB PeSPL is being used.

The fact that the latencies of the peaks of the ABR increase with increasing stimulus repetition rate is not important for the selection of the stimulus repetition rate for ABR in the operating room because in the operating room, the patient's own ABR serve as the reference (baseline), provided that the same repetition rate is used for monitoring as was used for obtaining the baseline recording.

Sound Delivery. Several kinds of insert earphones are suitable for use in the operating room to deliver sound stimuli for recording ABR. The miniature earphones used with, for instance, typical MP3 players, have a broad frequency response and can easily be fitted into the ear of a patient in the operating room. This author has used similar earphones (Radio Shack[1]) routinely in the operating room for many years. The earphones are normally driven by rectangular waves of 100-microsecond (μs) duration. These earphones deliver a narrow sound impulse and have a maximal sound output of approximately 110 dB PeSPL and deliver clicks of 105 dB PeSPL without any noticeable differences in amplitudes or waveforms of rarefaction and condensation clicks (corresponding to ~65 dB HL when presented at a rate of 20 pps). The frequency spectrum of the clicks that are generated by these earphones is relatively flat over a large range of frequencies (100–7,000 Hz±8 dB) with a broad peak around 5 kHz when measured at the entrance of the ear canal. The sound spectrum is the product of the frequency transfer function of the earphone and the spectrum of the electrical impulses used to drive the earphone. When using a square wave of 100 μs duration, there is a dip in the spectrum of the sound at 10 kHz because of the spectrum of the electrical input to the earphone. The spectrum of a square wave of 100 μs duration has a cutoff at 8,000 Hz (6 dB), and its energy is zero at 10 and 20 kHz causing dips in the spectrum of the sound at these two frequencies (22). In fact, the commonly used duration of the rectangular impulses of 100 μs is not ideal; both longer and shorter durations are more suited for driving the sound generators used for eliciting ABR (see (22)).

When such a miniature stereo earphone is placed in the ear of a patient, it should be placed so that its sound-radiating (flat) surface faces the ear canal and that the earphone does not just rest in the pinna. This is particularly important to consider when such an earphone is placed in the ear of patients who have large outer ears (pinna), which is often the case in elderly men. The earphone must be carefully secured in place with several layers of a

---

[1] Radio Shack Corporation, Ft. Worth, Texas 76102.

good-quality plastic adhesive tape (e.g., 3 M Company[2] Blenderm[R]) in such a way that fluid cannot reach the earphone just in case the area around the ear should get wet. The cord to the earphone must be secured with adhesive tape to the side of the patient's face and to the head-holder (or operating table) so that the earphone is not accidentally dislodged from the ear if the cable is accidentally pulled.

Some of the modern insert earphones usually have the transducer connected to the ear by means of a plastic tube of various lengths. When driven by the standard rectangular wave of 100 μs duration, some earphones deliver a sound with a relatively flat spectrum up to ~6 kHz, which is similar to the spectrum delivered by the earphones used in audiometry and those often used in clinical ABR testing. The fact that insert earphones deliver sound through a long (plastic) tube results in a delay between the delivery of the electrical impulse that drives the earphone and the arrival of the sound at the ear. Sound travels at a speed of about 340 m/s, corresponding to a delay of 1 ms/34 cm, thus the delay is slightly less than 1 ms for each foot of tubing. A delay of 1 ms makes the (electrical) stimulus artifact appear 1 ms ahead of the sound's arrival at the ear and thus, reduces interference from the stimulus artifact with the ABR (see also Chap. 18 regarding how to reduce stimulus artifacts).

Electrode Placement. The electrodes used for recording ABR should be placed so that the amplitude of the recorded potentials is as high as possible and so that the components of the ABR that are of interest appear as clearly as possible. The traditional way of recording ABR is by connecting one of the two inputs of a differential amplifier to an electrode placed on the vertex and connecting the other input to an electrode placed on the ipsilateral earlobe or the ipsilateral mastoid.

As mentioned above, this placement of recording electrodes for ABR recordings is not ideal for obtaining the largest possible

potentials. Instead, recordings should be made in accordance with the orientations of the dipoles that represent the different components of the ABR. Scherg and von Cramon (*23*) showed that the generation of the different components of the ABR could be synthesized by six dipoles that were approximately located in the coronal plane (a vertical plane that is perpendicular to the saggital plane). Dipole of peaks I and III are approximately oriented horizontally, and peak V is nearly vertically oriented (**Fig. 7.2**). The negative troughs that follow peak I and peak III are oriented slightly differently. This means that electrodes placed in the horizontal plane record peaks I and III optimally, and peak V is best recorded by electrodes placed in the vertical plane. Using two separate recording channels, one recording differentially between electrodes placed at the vertex and on the dorsal upper neck (a noncephalic reference) and the other recording differentially from

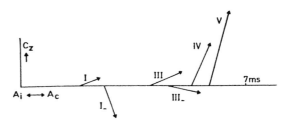

Figure 7.2: Orientation and strength of the six dipoles identified from recordings from electrodes placed in three planes. The horizontal line is a line between the two ears, and it is also the time axis. The vertical axis is a line between the middle of that line and the vertex. The origin of the vectors is the latency of the first peaks and the length is the relative strength of the dipoles. (Reprinted from (*23*), with permission from Elsevier).

---

[2] 3M™ Blenderm™ Surgical Tape, 3M Global Headquarters 3M Corporate Headquarters 3M Center) St. Paul, MN 55144-1000.

electrodes placed on the two earlobes, thus record peak V optimally and peaks I–III optimally. This way of recording ABR provides a record in which peak V appears more distinctly in the recording from the vertex–neck placement of the electrode, and peaks I and III are better represented in the recording from the earlobes than that which can be seen in the traditional way of recording ABR from electrodes placed at the vertex and on the ipsilateral earlobe.

Recording in two independent channels offers two alternative ways to detect changes in auditory function during an operation, and it makes it possible to continue monitoring using only one channel if one of the electrodes should malfunction during an operation.

If the recordings in one of these channels change noticeably, the surgeon should be informed. This does not need to be an alarm, as it is now popular to define a certain change in the recorded potentials as a warning. Any change that is larger than the normal small fluctuations should be reported to the surgeon because such changes mean that some structure has been affected.

> The equivalent dipoles shown in Fig. 7.2 were derived from recordings in three channels from three pairs of electrodes placed orthogonally on the scalp (24–26). Each pair of electrodes is connected to the two inputs of three independent differential amplifiers. The recorded potentials are then plotted as a function of each other to form a three dimensional display with time as a parameter.
>
> An example of recordings of the ABR in three orthogonal planes is shown in Fig. 7.3A. When combined, such recordings are known as three-channel Lissajous' trajectory as shown in Fig. 7.4B. Such recordings, which provide a complete description of the ABR, have been used to determine the neural generators of the ABR (27).
>
> Such recordings provide information about the anatomical location of the neural generators of the various components of the ABR in the head because they take into account the orientation of the different dipoles. There is, however, some uncertainty regarding the interpretation of the

potentials when they are recorded in this way. This type of recording is not commonly used in intraoperative monitoring, but has been used for research purposes in the operating room (28) and may find use in intraoperative monitoring in the future.

Types of Electrodes. When ABR are recorded for clinical diagnostic purposes, it is convenient to use surface electrodes to record the responses, but in the operating room, needle electrodes or wire hook electrodes are more suitable for several reasons. When held in place with a good-quality plastic adhesive tape (for instance, 3M, Blenderm[R2]), needle electrodes or wire electrodes provide a more stable recording over a longer period of time than do surface electrodes. Platinum subdermal electrodes (or disposable electrodes that are available from numerous sources) are suitable. The same is the case for wire hook electrodes. Inserting needle electrodes or wire hook electrodes are usually applied in the operating room after the patient is anesthetized, and there is no discomfort associated with placing such needles on anesthetized patients. At the end of the operation, the electrodes should be taken out before the patient is awake.

> All precautions should be taken to avoid failure of any recording electrodes during an operation. It is, thus, important that the electrodes be inserted properly and secured well to reduce the risk that they become dislodged should the electrode wires be accidentally pulled or should the area where the electrodes are placed be manipulated during the operation. The electrode placed on the vertex for recording ABR must be inserted deep in the tissue, and the electrode wire must be drawn toward the forehead and placed under the hair as close to the skin as possible and then secured to the forehead with adhesive tape. When recording from a person with much hair, the movements of the drape can make the hair move, and if the electrode wire is resting on top of the hair, it too moves and results in a noisy recording or a dislodged electrode.
>
> For these reasons, surface electrodes are not suitable for ABR recordings. In operations in which skin incisions are made near the earlobe,

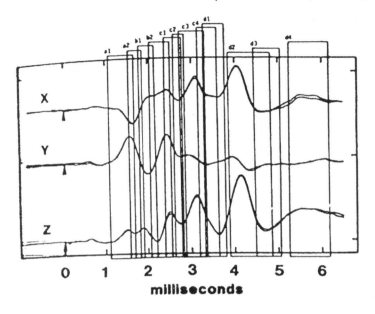

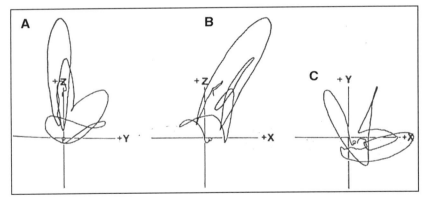

Figure 7.3: (**A**) Illustration of recordings for the three-channel Lissajous trajectory. (**B**) Three two-dimensional trajectories, with time along the line and each point representing the voltage at any given time after the stimulus. (Reprinted from (*27*) with permission from Elsevier).

the earlobe electrode may be pulled out if it is not sufficiently secured with adhesive tape or with sutures.

Processing of Recorded ABR

Because mainly changes in the latency of peak V (and to some extent of peak III) are used in connection with intraoperative monitoring, it is important that these peaks appear as clearly as possible in the recordings. The

purpose of processing recorded ABR is, therefore, to enhance these peaks (III and V) so they can be clearly identified and their latency can be measured. This can be performed by two methods: (1) averaging the responses to a sufficient number of stimuli, and (2) suitable filtering of the responses. Signal averaging increases signal-to-noise ratio (SNR) by adding responses to many stimuli. The purpose of filtering is to attenuate signals that are not wanted (noise) and to

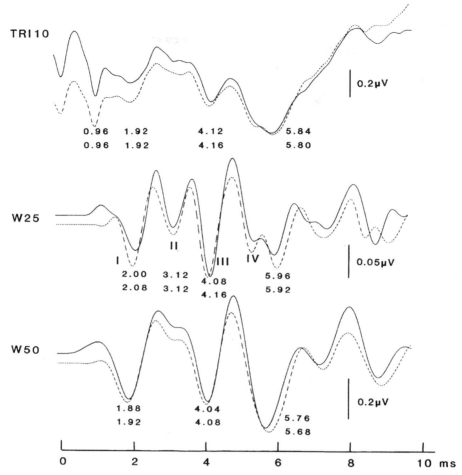

Figure 7.4: The effect of different kinds of digital filtering of an ABR recorded in the traditional way (differentially between vertex and mastoid) in an individual with normal hearing. Each curve is the average of 8,192 responses. *Solid lines*: response to rarefaction click, *dashed lines*: response to condensation clicks. The recordings were first filtered only by analog filters (10–3,400 Hz), after that, by three different digital filters: Tri 10: A triangular weighting function. W25: Digital filtering with a weighting function that provided band-pass characteristics. This filter enhances all peaks. W50: Digital filtering with a filter that has a wider weighting function. This filter enhances only peak I, III, and V. The filters are described by their weighting functions (Chap. 18, Figure 18.7).

enhance features of the recorded potentials that are important for their interpretation. The latter can be performed either at the same time that the responses are recorded using analog filters or after the responses have been averaged using computer programs using digital filters (see Chap. 18).

Filtering of Recorded Potentials. There are several reasons for filtering recorded potentials such as ABR. As is discussed in Chap. 18, high-frequency energy must be attenuated before the recorded signals are sampled and converted to a stream of digits. Another reason for filtering is to suppress background noise as much as possible. A third reason is to enhance important factors of recorded potentials.

Recorded ABR are, therefore, always subjected to some form of spectral filtering; analog filtering is used before the recorded responses are digitized for signal averaging to avoid aliasing (see Chap. 18). After being converted to a digital form, the recorded potentials may be filtered by digital filters, which are computer programs that perform the filtering. Digital filters and their use in filtering evoked potentials are described in Chap. 18. Digital filters have many advantages over analog filters for attenuating noise and for enhancing the waveform of evoked potentials, such as ABR, as illustrated in **Fig. 7.4**.

The purpose of processing the recorded ABR is to obtain a record that is as clear as possible and to enhance features that are of interest, an example of which is seen in **Fig. 7.5**. The techniques that are suitable for processing ABR are similar to commonly utilized methods for processing other evoked potentials (for details see Chap. 18).

In the recordings illustrated in **Fig. 7.4**, analog filters were set at rather "open" values; 10 Hz high-pass and 3-kHz (kilohertz) low-pass, and the slope of the high-pass filter was 6 dB/octave and that of the low-pass filter was 24 dB/octave. The digital filters were zero-phase finite impulse response filters as described in Chap. 18 (*29, 30*). The TRI 10 filter only smoothes the recordings, but the filters used for the lower two traces enhance the peaks, and the ABR shown in the two lower graphs have a much clearer definition of the peaks than the ABR that were only subjected to analog filtering. (The use of zero-phase finite impulse digital filters is discussed later in this book, Chap. 18).

Quality Control. Quality control of recorded potentials is important. In the clinic, quality control is performed by response replication. This is not a suitable method for intraoperative monitoring because having to make two recordings extends the time to get an interpretable recording. Methods that do not require repeating the response, and thus, do not take any additional time, are described in Chap. 18.

Display of ABR in the Operating Room

When monitoring ABR in the operating room, several tracings should be displayed, namely, the digitally filtered, averaged ABR recorded on two channels. One is recorded differentially between electrodes placed on the vertex and the dorsal neck, and the other channel should be recorded differentially between the two earlobes. The filtered ABR should be superimposed on a baseline recording on both of these channels. It is also important to have a display of the direct output of the amplifiers of the ABR in order to be able to evaluate background noise. If the output of the amplifier is not monitored, suddenly occurring interference would only be detected by an increase in the number of rejected responses, and that does not provide information about the kind of interference. Only by continuously observing the output from the amplifier is it possible to identify the source of interference (see Chap. 17 for details).

RECORDING OF NEAR-FIELD POTENTIALS

Recordings of near-field potentials from structures of the ascending auditory pathways in humans were first made for research purposes (*11, 31–37*), but have later found practical application in intraoperative monitoring, particularly for reducing the risk of injures to the auditory nerve (*4, 5, 7, 38*). Recordings from the exposed auditory nerve or from the surface of the cochlear nucleus are valuable in monitoring neural conduction in the auditory nerve (*9*).

Direct Recording from the Eighth Cranial Nerve

Recordings of CAP from the auditory nerve in such operations can be performed by placing an electrode on the exposed CN VIII. In response to transient sounds (clicks or tone bursts), such recordings yield CAP with amplitudes of a few microvolts in patients with normal hearing (*31, 32, 37, 39*). These potentials can, therefore, be displayed directly or after only a few responses have been averaged. This method provides a much more

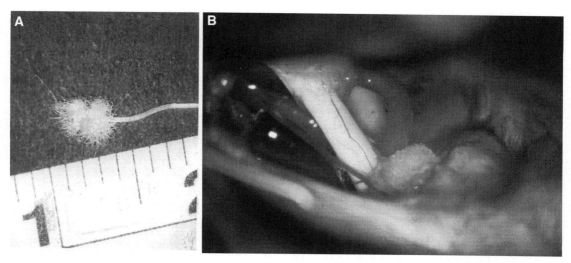

Figure 7.5: (**A**) The wick electrode used to record CAP from the auditory nerve. The electrode is made from a Teflon insulated silver wire with the cotton wick sutured to its uninsulated tip. (**B**) The electrode shown in (**A**) is placed on the exposed eighth cranial nerve to record CAP from the auditory nerve.

rapid way to detect injuries to the auditory nerve than monitoring ABR in MVD operations to move blood vessels off different cranial nerves in disorders, such as hemifacial spasm, trigeminal neuralgia, tinnitus disability, and in monitoring of operations to remove vestibular schwannoma (*4, 5, 7, 31*).

A fine, malleable, single-strand, Teflon-insulated silver wire (Medwire Corporation[3] Type Ag 7/40 T) (31) has been used by the author for many years. About 2 mm of the insulation is removed from the tip of this wire; the bare wire is then bent, and a small piece of cotton is sutured to the tip using a 5-0 silk suture. The cotton is then trimmed using microscissors to produce the finished electrode shown in Fig. 7.5. It is important that the cotton wick is securely sutured to the wire, since the electrode is to be placed on the exposed eighth nerve and losing a piece of cotton in the CPA can have serious consequences. Shredded Teflon® offers the same advantage as cotton but creates a less adverse reaction if accidentally lost intracranially. After the cotton, wick is sutured to the silver wire, it is soldered to a PVC-insulated and electrostatically shielded wire that connects the electrode to the input of the amplifier (electrode box).

In operations in the CPA, the recording electrode wire is tucked under one of the sutures that holds the dura open. In addition, the electrode wire is clamped to the drape near the incision to secure it in place.

The wire from the recording electrode should be connected to the inverting inputs of a differential amplifier so that a negative potential causes an upward deflection on the screen. The shield of the wire should be grounded to the iso-ground of the amplifier. The reference electrode for the intracranial recordings can be placed in the opposite earlobe.

The Anatomy of CN VIII. CN VIII comprises the vestibular nerve and the auditory (or cochlear) nerve. The arrangement of the different components of the eighth nerve is seen in a cross-sectional view, illustrated in **Fig. 7.6**, which shows the eighth cranial nerve inside the internal auditory meatus. The auditory nerve is located on the caudal side of the eighth

---

[3] Medwire Corporation, 121 South Columbus Avenue, Mt. Vernon, New York 10553.

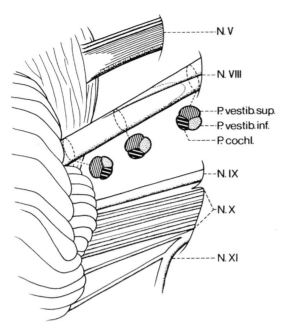

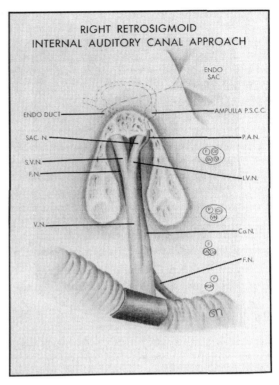

Figure 7.6: Schematic drawing showing the CPA viewed from the dorsal side with a cross-section of the eighth nerve to illustrate the anatomical organization of the different portions of the eighth nerve and its relationship with the other cranial nerves. (Reprinted from (*57*) with the permission from Elsevier).

Figure 7.7: Drawing of the anatomy of the internal auditory canal as seen from a retrosigmoid approach. The posterior wall of the internal auditory meatus has been removed so that its contents are visible. *IVN* inferior vestibular nerve, *SVN* superior vestibular nerve, *FN* facial nerve, *VN* vestibular nerve, *CoN* cochlear nerve (auditory nerve). (Reprinted from (*58*) with the permission from Elsevier).

nerve near the brainstem and anterior ventral to the eighth nerve near the porus acousticus. The nerve is rotated as it passes from the ear to the brain stem (**Fig. 7.6 and 7.7**).

The CAP that can be recorded from the auditory nerve in a patient with normal or near normal hearing – with the recording electrode placed on the nerve near the porus acousticus – has a triphasic waveform (**Fig. 7.8A**). An initial (small) positive peak is followed by a large negative peak, which in turn is followed by another small, positive peak. This is what may be expected when recording from a long nerve using a monopolar electrode (see Chap. 3). The amplitude and the waveform of the CAP depend on the stimulus intensity (**Fig. 7.9A**) and on the placement of the electrode along the auditory nerve (**Fig. 7.9B**).

The size of the recorded potentials is largest when the recording electrode is placed on the auditory portion of the eighth nerve, but even when placed on the vestibular portion of the eighth nerve, the recorded potentials (CAP) are normally several microvolts (µV) and large enough to be visible directly on a computer screen (or after averaging only a few responses). The reason that potentials of such large amplitude can be recorded, even when the electrode is placed on the vestibular portion of the eighth nerve, is that the vestibular nerve is a good conductor of electrical current.

The waveform of the normal CAP is essentially the same when using 2-kHz tone bursts as

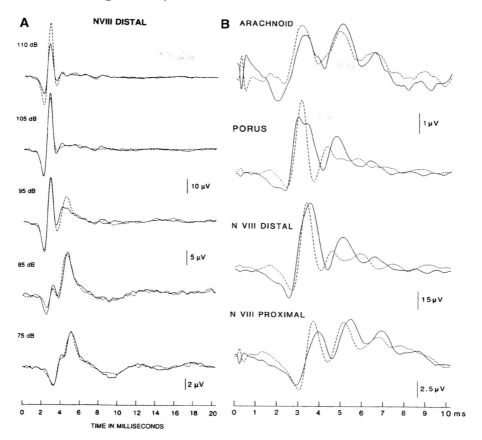

Figure 7.8: (**A**) CAP recorded from the eighth nerve near the porus acousticus in a person with normal hearing at different stimulus intensities (given in dB PeSPL). The responses were obtained in a patient undergoing MVD to relieve disabling positional vertigo (DPV), and the recording was made before manipulating the eighth cranial nerve. The sound stimuli were rarefaction clicks (*solid lines*) and condensation clicks (*dashed lines*). The sounds were delivered by a miniature earphone. (**B**) CAP recorded from different locations: near CN VIII (*top tracing*), from the porus acousticus, distally and proximally (*near the brainstem*). (Reprinted from (*38*) with the permission from Kugler Publications).

stimuli as when using clicks, but the changes in the responses as a result of pathologies affecting the ear or the auditory nerve may be different for click sounds than for tone bursts. The waveform of the CAP when recorded in the same way in patients with hearing loss (**Fig. 7.9**) may deviate noticeably from the waveform shown in **Fig. 7.9**.

Recording from the Vicinity of the Cochlear Nucleus

The value of monitoring directly recorded evoked potentials from the exposed auditory nerve is well documented as shown above. However, the difficulties in placing the electrode in the correct position on the eighth nerve are obstacles to the routine use of such directly recorded evoked potentials. The recording electrode must be placed proximal to the location on the nerve where it is at risk of being injured, and it may be difficult to keep the recording electrode in the correct position at times during an operation. These problems hamper the general use of recording directly from the auditory nerve.

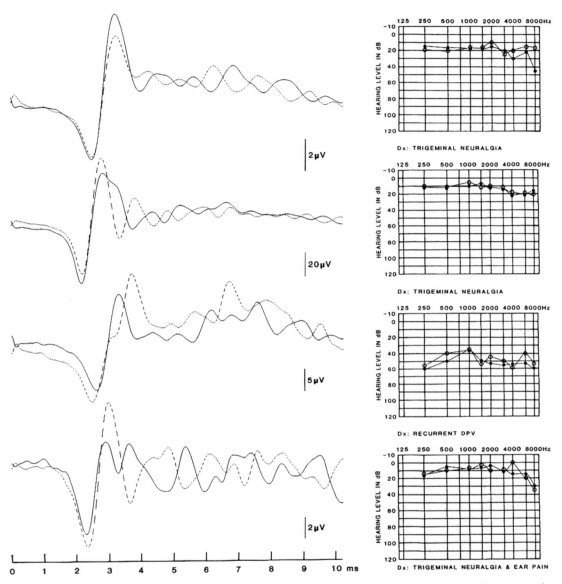

Figure 7.9: Examples of CAP recorded from patients with different degrees of preoperative hearing loss as seen in the preoperative pure tone audiograms shown to the *right*. (Reprinted from (*44*) with permission from Elsevier).

Recording from the vicinity of the cochlear nucleus (*11, 12*) can overcome many of the practical difficulties associated with recording directly from the exposed eighth nerve, and it has similar advantages as recording CAP directly from the eighth nerve (*8, 9*). The coch-lear nucleus forms the floor of the lateral recess of the fourth ventricle (*8, 40*), and recording from the vicinity of the cochlear nucleus can be performed by placing a recording electrode in the lateral recess of the fourth ventricle (*8, 9*) (**Fig. 7.10A**).

The same type of wick electrode (Fig. 7.5A) as used to record from the exposed eighth nerve can be used for recording from the surface of the cochlear nucleus. The opening of the lateral recess of the fourth ventricle, known as the foramen of Luschka, is found just anterior to the entrance of the CN IX/CN X complex into the brainstem. The foramen of Luschka may be identified by locating the choroid plexus that normally protrudes from the foramen. Elevating the cerebellum over the CN IX/CN X complex provides access to the foramen of Luschka. By following the choroid plexus into the lateral recess of the fourth ventricle, the recording electrode may be placed deep into the lateral recess (8). The wire of the recording electrode should be tucked under the sutures that hold the dura open so that it cannot be easily moved during the operation (Fig. 7.10A). The recording electrode should be connected to the inverting input of the amplifier just as it is connected when recording from the exposed CN VIII. The opposite earlobe is a suitable location for the reference electrode for such recordings.

Recorded potentials from the surface of the cochlear nucleus consist of an initial sharp, positive–negative deflection that is generated by the termination of the auditory nerve in the cochlear nucleus. This peak is followed by a slow wave that may last tenths of milliseconds and which has several waves riding upon it (**Fig. 7.10B**). The waveform of the potentials recorded from the surface of the cochlear nucleus (or its vicinity) resembles that which is normally recorded from a nucleus (see Chap. 2, **Fig. 2.7**). As seen from **Fig. 7.10B** and C, preoperative hearing loss affects the waveforms of the potentials that are recorded from the surface of the cochlear nucleus.

Recordings of evoked potentials from the cochlear nucleus or its vicinity represent evoked potentials that are generated by structures located proximal to the auditory nerve. Changes in these potentials are, therefore, good indications of changes in the function of the auditory nerve such as those that may occur when the nerve is being manipulated, such as in MVD

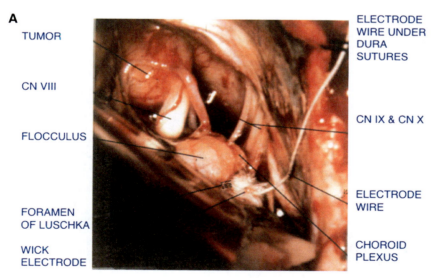

A

TUMOR

CN VIII

FLOCCULUS

FORAMEN OF LUSCHKA

WICK ELECTRODE

ELECTRODE WIRE UNDER DURA SUTURES

CN IX & CN X

ELECTRODE WIRE

CHOROID PLEXUS

Figure 7.10: (**A**) Placement of the recording electrode in the lateral recess of the fourth ventricle in a patient with a vestibular schwannoma. The *solid lines* are the responses to rarefaction clicks and the *dashed lines* are the responses to condensation clicks. (Reprinted from (59) with the permission from McHraw Hill). (**B, C**) Examples of recordings from the vicinity of the cochlear nucleus in patients with varying degree of hearing loss. The patients were operated upon for hemifacial spasms (HFS) and disabling positional vertigo (DPV).

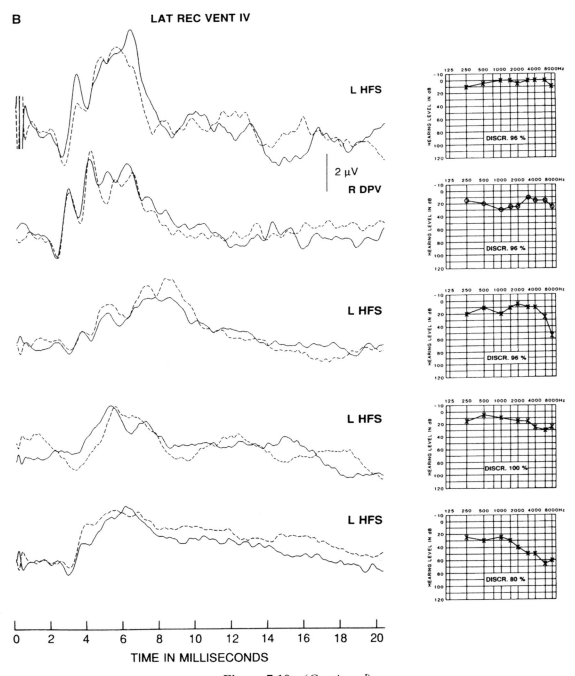

Figure 7.10: (*Continued*)

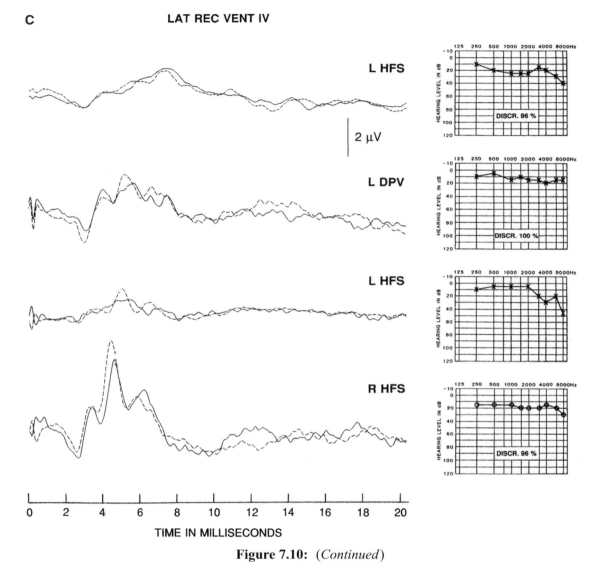

Figure 7.10: (*Continued*)

operations. Recordings from the cochlear nucleus are, however, perhaps of the greatest importance in connection with the removal of vestibular schwannoma in patients who have useful hearing preoperatively and in whom hearing preservation is being attempted during the removal of the tumor (see page 137).

The fast components of the response from the cochlear nucleus are generated where the auditory nerve terminates in the cochlear nucleus, and the slow components are generated by dendrites. The fast components are, thus, directly associated with neural transmission in the auditory nerve and signal arrival of neural activity in its target neurons. The fast components are, therefore, probably the best indicators of injury to the auditory nerve, and they are the components that should be watched in intraoperative monitoring of the auditory nerve.

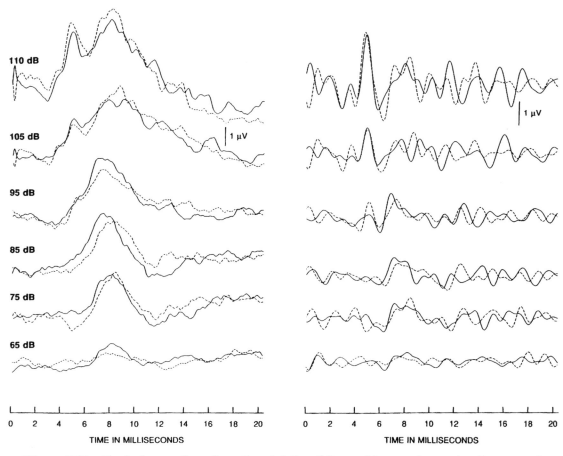

Figure 7.11: Typical recordings from the vicinity of the cochlear nucleus using the same electrode placement shown in Figure 7.10 A. *Left column*: Unfiltered responses. *Right column*: Same recordings after digital filtering to enhance the narrow peaks. The recordings were made consecutively, and each record is the average of 250 responses. The dashed line curves represent the baseline. (Reprinted from (*8*) with the permission from the Journal of Neurosurgery).

Digital filters can be used to enhance the fast peaks of the responses and suppress the slow components (**Fig. 7.11**). Changes in the stimulus intensity affect the fast (initial) and the (later) slow potentials differently. The amplitude of the main peak of the fast response that occurs with a latency of ~4 ms decreases rapidly when the stimulus intensity is decreased, while the slow components that dominate the unfiltered response only change minimally with decreasing stimulus intensity (**Fig. 7.11**). It is not known which of these components, slow or fast, are the best indicators of injury to the auditory nerve, but it seems

likely that the fast components (such as the negative peak at 4 ms) would be more sensitive to changes in neural conduction in the auditory nerve than the slow components.

It may sometimes be difficult to place the recording electrode deep in the lateral recess of the fourth ventricle, but it is not necessary to penetrate the foramen of Luschka with the recording electrode to obtain satisfactory recordings; merely placing the recording wick electrode on CN IX and X where they enter the brainstem usually provides a satisfactory recording of the response from the cochlear nucleus. The amplitudes of these potentials may be slightly lower than those recorded from an electrode placed deep in the lateral recess, but the potentials that are recorded from the entrance of CN IX and CN X in the brainstem are usually several microvolts, and can, thus, be interpreted after only a few hundred responses are added. It is easier to place the recording electrode in this location than it is to place it on the eighth nerve, which is an advantage when monitoring operations for vestibular schwannoma.

It is practical to record ABR and the potentials from the lateral recess simultaneously to produce different traces on the display. The same stimuli used to elicit ABR are also suitable to elicit these directly recorded potentials from the surface of the cochlear nucleus.

INTERPRETATION OF CHANGES IN AUDITORY RESPONSES

The changes that occur during an operation should be related to specific manipulations, such as stretching, compressing or heating neural tissue, and the anatomical location of the structures whose functions have changed should be identified to the surgeon. Such events should be documented in the final report of the monitoring together with the recordings of the evoked potentials.

Interpretation of Changes in the ABR

In the operating room, the task is to detect changes in auditory evoked potentials from a baseline recording that is made after the patient is brought to the sleep stage of anesthesia, but before the operation has begun. Traditionally, it has been the latency of specific components (vertex positive peaks) of the ABR that has been used to indicate surgically induced injuries to the auditory nerve. Since peak V of the ABR is the most prominent and most easily identified peak, it seems natural to use changes in the latency of this peak as an indication of injury to the auditory nerve. It has often been assumed that any change in neural conduction

of the auditory nerve is equally reflected in the latencies of peak II and any one of the ABR peaks that follows peak II.

It is also of value to observe changes in the amplitude of the components of the ABR. It has been shown that inclusion of changes in the amplitude increases the value of the ABR for detecting changes in the function of the auditory nerve (18, 41).

However, changes in the amplitudes of peak III and peak V are not necessarily the same, and there are, therefore, reasons to monitor changes in the amplitudes of both peak III and peak V. Changes in the function of the auditory nerve may cause a smaller change in the amplitude of peak V than that of peak III. Peak V may, therefore, be less sensitive to injury to the auditory nerve than peak III or the CAP recorded directly from CN VIII or the cochlear nucleus. The amplitude of peak III may be a more reliable (clean) indicator of changes in neural conduction of the auditory nerve than peak V. Often the vertex-negative peak between peak III and peak IV–V complex is prominent, and in such cases, using this vertex-negative peak (valley) is just as suitable for monitoring purposes as peak III.

If the latency of peak V increases, but the latency of peak III remains unchanged, the interval between peaks III and V increases (increased interpeak latency, IPL, III–V). The reason for such a change is most likely altered functions of structures of the ascending auditory pathways that are located rostral to the generators of peak III (mostly the cochlear nucleus). Increased IPL III–V may also be caused by general changes in, for example, cerebral circulation or from changes in oxygenation (causing ischemia), which can have many causes. If this occurs in operations in the CPA, the anesthesiologist should be informed because ischemia may be a result of cardiovascular changes or other changes that the anesthesiologist can correct.

Interpretations of CAP from CN VIII and the Cochlear Nucleus

Changes in the CAP recorded directly from the proximal portion of the auditory nerve as a result of manipulation of CN VIII are more easily interpreted than changes in the ABR. The CAP recorded from CN VIII or the cochlear nucleus is probably also more sensitive to small changes in the function of the auditory nerve than are the ABR. Recording of ABR is, however, the only way to detect injuries to the auditory nerve that may occur before surgical exposure of the eighth nerve. Changes in the ABR may occur during retraction of the cerebellum that can stretch the auditory nerve, or it may be caused by surgical dissection to expose the auditory nerve.

The major advantage of recording directly from the exposed CN VIII or the cochlear nucleus is that changes in neural conduction in the auditory nerve can be detected almost at the moment they occur. The large amplitude of the CAP recorded directly from the auditory nerve allows the CAP to be viewed on a computer screen once a few responses have been averaged, making it possible to accurately identify which steps in an operation caused change in neural conduction in the auditory nerve. The rapid detection of change in neural conduction of the auditory nerve also provides a much better possibility to reverse a surgically induced change in the function of the auditory nerve, thus increasing the effectiveness of intraoperative monitoring. Assessment of neural conduction in the auditory nerve on the basis of changes in ABR takes a much longer time than from inspection of the CAP recorded directly from the auditory nerve or recordings from the cochlear nucleus.

The first CAP that are recorded should be used as a baseline to which successive recorded potentials can be compared. Any deviations in the components from the baseline recording should be regarded as a sign of an effect on neural transmission in the part of the auditory nerve that is located distal to the location of the recording electrode on the nerve. The recording electrode should, therefore, be placed as far proximal on the cochlear–vestibular nerve as possible, or it should be placed on the cochlear nucleus. Recordings from the cochlear nucleus reflect the neural conduction in the entire auditory nerve.

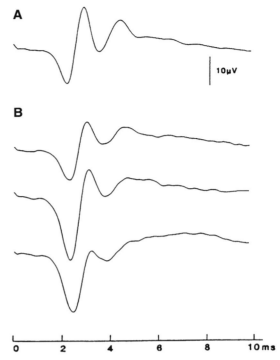

Figure 7.12: Typical alterations in the CAP recorded from the auditory nerve that resulted when heat from electrocoagulation was transmitted to the nerve. The sound stimuli were clicks at 110 dB PeSPL (Reprinted from (*28*)).

Heating from electrocoagulation can cause changes in the waveform of the CAP recorded from the exposed auditory nerves as illustrated in **Figs. 7.12** and **7.13**.

The change in the CAP recorded from the auditory nerve that may occur as a result of surgical manipulations or heating is a more or less marked decrease in the amplitude of the main negative peak of the CAP. In addition, an increased latency and increased amplitude of the initial positive wave may occur. The increased amplitude of the initial positive wave (downward deflection in **Figs. 7.12** and **7.13**) indicates that a conduction block has occurred in many nerve fibers. The recordings shown in **Fig. 7.13** illustrate changes that occurred after heating of the auditory nerve by electrocoagulation. Shortly after the eighth nerve was

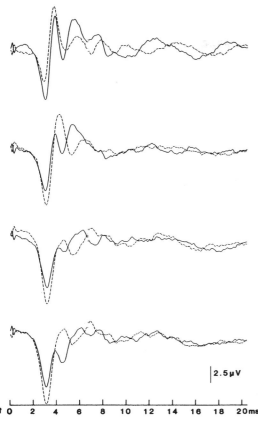

Figure 7.13: Examples of changes in the CAP recorded from the proximal portion of CN VIII at different times after surgical manipulations (probably heating). *Solid lines* are the CAP in response to rarefaction clicks and *dashed lines* are the responses to condensation clicks.

exposed, the recorded CAP had the normal triphasic waveform (**Fig. 7.13**), but after electrocoagulation of a nearby vein, it gradually changed and became a single positive wave (**Fig. 7.13**), which indicated that there was nearly total blockage of neural conduction in the auditory nerve.

In order to understand the nature of this kind of injury, the generation of the CAP from a long nerve, when recorded by a monopolar electrode, should be recalled. The initial positive deflection in the CAP is generated by a region of neural depolarization as it approaches the site of the recording electrode, and the negative peak in the

CAP is generated when the region of depolarization of auditory nerve fibers passes under the recording electrode (see Chap. 2). The near disappearance of the negative peak (**Figs. 7.12** and **7.13**) can be explained by the region of depolarization never reaching the location on the nerve where the recording electrode is placed. The amplitude of the initial positive peak in the CAP – which is generated when the region of depolarization of nerve fibers approaches the recording electrode – is normally decreased because the negative peak that normally follows pulls up the positive peak. When the amplitude of the negative peak decreases, this "pull" of the negative peak on the positive peak upward decreases, and therefore, the positive peak appears to have become larger in amplitude.

Examples of changes in the CAP caused by the retraction of the cerebellum are seen in **Fig. 7.14**. The slight widening of the main negative peak in the CAP is an indication that the increase in latency (decreased conduction velocity) affected different nerve fibers of the nerve differently. That there is only a small decrease of the amplitude of the negative peak indicates that almost all of the fibers of the auditory nerve were conducting nerve impulses. Changes in neural conduction that cause increases in the latency of the main negative peak with little change in amplitude indicate that the only effect of the surgical manipulation was an increase in neural conduction time (decrease in conduction velocity). Changes that consist of broadening of the negative peak indicate that the latency of neural conduction has increased (decreased conduction velocity) unevenly for different nerve fibers (**Fig. 7.14**). We believe that this is what happens when the auditory nerve is stretched moderately. Provided that proper action is taken promptly to reverse the injury, such changes seem to be completely, or nearly completely, reversible so that the patient does not acquire hearing deficits when assessed by traditional measurements of hearing postoperatively.

Recordings from the Cochlear Nucleus

Less experience has been gained regarding the interpretations of recordings made from the

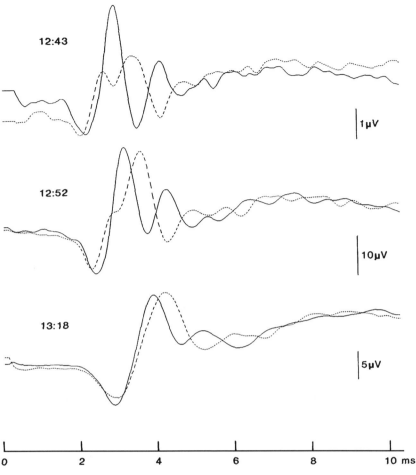

Figure 7.14: Examples of changes in the CAP recorded from the proximal portion of CN VIII as a result of surgical manipulations (stretching). The time the recordings were made are indicated on each record. *Solid lines* are the responses to rarefaction clicks and *dashed lines* are the responses to condensation clicks.

vicinity of the cochlear nucleus than those made from recording the auditory nerve. It is not known for certain which of the different components of the potentials that are recorded from the cochlear nucleus are most sensitive to changes in neural conduction in the auditory nerve.

The initial, fast component that signals the arrival of nerve activity at the cochlear nucleus may, therefore, be regarded to provide the same information about injury of the auditory nerve as CAP recorded from the exposed auditory vestibular nerve. The amplitudes of the slow components, however, decrease at a different rate than the initial, fast component when stimulus intensity is decreased (see page 140), which may mean that fast components are more sensitive to changes in neural conduction in the auditory nerve than are the slow components. Results from intraoperative recording during the removal of a vestibular schwannoma, such as those illustrated in **Fig. 7.15**, seem to support this hypothesis. The latencies of both the fast and slow components of these potentials, however, were prolonged as a result

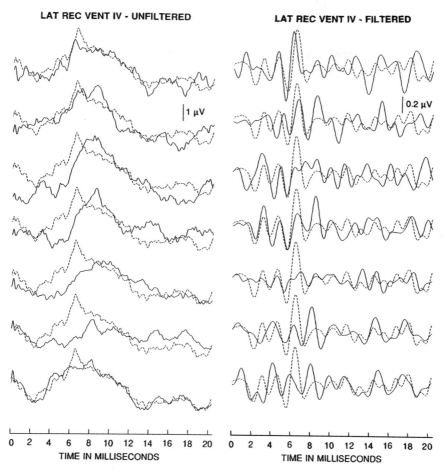

LAT REC VENT IV - UNFILTERED

LAT REC VENT IV - FILTERED

1 µV

0.2 µV

0 2 4 6 8 10 12 14 16 18 20
TIME IN MILLISECONDS

0 2 4 6 8 10 12 14 16 18 20
TIME IN MILLISECONDS

Figure 7.15: Recordings from the surface of the cochlear nucleus (lateral recess of the fourth ventricle) in a patient undergoing the removal of a 3 cm vestibular schwannoma. The *left column* shows the recorded potentials before filtering, and the *right column* shows the same recordings after digital filtering (W50 filter, see page 367). The *dashed lines* in all recordings are baseline recordings obtained before tumor removal. The patient had normal hearing before the operation, and his hearing threshold and speech discrimination did not change noticeably after the operation.

of surgical manipulation. This indicates that the latencies (but perhaps not the amplitudes) of either slow or fast components may be valid indicators of changes in neural conduction in the auditory nerve.

Effect of Injury to the Auditory Nerve on the ABR

It has traditionally been the latency of the different components of the ABR that has been used as a criterion for altered neural conduction

in the auditory nerve. As discussed above, the amplitude of the CAP that can be recorded from a nerve is proportional to the number of nerve fibers that are conducting nerve impulses, and a loss of conduction in some nerve fibers causes a decrease in the amplitude of the recorded CAP. Presumably, this means that the amplitudes of the different components of the ABR also change when neural conduction in the auditory nerve is altered. It would, therefore be expected that monitoring amplitudes of the different components of the ABR in addition to monitoring latencies would be of value, and studies have supported this assumption (*18*).

One of the reasons why latency changes have been favored over amplitude changes as indicators of injury to the auditory nerve is that the latencies of ABR peaks are less variable than the amplitudes of the different peaks of the ABR. The reason for the greater variability of the amplitudes of the different peaks is not known, but changes in recording conditions may contribute to this variability. The noise that is always superimposed on ABR recordings also contributes to the variability of the amplitudes of the components (peaks) of the ABR.

One reason for a decrease in the amplitude of the recorded ABR is that the amplitude of the recorded potentials does actually decrease, but this is not the only reason. Another reason for a decrease in amplitude is associated with the use of signal averaging. When many responses are added, the amplitude of the resulting averaged recording decreases if the latencies of the different components (peaks) of the ABR change during the time that the responses are being collected, and the averaged response, therefore, becomes less than what it would have been if all the responses included in the average were identical.

Change in the latency of the responses that compose ABR during the time in which the evoked potentials are being collected also causes changes in the waveform of the averaged response, and the waveform of the averaged response is different from that of any waveform of the individual responses that were added to make up the averaged response. These effects of the averaging process increase when more responses are added, thus taking more time to complete the averaged response. This problem worsens as the number of changes that occur in the responses increase during the time of data acquisition. However, studies have suggested that monitoring the amplitudes of the peaks of the ABR during operations where the auditory nerve is being manipulated is valuable in detecting changes in the function of the auditory nerve (*18*).

Relationship Between Changes in ABR and in CAP from the Auditory Nerve and the Cochlear Nucleus

The CAP recorded from the exposed CN VIII have specific relationships to the waveform of the ABR as discussed above (page 141). Surgical manipulations of the auditory nerve that cause changes in the waveform of the CAP recorded from the exposed CN VIII also cause changes in the ABR, but the changes in the ABR are less specific and, therefore, more difficult to interpret (**Fig. 7.16**). Examination of the CAP recorded from the exposed CN VIII shows an increase in latency and widening of the negative peak of the CAP after surgical manipulation of CN VIII. These changes indicate that the increase in neural conduction time is different for different auditory nerve fibers, but similar information cannot be obtained from inspection of the ABR.

Surgically induced injuries to the auditory nerve result in an increase in the latency of the later (slow) components recorded from the cochlear nucleus. This change in latency is not necessarily seen in the CAP recorded from CN VIII. The same can be said for the later components of the ABR (peaks III and V). The amplitudes of these different components of auditory evoked potentials do not necessarily change to the same degree as a result of injury to the auditory nerve as do the CAP amplitudes.

One reason that the different components of the far-field response (ABR) may change in a different way than the near-field response (CAP from the auditory nerve or cochlear nucleus) is that the different components of the ABR are less dependent on the temporal coherence of neural activity than are the responses that are recorded directly from the auditory nerve. This is especially the case for the later peaks in the ABR (peaks III and V), which seem to be less dependent on temporal coherence of neural activity than the earlier peaks (peaks I and II). Thus, a large reduction in the temporal coherence of neural activity in auditory nerve fibers, which manifests as a large reduction in the response from the auditory nerve, may cause much less reduction in

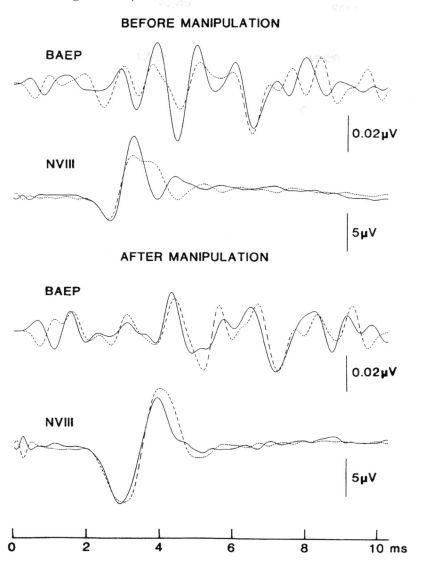

Figure 7.16: ABR recorded simultaneously with the CAP recorded from the exposed eighth nerve. Each recording of the ABR represents about 2,000 responses, and the averaged responses were filtered with a zero-phase digital filter (see Chap. 18). (The directly recorded responses from CN VIII were not digitally filtered.) (Reprinted from (2) with the permission of the Journal of Neurosurgery).

the amplitude of the later peaks in the ABR. This is also why the amplitude of the CAP recorded from the auditory nerve are probably more sensitive to surgically induced injuries than later peaks of the ABR such as peak V. While the CAP recorded from the auditory nerve usually have much lower amplitudes in patients with hearing loss caused by auditory nerve injuries; the amplitude of wave V in patients with this kind of hearing loss may be closer to that of patients with normal auditory nerve function. Thus, the later peaks of ABR, particularly peak V, are often less affected by injuries to the auditory nerve than earlier peaks. This means that also the CAP recorded directly from the auditory nerve are likely to be more sensitive to injury of the auditory nerve than is peak V of the ABR. This is the reason that the CAP recorded directly from CN VIII (and the initial components of the response from the cochlear nucleus) may be better indicators of injury of the auditory nerve and thus, more suitable for use in intraoperative monitoring during operations in which the eighth nerve is manipulated than recordings of the ABR when changes in peak V are used.

It was mentioned in Chap. 5 that excitation of the hair cells in the basal portion of the cochlea evokes more synchronized discharges than does excitation of hair cells that are located in the low-frequency (apical) portion of the basilar membrane. Excitation of low-frequency hair cells, therefore, contributes little to the CAP and ABR elicited by wideband click sounds. In a similar way, it may be assumed that the loss of low-frequency nerve fibers may not affect the responses to wideband click sounds noticeably, and it is possible that low-frequency hearing loss may escape detection by intraoperative monitoring when click sounds are used as stimuli.

Other Causes of Injury to the Auditory Nerve

It was discussed above how retraction and heating of the auditory nerve are probably the most common causes of injury to the auditory nerve during surgical operations in the CPA. However, there are other causes of injury that can occur during an operation. One type results from irrigating the surgical area, but there are also unknown causes of injury to the auditory nerve.

Injury to the Auditory Nerve from Irrigating. Results of intraoperative monitoring of ABR have shown evidence that irrigation of the CPA in the region of CN VIII can cause severe injury to the auditory nerve and possibly lead to permanent hearing impairment and even deafness. It was first believed that a strong stream of fluid from a syringe used for irrigation could injure the auditory nerve, but

later it was found that even a low velocity flooding of saline into the CPA could injure the auditory nerve. These experiences changed the way irrigation in the CPA was performed, and saline was gently poured on the cerebellum and never directly into the CPA.

These are examples of how intraoperative neurophysiological monitoring can improve operative techniques.

Unknown Causes of Injury to the Auditory Nerve. Experience from intraoperative monitoring of auditory evoked potentials in MVD operations of cranial nerves has shown that there may be causes for injury to the auditory nerve other than direct and known surgical manipulations or heating from electrocoagulation.

An example of one such unknown cause of injury was a case where a patient lost hearing after an operation in the CPA during which there were no remarkable changes in the auditory evoked potentials. ABR were not monitored in the operating room after the dura was closed because it was believed then that the risk of injury to the auditory nerve had passed when the dura was closed. However, the ABR in this patient were recorded automatically to the end of the operation as a part of a research project. After it was discovered that the patient had suffered a total hearing loss, examination of the records revealed a steadily increasing latency of peak V of the ABR after the dura was closed (Fig. 7.17A). Obviously, something happened after closing the dura that caused the auditory nerve to be stretched or affected in some other way. This experience taught us to always monitor ABR until skin closure. On several occasions after this experience, once the dura was closed, large changes in the ABR occurred in similar operations. In each of these patients, reopening the dura and releasing fluid and irrigating the CPA caused the ABR to recover and thus, seemingly resolved the problem. However, it was not possible to pinpoint the exact cause of these ABR changes. None of these patients suffered permanent hearing impairment.

In similar operations in which changes in the ABR during the operation were due to operative

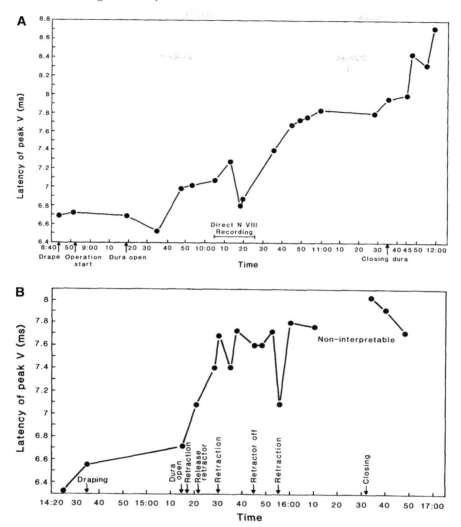

Figure 7.17: Changes in the latency of peak V during MVD operations to relieve cranial nerve disorders. (**A**) Results from a patient who was operated on to relieve HFS and who acquired a postoperative hearing loss that became partly resolved over a 3-month period. (**B**) Graph similar to that in (**A**), but showing an increase in the latency of peak V after the dura was closed. This patient lost hearing permanently. (Reprinted from (*3*) with the permission from Lippincott Williams & Wilkins).

difficulties, the latency of peak V of the ABR typically decreased toward normal values during the wound closure. Fig. 7.17B shows results from a patient who experienced large changes in evoked potentials during the operation, but the latency of peak V decreased during wound closure. The patient had a moderate postoperative hearing impairment, but the hearing improved within a 3-month period.

PRACTICAL ASPECTS REGARDING MONITORING AUDITORY EVOKED POTENTIALS IN OPERATIONS FOR VESTIBULAR SCHWANNOMA

Most of the examples of results of intraoperative monitoring of auditory evoked potentials that were given earlier in this chapter were from monitoring of patients who underwent MVD of cranial nerves to relieve TGN, HFS, DPV, or tinnitus. It was shown that intraoperative monitoring of auditory evoked potentials could decrease the risk of postoperative hearing loss in such patients (*3*). MVD operations are rare, but similar methods to preserve hearing can be used in other operations in the CPA, such as those to remove vestibular schwannoma. Such operations are much more common than MVD operations. Diagnostic methods for identifying vestibular schwannoma continue to improve, and such tumors can now be identified while still small. Many surgeons recommend surgery for small vestibular schwannoma in patients that have usable hearing to help them retain the greatest degree of this sensory function. For that, intraoperative monitoring of the function of the auditory nerve is essential.

Four different ways of monitoring auditory function in surgical operations to remove vestibular schwannoma have been described: recording of far-field auditory evoked potentials (ABR), recording of near-field auditory elicited potentials from the ear (ECoG), CAP from the auditory nerve, and CAP from the surface of the cochlear nucleus.

Recording of ABR

An example of ABR recorded during an operation to remove a vestibular schwannoma in a patient who had good hearing before the operation (96% speech discrimination) is shown in **Fig. 7.13**. Despite variations in the ABR during the operation – there was an almost 1-ms prolongation of the latency of peak III in the early phase of the tumor resection procedure – the ABR obtained at the time of closure were remarkably similar to those obtained preoperatively (**Fig. 7.18**). Postoperatively, the patient's speech discrimination score was 96% (recorded speech material), and his pure tone audiogram showed no significant hearing loss (except at 4 and 8 kHz) as a result of the operation.

If peak I of the ABR changes or disappears during an operation and there also is a change in all other peaks (or total obliteration of the ABR), it is a sign that the blood supply to the ear (cochlea) has been compromised. If peak I is largely unchanged while there are changes in peaks III or V, it is likely that there has been injury to the intracranial portion of the auditory nerve with the blood supply to the cochlea remaining intact. (In some patients, no peak III can be identified, as is the case in the patient whose recordings are seen in **Fig. 7.18**) If there is a change in peak V, but peak III is unchanged, there is reason to assume that the brainstem has been affected by surgical manipulations, or that there is ischemia due to impaired blood supply to the brainstem. If it is not possible to clearly identify peak I, a judgment about the cause of a change in, for instance, peak V of the ABR, cannot be made with certainty, and the anatomical location of the injury is less obvious.

Patients who undergo operations to remove vestibular schwannoma often have abnormal ABR before the operation (as the one seen in **Fig. 7.18**) because the tumor affects the neural conduction in the auditory nerve, and the components of the ABR other than peak I are delayed and often have much smaller amplitudes than normal. This results in the need to average more responses in order to obtain an interpretable recording and consequently makes it more difficult to use ABR to detect injury to the auditory nerve.

Patients undergoing operations to remove vestibular schwannoma are usually not paralyzed during the operation because the administration of muscle relaxants prevent monitoring of the facial nerve, which is critical to preserving facial nerve function. The small EMG activity of the head muscles that may occur spontaneously, or when the facial nerve is manipulated, acts as noise that contaminates the ABR recordings. This impairs the SNR of the recorded ABR and thus, increases the time required to obtain an interpretable record. There is, therefore, a great need to optimize the way ABR are recorded and processed, such as utilizing optimal stimulus and recording parameters, aggressive filtering, and an efficient quality control system that does not require any additional time for data collection (Chap. 18). By taking these matters into proper consideration,

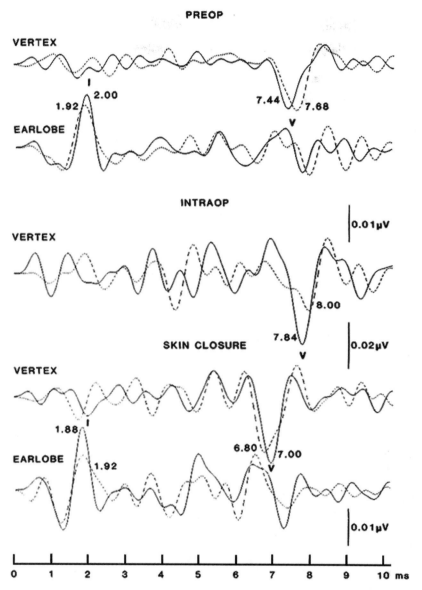

Figure 7.18: Samples of ABR recordings made on two channels from a patient undergoing the removal of a vestibular schwannoma. The *upper tracing* shows potentials recorded from electrodes placed on the vertex and the upper neck, and the *lower tracings* were obtained by differential recordings between electrodes placed on the ear lobes. The stimuli were clicks presented to the ear on the side of the tumor at a rate of 20 pps. The recorded potentials were digitally filtered with a W50 filter (see Chap. 18) that enhances peak V.

it is possible to obtain interpretable ABR and detect changes in ABR by recording for about 1–3 min, at least in patients with reasonably good ABR.

Recording from the Vicinity of the Ear

Some investigators have monitored auditory evoked potentials recorded from the ear in operations to remove vestibular schwannoma (*15, 42*).

For direct recording from the cochlear capsule, a recording electrode must be passed through the tympanic membrane, which is an invasive procedure that takes considerable skill to perform safely. An electrode placed on the cochlear capsule not only records CAP from the distal portion of the auditory nerve, but it also records the cochlear microphonics (CM) potential and the summating potential (SP). These three different kinds of auditory evoked potentials are known as the electrocochleographic potentials (ECoG) (**Fig. 7.19**). Only one of the components of the ECoG is of interest in intraoperative monitoring for vestibular schwannoma, namely, the CAP from the auditory nerve.

The CAP from the auditory nerve that is recorded from the cochlear capsule usually has amplitudes within the range of several microvolts (*43*) and can, therefore, be evaluated with very little signal averaging (**Fig. 7.14A**). This makes it possible to detect changes in CAP with practically no delays.

ECoG potentials can also be recorded from a (wick) electrode placed on the tympanic membrane (**Fig. 7.19B**) (*43*) or from an electrode placed in the ear canal. However, the amplitude of the CAP component recorded this way is much smaller than those recorded from the cochlear capsule, and a considerable number of responses must be averaged before an interpretable record can be obtained.

There are, unfortunately, several problems associated with the use of ECoG potentials recorded from the ear, or its vicinity, for intraoperative monitoring of hearing in patients undergoing vestibular schwannoma surgery. These problems are related to the fact that the CAP recorded from the ear originate from the very distal portion of the auditory nerve (where it exits the cochlea), and, therefore, the ECoG potentials do not show change when the intracranial portion of the auditory nerve has actually been injured. In fact, the intracranial portion of the eighth nerve can be severed without any noticeable change occurring in the CAP recorded from the ear. Because it is the intracranial portion of the auditory nerve that

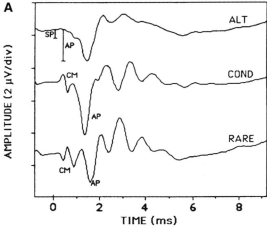

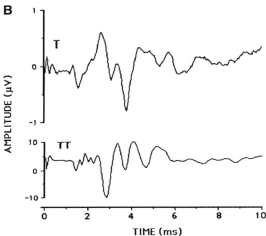

Figure 7.19: (**A**) Normal ECoG potentials recorded from the promontorium of the cochlea. *Top tracing* shows the response to clicks of alternating polarity, and the *middle* and *lower tracings* show the responses to condensation and rarefaction clicks, respectively. Note that negativity is shown as a downward deflection. (**B**) Comparison between ECoG potentials obtained from a wick electrode placed on the tympanic membrane (*upper tracing*) and on the promontorium (*lower tracing*). Note the much higher (about ten times) amplitude of the response recorded from the promontorium than that recorded from the tympanic membrane. (Reprinted from (*43*) with the permission of Elsevier).

is most likely to be injured during the removal of vestibular schwannoma, recordings of ECoG potentials are, therefore, not suitable for monitoring purposes in connection with operations for vestibular schwannoma because they do not detect injuries to the intracranial portion of the auditory nerve. Recording ECoG potentials makes it possible, however, to detect if the blood supply to the cochlea has been compromised. Blood supply compromise can also be detected by methods that are useful in monitoring nerve conduction in the intracranial portion of the auditory nerve such as recording from the intracranial portion of CN VIII, the cochlear nucleus, or the ABR where peak I is an indicator of the function of the ear (**Fig. 7.18**).

Recording CAP Directly from the Exposed Eighth Cranial Nerve

The ABR of patients with vestibular schwannoma often have small amplitudes, which, consequently, makes obtaining an interpretable record a time-consuming activity. This makes it important to be able to record CAP from the auditory nerve or the response from the cochlear nucleus because both have large amplitudes and are not easily contaminated by EMG activity. The CAP can be observed after only a few responses.

It is relatively easy to place a recording electrode on the proximal portion of the eighth nerve in operations on small vestibular schwannoma when there is a segment of the eighth nerve near the brainstem that is free of tumor (4–7). Click-evoked CAP from the eighth nerve can provide a prompt indication of injury to the auditory nerve thereby aiding in the preservation of hearing. The situation is even more apparent in operations on larger tumors where the tumor has reached the brainstem. In such operations, it is not possible to place an electrode on the proximal portion of the eighth nerve, at least not until some of the tumor has first been removed (because the eighth nerve in such cases is embedded in the tumor or is underneath it).

Recording from the Vicinity of the Cochlear Nucleus

Recording from the vicinity of the cochlear nucleus can to a great extent solve these practical problems as described above (page 135). An electrode can be placed in the lateral recess of the fourth ventricle even when operating on large vestibular schwannoma (see **Fig. 7.10**). More importantly, an electrode placed in or near the foramen of Luschka is far away from the operative field, and the electrode is not as easily dislodged as may be the case when it is placed on CN VIII. This technique is an effective way of monitoring neural conduction in the auditory nerve.

Effect of Drilling of Bone

There are three ways that drilling of the bone for exposing the content of the internal auditory meatus in operations such as those for vestibular schwannoma can affect the ABR or the potentials recorded from the auditory nerve or the cochlear nucleus.

1. The response may decrease or even disappear totally because the bone-conducted noise masks the sounds used to elicit the auditory evoked potentials. This noise is transmitted to the cochlea through vibrations in the skull bone (bone conduction) rather than via the normal route for airborne sound (through the middle ear). Although sealing the ear canal reduces the airborne noise that reaches the tympanic membrane, it does not reduce the noise from drilling that reaches the cochlea through bone conduction. In fact, a closed ear canal may enhance the transmission of bone-conducted sound to the cochlea, although this effect is slight. In any event, the stimulation of the cochlea from the noise produced by drilling is usually so strong that it is impossible to record auditory evoked potentials during drilling.

2. Intensive drilling of the internal auditory meatus may cause impairment of the function of the cochlea that may in turn cause a temporary (or permanent) threshold shift

because the drilling noise overloads the cochlea. This may cause alterations in the ABR, and other auditory evoked potentials may be affected for some time after termination of the drilling or permanently.

3. The drilling may heat the bone, and that heat may be transmitted to the auditory nerve in the internal auditory meatus where it may cause temporary or permanent injury to the auditory nerve. This damage is revealed in changes in ABR, CAP recorded from the cochlear nucleus, as well as in the CAP recorded from the exposed auditory nerve. It is, therefore, important to monitor auditory evoked potentials during pauses in the drilling.

FACTORS OTHER THAN SURGICAL MANIPULATION THAT MAY INFLUENCE AUDITORY EVOKED POTENTIALS

Monitoring of ABR and CAP from CN VIII or the cochlear nucleus is affected by the conditions of the ear and the auditory nervous system of individual patients before the operation. Prior operations affecting the same structures, such as CN VIII, and the patient's general health condition can affect the recorded evoked potentials. The presence of other disorders, such as cardiovascular disorders, can also affect auditory evoked potentials.

Effects of Preoperative Hearing Loss on ABR and CAP from the Auditory Nerve

The presence of preoperative hearing loss may affect click-evoked ABR as well as the CAP that can be recorded from the exposed CN VIII or the vicinity of the cochlear nucleus. The effect depends on the degree and type of hearing loss. Hearing loss that is caused by an impairment of conduction of sound to the cochlea (affecting the ear canal, ear drum, middle ear) (30) affects the ABR and CAP from the auditory nerve and the cochlear nucleus in a similar way as does a decrease in the intensity of the stimulus sound. Different forms of con-

ductive hearing loss may affect sound transmission for different frequencies differently and may, thereby, affect the recorded responses dissimilarly. Evoked responses from the auditory nervous system to broad spectrum sounds, such as click sounds, may, therefore, differ between a person with hearing loss and a person with normal hearing, even when the stimulus intensity has been elevated to compensate for the loss in sound transmission to the cochlea.

The high-frequency spectral components of broadband sounds (such as click sounds) are most important for eliciting auditory evoked responses. Low-frequency hearing loss of the conductive type may, therefore, not affect the ABR noticeably, and individuals with such hearing loss may have ABR that are similar to those of individuals with normal hearing. The intensity of the click sound that is used to elicit ABR intraoperatively in a patient with conductive hearing loss should, therefore, only be increased if the hearing loss includes the high-frequency range of hearing (above 4 kHz). If a true conductive hearing loss involves the high-frequency range of hearing, the stimulus sound level can be increased by an amount equal to the conductive hearing loss for high frequencies (4–8 kHz) in order to obtain an interpretable ABR recording. It is, however, unusual that conductive hearing loss extends to the high-frequency range of hearing.

A moderate sensorineural hearing loss caused by cochlear deficits has minimal effects on the ABR. Sensorineural hearing loss often occurs in elderly individuals (presbycusis), but may also be present in younger individuals and is often caused by noise exposure (NIHL) or administration of ototoxic drugs, such as aminoglycoside antibiotics. These factors all affect auditory sensitivity to sounds of higher frequencies more than they affect sounds of lower frequencies. Cochlear hearing loss is caused by the loss of outer hair cells, primarily, in the basal portion of the cochlea and thus, mostly affecting high-frequency hearing. More important perhaps is the fact that the loss of outer hair cells affects the cochlear amplifier, which is most important for sounds of low intensity, but the loss usually does not affect cochlear function noticeably at the high sound levels used for recording auditory evoked potentials (*30*). While hearing loss of cochlear origin can affect the waveform of ABR, there is no reason to increase the stimulus intensity used to elicit auditory evoked potentials in patients who have a cochlear type of hearing loss.

Such hearing loss may also affect the CAP recorded from the exposed CN VIII to an extent that depends on the severity of the hearing loss (see **Fig. 7.9**). The CAP that are recorded from patients with such hearing loss often has a more complex waveform than in individuals with normal hearing with several peaks (*44, 45*).

In the extreme situation in which a disorder of the ear or of the auditory nervous system is so severe that it is not possible to obtain an interpretable ABR recording from the patient before the operation; it is not possible to perform intraoperative monitoring of auditory evoked potentials. If the person in charge of monitoring did not know before the operation that such a patient had a severe hearing loss, a tedious search for technical causes for the failure to obtain reproducible ABR in the operating room would ensue. On the other hand, if the patient had reproducible ABR preoperatively, but it is not possible to obtain a response in the operating room, then it is obvious that the cause of the failure to obtain reproducible ABR in the operating room is a technical problem that must be solved before the operation can begin.

Previous Injuries to CN VIII

The ABR recorded from people with hearing losses caused by injury to the auditory nerve may have complex abnormalities, including increased interpeak latencies, and the waveforms of the recorded potentials are different from those that are seen in patients with normal hearing. Injury to the auditory nerve is typically present before the operation in patients with vestibular schwannoma and in patients who have undergone previous surgical operations in which injury to the auditory nerve has occurred. Such conditions affect the ABR in a different way than do lesions to the cochlea. Injuries to

the auditory nerve typically result in ABR with low amplitudes and complex waveforms. The CAP recorded from the exposed CN VIII in patients with an injured auditory nerve is likely to have complex waveforms (**Fig. 7.9**).

Slight injury to the auditory nerve may decrease the temporal coherence of discharges in different nerve fibers because the conduction velocity in different fibers may be affected differently as a result of such injury. The complex waveform and low amplitude of the CAP in patients with an injured auditory nerve is a result of a difference in the conduction velocity of the nerve fibers that make up the auditory nerve.

RELATIONSHIP BETWEEN AUDITORY EVOKED POTENTIALS AND HEARING ACUITY

It is important to remember that changes in auditory evoked potentials do not measure changes in hearing. The effects on hearing thresholds from injuries to the auditory nerve can, therefore, *not* be predicted directly on the basis of knowledge about the changes in the CAP recorded from the auditory nerve in response to loud click sounds, as is commonly the case for eliciting the response in the operating room. The ability to understand speech, which is more important than the hearing threshold, is even more difficult to predict on the basis of evoked potentials. While there is a correlation between hearing threshold (audiogram) and speech discrimination scores when the hearing loss is caused by damage to the sensory cells in the cochlea, such a relationship does not exist for damage to the auditory nerve.

Individuals in whom the intracranial portion of the auditory nerve has sustained surgically induced injury often have severely impaired speech discrimination, with only a moderate reduction in hearing threshold, as revealed by pure tone audiograms (**Fig. 7.20**). This is probably because injuries to the auditory nerve impair the timing of auditory nerve activity and synchronization of neural activity

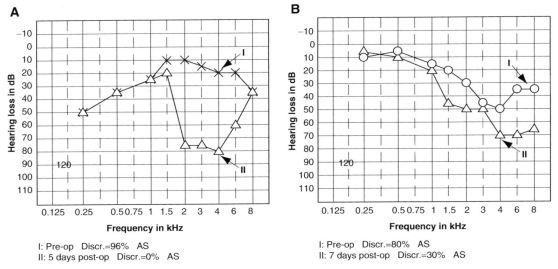

Figure 7.20: Pure tone audiograms obtained before and after operations where the auditory nerve had been manipulated illustrating the effect on the tone threshold and speech discrimination from iatrogenic injury to the auditory nerve. (**A**) Audiograms obtained before (I) and 5 days after (II) an operation in the cerebellopontine angle where the eighth cranial nerve was manipulated. The speech discrimination decreased from 96% before the operation to 0% after the operation. (**B**) Similar data as in (**A**), obtained in another patient who had large changes in speech discrimination with relatively small changes in the pure tone audiogram. I: Preoperative audiogram, II: audiogram obtained 7 days after an operation in the cerebellopontine angle where the eighth cranial nerve was manipulated. The speech discrimination decreased from 80% to 30% after the operation.

in the auditory nerve is important for speech discriminations, but has less effect on pure tone thresholds reflected in the audiogram. Individuals who have suffered injuries to their auditory nerve often have severe tinnitus, which causes a severe reduction of the quality of life. After injury to the auditory nerve, it is not known if deterioration of the earliest peaks of the ABR with a preservation of peak V means that the patient's ability to understand speech will be impaired, or if also peak V must be noticeably affected before a functional change in hearing may occur.

Even though changes in neural conduction that occur during manipulation of the auditory nerve (as revealed by changes in the CAP recorded from the exposed auditory nerve) may have been totally reversed, the auditory nerve

may still have suffered some injury. Thus, studies in animals indicate that the injury that is caused by a partial dislocation of the transition zone between the peripheral and central myelin of the auditory nerve (Obersteiner–Redlich zone, or O–R zone) (46–48) may be reversible, but still may imply permanent injury. This may impair speech discrimination without causing any noticeable abnormality in auditory evoked potentials and without noticeable change in hearing, thresholds as reflected in the audiogram.

Injuries to the auditory nerve from surgical manipulations often produce a greater loss in speech discrimination than would have been inferred from the threshold elevation to pure tones, (pure tone audiograms) (**Fig. 7.20** (*3, 30*)). The likely reason is that slight injuries to the auditory nerve may cause reduced temporal coherence of neural firing in auditory nerve fibers without affecting the threshold to pure tones (thus having a normal pure tone audiogram). Deterioration of the timing of neural discharges, which may occur from injury to the auditory nerve, is known to affect the ability to discriminate speech.

The effects of injuries to the auditory nerve on everyday use of hearing (such as for speech communication) are not well described by the pure tone audiogram because injury to the auditory nerve is likely to cause a considerable decrease in the speech discrimination score even when the pure tone threshold is only slightly affected as indicated by the conventional audiogram (30, 49). Since speech discrimination can deteriorate to a considerable degree with little or only moderate changes of the pure tone audiogram (30, 48), the pure tone audiogram alone is not a suitable measure of (functional) hearing loss in patients whose CN VIII has been injured; speech discrimination tests should instead be used to evaluate injuries to the auditory nerve (49).

OTHER ADVANTAGES OF RECORDING AUDITORY EVOKED POTENTIALS INTRAOPERATIVELY

Studies of the changes in auditory evoked potentials have provided information that have resulted in the development of better surgical methods, which are important for the surgeon performing the surgical procedure and for the individual patient in whom monitoring was performed. Thus, there are advantages from recording of CAP directly from the auditory nerve other than for reducing the risk of hearing loss in the individual patient. Recordings of CAP directly from the exposed eighth nerve or the vicinity of the cochlear nucleus during operations in the CPA have not only been valuable in reducing injuries due to surgical manipulations in individual patients, but they have also contributed to our understanding of how injuries to nerves from surgical manipulations

may come about. The ability to detect changes in neural conduction, almost instantaneously, has made it possible to detect such changes early enough to be able to identify exactly which step in an operation caused an adverse effect on neural conduction. For example, this technique has made it possible to relate the effects to specific surgical events, such as electrocoagulation to injury of the auditory nerve, because recording of the CAP from the auditory nerve or the cochlear nucleus has made it possible to determine exactly which step in an operation caused a change in function of the auditory nerve. Such observation showed that the risk that a nerve can be damaged by the heat used in electrocoagulation of blood vessels is greater than earlier believed. Such studies would not have been possible using recordings of ABR because of the time it takes to obtain an interpretable record.

Experience has demonstrated that the auditory nerve can be seriously injured by the normal use of bipolar electrocoagulation when performed close to the auditory portion of CN VIII. The adverse effect on the auditory nerve is not caused by a spread of high-frequency current (which was a serious problem when monopolar coagulation was used), but rather by the spread of heat. Since all electrocoagulation is based on heating the tissue in question (usually a vein), such heat may spread to neural tissue located close to the site that is undergoing coagulation. Electrocoagulation using the bipolar technique may, thus, injure neural tissue from the spread of heat used to coagulate nearby tissue, even though the spread of high-frequency current may be negligible.

These findings have prompted a change in the way electrocoagulation is performed near the eighth nerve, namely, to use the lowest possible current, to do electrocoagulation in bursts of only a few seconds duration and to allow time for the tissue to cool between periods of electrocoagulation. These changes in the way blood vessels are coagulated have reduced the risks of injury to neural tissue from electrocoagulation in general.

Recordings of CAP have also provided information on how the auditory nerve may be injured by stretching, and how the nerve is highly sensitive to heat (from electrocoagulation).

Recording of the CAP from the auditory nerve has also shown that there are considerable differences in individual susceptibility to mechanical manipulation of the auditory nerve. In operations in the CPA using the retromastoid approach, manipulations of the eighth nerve may occur, for instance, when the cerebellum is retracted. It has been indicated in earlier studies that medial-to-lateral retraction (*50, 51*) places the eighth nerve at greater risk than does retraction in a caudal-to-rostral direction. This hypothesis has been confirmed by studies of CAP recordings from the auditory nerve (*2*).

Animal experiments have helped to understand how certain surgical manipulations can cause injury to the auditory nerve, and it has been shown that injuries are likely to occur where the auditory nerve passes through the cribriform plate (*46, 47, 52*).

Experience from intraoperative monitoring has also shown that the arachnoid membrane that covers CN VIII may be stretched by retracting the cerebellum and thereby, stretch the eighth nerve. It was found that changes in auditory evoked potentials that occur during MVD operations can be reduced by opening the arachnoid membrane widely as soon as possible after it has been exposed (Jho and Møller, unpublished observation 1990) even in operations in which only CN V must be exposed in order to carry out the operation. The reason that it is beneficial to make a large opening in the arachnoid membrane is probably that tensions along the edge of the opening are reduced. It is also possible that the arachnoidal membrane that is connected to CN VIII can stretch the auditory nerve when, for example, the cerebellum is retracted.

These are examples of how intraoperative neurophysiological monitoring can promote the development of surgical methods that are more effective and have less risk.

Recording of ABR can also be useful for other purposes than monitoring the auditory system. The use of recordings of ABR has been shown to be of value for detecting brainstem manipulations that affect control of blood pressure and heart rate (Chap. 11, **Figs. 11.9 and 11.10**).

Furthermore, recordings of auditory evoked potentials have provided important basic information about the function of the normal auditory system and about some pathological conditions such as tinnitus.

ANESTHESIA REQUIREMENTS

Although slight changes in ABR have been reported as a result of the administration of certain anesthetic agents (*53, 54*), the ABR are remarkably insensitive to anesthesia. The type of anesthesia can be chosen without any consideration as to whether or not ABR are to be monitored. However, it has been noted that the patient's body temperature has a significant effect on the latency of ABR. When the body temperature drops below 35.0°C, there is a noticeable increase in the latency of the peaks of the ABR (*55*). This should be remembered when interpreting slow changes in ABR.

REFERENCES

1. Grundy B (1983) Intraoperative monitoring of sensory evoked potentials. Anesthesiology 58:72–87.
2. Møller AR and PJ Jannetta (1983) Monitoring auditory functions during cranial nerve microvascular decompression operations by direct recording from the eighth nerve. J. Neurosurg. 59:493–9.
3. Møller AR and MB Møller (1989) Does intraoperative monitoring of auditory evoked potentials reduce incidence of hearing loss as a complication of microvascular decompression of cranial nerves? Neurosurgery 24:257–63.
4. Colletti V, A Bricolo, FG Fiorino et al (1994) Changes in directly recorded cochlear nerve compound action potentials during acoustic tumor surgery. Skull Base Surg. 4:1–9.

5. Silverstein H, H Norrell and S Hyman (1984) Simultaneous use of CO2 laser with continuous monitoring of eighth cranial nerve action potential during acoustic neuroma surgery. Otolaryngol. Head Neck Surg. 92:80–4.

6. Fischer C (1989) Brainstem auditory evoked potential (BAEP) monitoring in posterior fossa surgery, in *Neuromonitoring in Surgery*, J Desmedt Editor. Elsevier Science Publishers: Amsterdam. 191–218.

7. Linden R, C Tator, C Benedict et al (1988) Electro-physiological monitoring during acoutic neuroma and other posterior fossa surgery. J. Sci. Neurol. 15:73–81.

8. Kuroki A and AR Møller (1995) Microsurgical anatomy around the foramen of Luschka with reference to intraoperative recording of auditory evoked potentials from the cochlear nuclei. J. Neurosurg. 82:933–9.

9. Møller AR, HD Jho and PJ Jannetta (1994) Preservation of hearing in operations on acoustic tumors: An alternative to recording BAEP. Neurosurgery 34:688–93.

10. Raudzens PA (1982) Intraoperative monitoring of evoked potentials. Ann. N.Y. Acad. Sci. 388:308–26.

11. Møller AR and PJ Jannetta (1983) Auditory evoked potentials recorded from the cochlear nucleus and its vicinity in man. J. Neurosurg. 59:1013–8.

12. Møller AR, PJ Jannetta and HD Jho (1994) Click-evoked responses from the cochlear nucleus: A study in human. Electroencephalogr. Clin. Neurophysiol. 92:215–24.

13. Sekiya T, T Iwabuchi, T Hatayama et al (1991) Vestibular nerve injury as a complication of microvascular decompression. Neurosurgery 29:773–5.

14. Levine RA, WW Montgomery, RG Ojemann et al (1978) Evoked potential detection of hearing loss during acoustic neuroma surgery. Neurology 28:339.

15. Levine RA, RG Ojemann, WW Montgomery et al (1984) Monitoring auditory evoked potentials during acoustic neuroma surgery. Ann. Otol. Rhinol. Laryngol. 93:116–23.

16. Sekhar LN and AR Møller (1986) Operative management of tumors involving the cavernous sinus. J. Neurosurg. 64:879–89.

17. Møller AR (1987) Electrophysiological monitoring of cranial nerves in operations in the skull base, in *Tumors of the Cranial Base: Diagnosis and Treatment*, LN Sekhar and VL Schramm Jr,

Editors. Futura Publishing Co: Mt. Kisco, New York. 123–32.

18. Hatayama T and AR Møller (1998) Correlation between latency and amplitude of peak V in brainstem auditory evoked potentials: Intraoperative recordings in microvascular decompression operations. Acta Neurochir. (Wien) 140:681–7.

19. Chiappa K, KG Gladstone and RR Young (1979) Brainstem evoked responses: Studies of waveform variations in 50 normal human subjects. Arch. Neurol. 36:81–6.

20. Campbell KCM and PJ Abbas (1987) The effect of stimulus repetition rate on the auditory brainstem response in tumor and non-tumor patients. J. Speech Hear. Res. 30:494–502.

21. Pratt H and H Sohmer (1976) Intensity and rate functions of cochlear and brainstem evoked responses to click stimuli in man. Arch. Otol. Rhinol. Laryngol. 212:85–92.

22. Møller AR (1986) Effect of click spectrum and polarity on round window N_1N_2 response in the rat. Audiology 25:29–43.

23. Scherg M and D von Cramon (1985) A new interpretation of the generators of BAEP waves I V: Results of a spatio temporal dipole. Electroencephalogr. Clin. Neurophysiol. 62:290–9.

24. Jewett DL (1987) The 3 channel Lissajous' trajectory of the auditory brain stem response. IX. Theoretical aspects. Electroencephalogr. Clin. Neurophysiol. 68:386–408.

25. Gardi JN, YS Sininger, WH Martin et al (1987) The 3-channel Lissajous' trajectory of the auditory brain-stem response. IV. Effect of lesions in the cat. Electroencephalogr. Clin. Neurophysiol. 68:360–7.

26. Pratt H, Z Har'el and E Golos (1984) Geometrical analysis of human three-channel Lissajous' trajectory of auditory brain stem evoked potentials. Electroencephalogr. Clin. Neurophysiol. 58:83–8.

27. Pratt H, N Bleich and WH Martin (1985) Three channel Lissajous' trajectory of humans auditory brain stem evoked potentials. I. Normative measures. Electroencephalogr. Clin. Neurophysiol. 61:530–8.

28. Møller AR (1988) *Evoked Potentials in Intraoperative Monitoring*. Williams and Wilkins: Baltimore.

29. Møller AR (1988) Use of zero-phase digital filters to enhance brainstem auditory evoked

potentials (BAEPs). Electroencephalogr. Clin. Neurophysiol. 71:226–32.

30. Møller AR (2006) *Hearing: Anatomy, Physiology, and Disorders of the Auditory System*, 2nd Ed., Academic Press: Amsterdam.

31. Møller AR and PJ Jannetta (1981) Compound action potentials recorded intracranially from the auditory nerve in man. Exp. Neurol. 74:862–74.

32. Hashimoto I, Y Ishiyama, T Yoshimoto et al (1981) Brainstem auditory evoked potentials recorded directly from human brain stem and thalamus. Brain 104:841–59.

33. Hashimoto I (1982) Auditory evoked potentials recorded directly from the human VIIIth nerve and brain stem: Origins of their fast and slow components. Electroencephalogr. Clin. Neurophysiol. Suppl. 36:305–14.

34. Hashimoto I (1982) Auditory evoked potentials from the humans midbrain: Slow brain stem responses. Electroencephalogr. Clin. Neurophysiol. 53:652–7.

35. Møller AR, PJ Jannetta and MB Møller (1981) Neural generators of brainstem evoked potentials. Results from human intracranial recordings. Ann. Otol. Rhinol. Laryngol. 90:591–6.

36. Møller AR and PJ Jannetta (1982) Evoked potentials from the inferior colliculus in man. Electroencephalogr. Clin. Neurophysiol. 53:612–20.

37. Spire JP, GJ Dohrmann and PS Prieto (1982) *Correlation Of Brainstem Evoked Response with Direct Acoustic Nerve Potential*, J Courjon, F Manguiere and M Reval, Editors. Vol. 32. Raven Press: New York.

38. Møller AR (1993) Direct eighth nerve compound action potential measurements during cerebellopontine angle surgery, in *Proceedings of the First International Conference on ECoG, OAE, and Intraoperative Monitoring*, D Höhmann, Editor. Kugler Publication: Amsterdam, The Netherlands. 275–80.

39. Møller AR and PJ Jannetta (1982) Auditory evoked potentials recorded intracranially from the brainstem in man. Exp. Neurol. 78:144–57.

40. Terr LI and BJ Edgerton (1985) Surface topography of the cochlear nuclei in humans: Two and three-dimensional analysis. Hear. Res. 17:51–9.

41. Hatayama T, T Sekiya, S Suzuki et al (1999) Effect of compression on the cochlear nerve: A short- and long-term electrophysiological and histological study. Neurol. Res. 21:591–610.

42. Ojemann RG, RA Levine, WM Montgomery et al (1984) Use of intraoperative auditory evoked potentials to preserve hearing in unilateral acoustic neuroma removal. J. Neurosurg. 61:938–48.

43. Winzenburg SM, RH Margolis, SC Levine et al (1993) Tympanic and transtympanic electrocochleography in acoustic neuroma and vestibular nerve section surgery. Am. J. Otol. 14:63–9.

44. Møller AR and HD Jho (1991) Effect of high frequency hearing loss on compound action potentials recorded from the intracranial portion of the human eighth nerve. Hear. Res. 55:9–23.

45. Møller AR and HD Jho (1991) Compound action potentials recorded from the intracranial portion of the auditory nerve in man: Effects of stimulus intensity and polarity. Audiology 30:142–63.

46. Sekiya T and AR Møller (1987) Avulsion rupture of the internal auditory artery during operations in the cerebellopontine angle: A study in monkeys. Neurosurgery 21:631–7.

47. Sekiya T and AR Møller (1987) Cochlear nerve injuries caused by cerebellopontine angle manipulations. An electrophysiological and morphological study in dogs. J. Neurosurg. 67:244–9.

48. Møller AR (2006) *Neural Plasticity and Disorders of the Nervous System*. Cambridge: Cambridge University Press

49. Møller AR (1993) Late waves in the response recorded from the intracranial portion of the auditory nerve in humans. Ann. Otol. Rhinol. Laryngol. 102:945–53.

50. Gardner WJ (1962) Concerning the mechanism of trigeminal neuralgia and hemifacial spasm. J. Neurosurg. 19:947–58.

51. Jannetta P, (1981) Hemifacial spasm, in *The Cranial Nerves*, M Samii and P Jannetta, Editors. Springer: Heidelberg, West Germany. 484–93.

52. Møller AR and T Sekiya (1988) Injuries to the auditory nerve: A study in monkeys. Electroencephalogr. Clin. Neurophysiol. 70:248–55.

53. Cohen MS and RH Britt (1982) Effects of sodium pentobarbital, ketamine, halothane, and chloralose on brain stem auditory evoked responses. Anesth. Analg. 61:338–43.

54. Thornton C, DM Catley, C Jorden et al (1981) Enflurane increases the latency of early components of the auditory evoked response in man. Br. J. Anaesth. 53:1102–3.

55. Stockard JJ, F Sharbrough and J Tinker (1978) Effects of hypothermia on the human brain stem auditory response. Ann. Neurol. 3:368–70.
56. Martin WH, H Pratt and JW Schwegler (1995) The origin of the human auditory brainstem response wave II. Electroencephalogr. Clin. Neurophysiol. 96:357–70.
57. Lang J (1985) Anatomy of the brainstem and the lower cranial nerves, vessels, and surrounding structures. Am. J. Otol. Suppl, Nov:1–19.
58. Silverstein H, H Norrell, T Haberkamp et al (1986) The unrecognized rotation of the vestibular and cochlear nerves from the labyrinth to the brain stem: Its implications to surgery of the eighth cranial nerve. Otolaryngol. Head Neck Surg. 95:543–9.
59. Møller AR (1994) Monitoring techniques in cavernous sinus surgery, in *Monitoring Techniques in Neurosurgery, Chap. 15*, CM Loftus and VC Traynelis, Editors. McGraw-Hill, Inc: New York. 141–55.

8

Monitoring Visual Evoked Potentials

Introduction
VEP as Indicator of Manipulation of the Optic Nerve and Optic Tract
Techniques for Recording VEP
Anesthesia Requirements for Visual Evoked Potentials

INTRODUCTION

Intraoperative monitoring of visual evoked potentials (VEP) during neurosurgical operations has been described by several investigators (1–5) for the purpose of preserving vision in operations in which the optic nerve or optic tract is being manipulated as well as in operations that involved the occipital cerebral cortex (6). It has been found difficult, however, to obtain reliable recordings of VEP in anesthetized patients who did not undergo intracranial procedures (7).

VEP AS INDICATOR OF MANIPULATION OF THE OPTIC NERVE AND OPTIC TRACT

Reports have, in general, been discouraging on the use of monitoring of VEP for detecting injuries that could develop into postoperative visual deficits (2, 3). The results are much less clear than those obtained using other sensory modalities, and all investigators have reported both false-positive (intraoperative changes in the VEP, but no postoperative deficits) and false-negative (no change in the

From: *Intraoperative Neurophysiological Monitoring: Third Edition*,
By A.R. Møller, DOI 10.1007/978-1-4419-7436-5_8,
© Springer Science+Business Media, LLC 2011

VEP intraoperatively, but postoperative deficits) results. One investigator (4) recorded several instances of convincing VEP changes during surgical manipulation of the optic chiasm and during episodes of hypotension, but without any postoperative evidence of pathology. However, although the results were generally difficult to interpret, Raudzens (4) found that when VEP remained unchanged throughout the operation there was no deterioration of vision as a result of the operation. Nevertheless, he also reported that patients with visual defects preoperatively could have normal VEP intraoperatively, so that the true value of monitoring VEP to identify intraoperative damage remains questionable. These studies were made using light-emitting diodes (LED) mounted in an eye patch (goggles), with red light flashes reaching the patient's eyes through closed eyelids.

Another group of investigators (3) found that the value of intraoperative monitoring of VEP for the purpose of preserving neural function of the visual system that is important to practical vision is small. This observation is in agreement with this author's own experience. The introduction of high-intensity flashes (8) as stimuli for monitoring VEP intraoperatively seems to have increased the reproducibility of such evoked potentials. The use of high-intensity light-emitting diodes mounted in goggles that deliver flash stimuli for evoking visual evoked potentials (8) may solve the problem of adequate stimulation in anesthetized patients, but more studies are needed before a conclusion can be realized. More recently, monitoring of VEP has been used in operations that involved the occipital cortex for treating epilepsy (6). These investigators, using strobe light to elicit the VEP, found such monitoring useful in preserving central vision.

It has been difficult to determine whether recording of evoked potentials directly from the optic nerve (5) has any advantages over the use of VEP recorded from the scalp, except for the probable lesser susceptibility of such subcortical responses to suppression from the use of inhalation anesthetics. This method of recording directly from the optic nerve or optic tract, however, does not seem to have advantages over recording of VEP from electrodes placed on the scalp with regard to being able to signal when manipulations of the optic nerve or tract may be causing injuries that will result in a postoperative neurological deficit (impaired vision). Again, the reason for this does not seem to be the way the VEP are recorded, but it may be that the stimuli used to evoke the response are inadequate. The poor correlation between flash-evoked VEP and visual deficits is in agreement with experience in using VEP for clinical diagnosis. Thus, it has been shown that flash-evoked VEP are much less specific in detecting neurological deficits of the visual system than are VEP elicited by a reversing checkerboard pattern (9). The reason for this is that the time pattern of light stimuli is not "important" to the visual system, compared to changes in contrast, and, therefore, VEP elicited by a reversing checkerboard pattern show more important deficits than do VEP elicited by repetitive flashes. Clearly, techniques utilizing VEP for preserving vision in operations near the optic nerve and the optic tract must be much more highly developed before they can be considered practical for intraoperative use. Additionally, it seems necessary to be able to focus some kind of a pattern on the retina of

patients if intraoperative monitoring of VEP is to be useful in detecting injuries that are important to vision. The introduction of high-intensity light flashes as stimuli may offer a solution to these problems (8). Despite these shortcomings, VEP are indeed used in intraoperative monitoring in some kinds of operations.

Techniques for Recording VEP

VEP that are recorded intraoperatively are generally recorded using electrodes placed on the scalp at C_z and O_z locations. The analog filters in the amplifiers are typically set to cut off frequencies of 5 and 500 Hz for the high-pass and low-pass filters, respectively. The flash stimuli are generated by a stroboscope type of flash generator or by light-emitting diodes that are bonded to a contact lens (5).

Light-emitting diodes that are bonded to contact lenses and placed on the eye of the patient (5, 10) have a low risk of injuring the cornea when contact lenses that are designed for protection of the eye are used, but great care must be taken to avoid injuring the cornea when the contact lenses are placed on the eyes. Techniques of VEP intraoperative monitoring using light-emitting diodes that are placed in a goggle type of arrangement have also been described. The red light stimuli are transmitted through the closed eyelids of the patient. Although the intensity of the light that reaches the eye may be adequate to elicit an interpretable response, it may not be optimal to use red light for intraoperative monitoring during long operations, since it is likely to be the only light that reaches the patient's eye during the operation, and, therefore, the patient's eyes may become dark-adapted during the operation (11). This adaptation will change the response gradually, which may be interpreted as a pathologic change. Thus, it may be better to use green light, which will not produce such an evident adaptation effect. Light stimulators that utilize high-intensity, light-emitting diodes mounted in goggles (8) may avoid these problems.

ANESTHESIA REQUIREMENTS FOR VISUAL EVOKED POTENTIALS

Any recording of evoked potentials that rely on cortical responses is altered significantly by the use of inhalation anesthesia. This must be considered when using VEP recorded from scalp electrodes for intraoperative monitoring and is similarly evidenced for other cortical responses such as somatosensory evoked potentials (SSEP). In a recent study, the use of TIVA did not seem to increase the reliability of monitoring of VEP (7), and stable recordings were difficult to obtain. It is not known to what extent short-latency VEP, such as near-field potentials that can be recorded from the optic nerve or optic tract, are affected by inhalation anesthesia.

REFERENCES

1. Wilson WB, WM Kirsch, H Neville et al (1976) Monitoring of visual function during parasellar surger. Surg Neurol 5:323–9.
2. Cedzich C, J Schramm and R Fahlbusch (1987) Are flash-evoked visual potentials useful for intraoperative monitoring of visual pathway function? Neurosurgery 21:709–15.
3. Cedzich C, J Schramm, CF Mengedoht et al (1988) Factors that limit the use of flash visual evoked potentials for surgical monitoring. Electroencephalogr Clin Neurophysiol 71:142–5.
4. Raudzens PA (1982) Intraoperative monitoring of evoked potentials. Ann N Y Acad Sci 388:308–26.
5. Møller AR (1987) Electrophysiological monitoring of cranial nerves in operations in the skull base, in *Tumors of the Cranial Base: Diagnosis and Treatment*, LN Sekhar and VL Schramm Jr, Editors. Futura Publishing Co: Mt. Kisco, New York. 123–32.
6. Curatolo JM, RA Macdonell, SF Berkovic et al (2000) Intraoperative monitoring to preserve central visual fields during occipital corticectomy for epilepsy. J Clin Neurosci 7:234–7.
7. Wiedemayer H, B Fauser, W Armbruster et al (2003) Visual evoked potentials for intraoperative neurophysiologic monitoring using total intravenous anesthesia. J Neurosurg Anesthesiol 15:19–24.
8. Pratt H, WH Martin, N Bleich et al (1994) A high-intensity, goggle-mounted flash stimulator for short-latency visual evoked potentials. Electroencephalogr Clin Neurophysiol 92:469–72.
9. Chiappa K (1997) *Evoked Potentials in Clinical Medicine*, 3rd ed. Lippincott-Raven: Philadelphia.
10. Sekhar LN and AR Møller (1986) Operative management of tumors involving the cavernous sinus. J Neurosurg 64:879–89.
11. Møller AR (2003) *Sensory Systems: Anatomy and Physiology*. Academic Press: Amsterdam.

MOTOR SYSTEMS

Loss of spinal motor function, either total or partial, always has severe consequences, as does loss or impairments of the function of the cranial motor systems. The risk of neural function loss can be significantly reduced with the use of intraoperative neurophysiological monitoring and development of better surgical methods. Monitoring of spinal and cranial motor systems has proven to be very effective in reducing the risks of motor deficits in many different kinds of operations, and it is an important part of intraoperative neurophysiological monitoring in general.

Surgical operations on the bony structures of the spine are corrective operations for congenital malformations, such as scoliosis and kyphosis, and operations necessitated by age-related changes or trauma. Most of the surgical operations on the spinal cord are for tumors of various kinds. Some disorders such as arteriovenous malformations (AVM) and arteriovenous fistula (AVF) are rare congenital abnormalities that may benefit from surgical treatment. Intraoperative neurophysiological monitoring is very important in such operations, and its introduction has reduced the complications considerably.

Operations to treat vertebral disks and constrictions of spinal foramina (spinal stenosis) that occur as a result of age-related changes are common, but in many cases, these operations provide questionable benefit to the patients. These kinds of operations are often carried out without the aid of intraoperative neurophysiological monitoring.

In order to fully utilize the possibilities that monitoring of spinal motor systems offers in reducing the risks of postoperative motor deficits, it is important that the persons who are responsible for such monitoring understand the basic anatomy and the normal function of the different motor systems as well as individual variations and abnormalities in anatomy and physiology.

Therefore, this section includes a detailed description of the anatomy and physiology of the cerebral cortex, basal ganglia, the thalamus, and other deep brain structures (Chap. 9), as well as a discussion of some of the disorders that are treatable by interventions aimed at these structures. The following chapter (Chap. 10) discusses practical aspects of monitoring spinal motor systems.

The cranial motor systems that are discussed in Chap. 11 differ in many ways from the spinal motor system, but intraoperative neurophysiological monitoring can also reduce the risk of many forms of deficits in connection with operations that affect the cranial motor system.

9

Anatomy and Physiology of Motor Systems

(continued)

From: *Intraoperative Neurophysiological Monitoring: Third Edition*
By A.R. Møller, DOI 10.1007/978-1-4419-7436-5_9,
© Springer Science+Business Media, LLC 2011

INTRODUCTION

The anatomy and the physiology of motor systems have been studied extensively in animal experiments. However, the animals used in the 1970s, when large studies of the function of the motor systems were performed, were mainly cats, the motor systems of which have considerable differences from that of humans. Even when monkeys were used later for studies of the motor system, it became evident that their motor systems were also different from that of humans. The limited possibilities of studying the neurophysiology of the human motor systems have framed our understanding of the human motor systems.

Although studies in the operating room, beginning as early as the 1930s with Penfield's systematic studies of the human motor cortex during neurosurgical operations (1), have contributed valuable information about the human motor system, it was not until much more recently that the implications of the differences between the cat's motor system and that in humans became evident. The anatomical basis for the two main parts of the motor system, the lateral system (corticospinal and rubrospinal systems) and the medial system (reticulospinal, vestibulospinal, and tectospinal systems), was described many years ago by the Dutch anatomist Kuypers (2), but the implications of the differences in the motor system in animals such as the cat and in humans were not completely recognized until much later.

Our current knowledge regarding the function of the basal ganglia is primarily based on

intraoperative studies of recent date. Interaction between the different motor cortical areas and the somatosensory system has also only been explored in recent studies performed in the operating room. Some aspects of the cranial motor systems were not understood until they were studied during neurosurgical operations.

This chapter provides a basic description of the anatomy and functional organization of the cranial and the spinal motor systems, and these systems will be discussed separately. When the information stems from studies in animals, the possible limitations in applying the results to humans will be pointed out.

It is important to keep in mind that motor control depends on feedback from sensors in muscles, tendons, joints, and the skin. Deficits in these unconscious proprioception systems that act as feedback systems have severe consequences for motor control. Although these sensory systems may be regarded as parts of the motor system, they are discussed separately in the chapter on somatosensory systems (Chap. 5) and later in this chapter.

GENERAL ORGANIZATION OF THE SPINAL MOTOR SYSTEMS

The spinal motor system can be divided vertically into upper and lower parts, and these can be divided horizontally into the lateral and medial systems, which are so classified because of the anatomical location of their descending tracts in the spinal cord (2).

Traditionally, the upper motoneuron relates to the motor cortex, but in this chapter, the basal ganglia (including the motor thalamus) and the cerebellum are included in the description of the upper motor system. The alpha motoneuron has traditionally been regarded as the lower motoneuron (the "common final pathway"). In this book, the neural circuitry in the ventral horn of the spinal cord will be included in descriptions of the lower part of the motor system.

Both systems have been divided into upper and lower systems (**Fig. 9.1**).

The lateral system comprises the corticospinal and the rubrospinal system, and activity in these systems controls muscles in distal limbs and allows fine movement control of extremities. The lateral system is also known as the pyramidal system. These descending tracts originate in the primary motor cortex (M1), the supplementary motor area (SMA), and the premotor areas (PMA), and they also have contributions from the primary somatosensory cortex (S1).

The medial system, comprising the reticulospinal, tectospinal, and vestibulospinal

descending pathways, controls proximal limb muscles and trunk muscles, and it is important for basic functions such as posture, walking, etc. The pathways originate in nuclei in the brainstem and in the reticular formation. The medial system is phylogenetically older than the lateral system.

In addition to the two main descending pathways, there is a third descending pathway, the noradrenaline (NA)–serotonin pathway, that belongs to a nonspecific system originating in the raphe nuclei, which project to the spinal cord.

The descending pathways from the motor nuclei in the brainstem (the medial system) terminate on neurons in the spinal cord, either directly or via an interneuron. These systems are important for posture, for many basic movements, and for controlling the excitability of alpha motoneurons, spinal reflexes, and other complex neural circuits in the spinal cord.

In fact, spinal reflexes play an important role in most kinds of movements and they are controlled by the brain. It is, therefore, important to point out that while the motor cortical areas are the sole generators of voluntary motor commands, motor control heavily depends on spinal (and brainstem) reflexes. Some circuits in the brainstem and the spinal cord can generate complex motor commands without input from the motor cortex. An example is the central pattern generator (CPG) that can allow motor behaviors such as walking without programming or central control from the brain, except for initiation and termination of the process.

The normal function of the motor system is dependent on modulation (facilitatory and inhibitory) from structures in the brainstem, such as the reticular formation or vestibular nuclei, which contribute to motor control and especially to the control of posture and balance. It should be noted that the motor systems of the head are different from the spinal motor system.

The gamma motor system is a separate part of the motor system and is different from the alpha motor system, which controls skeletal muscles. The gamma system controls the small muscles that can adjust the length of muscle spindles (the sensors that measure the length of muscles) that

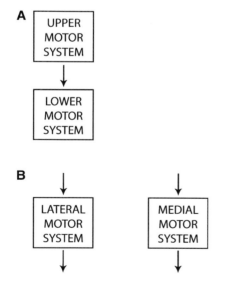

Figure 9.1: Two ways to divide the motor systems. (**A**) Structures that are activated consecutively form the upper and lower motor systems. (**B**) Parallel systems form the lateral and medial motor systems.

are innervated by gamma motor neurons. These muscles are known as the intrafusal muscles, and the skeletal muscles that are innervated by alpha motoneurons are known as the extrafusal muscles. Since intraoperative monitoring does not involve the gamma motor system, it will not be discussed further in this book.

The motor system is very complex and it receives input from many parts of the brain. It is, therefore, an oversimplification to lump the system into a few categories, such as the pyramidal and extrapyramidal systems, and although some textbooks (3) have stated that these terms are confusing, many still use these terms. The term extrapyramidal system was designated for the fiber tract system that does not pass through the pyramids, but for many, the extrapyramidal system is now known as the medial system. The extrapyramidal system was associated with the basal ganglia and brainstem motor nuclei. As we now have a better understanding of the role of the basal ganglia, the terminology pyramidal and extrapyramidal systems has become less relevant. However, the separation is still referred to clinically by neurologists because it characterizes two different groups of symptoms from the motor system.

Extrapyramidal symptoms include, for example, the inability to initiate movements. Disorders that are caused by abnormalities of the basal ganglia, certain brainstem nuclei, and the thalamus are referred to as "extrapyramidal signs" by neurologists.

Pyramidal signs are related to disorders of the corticospinal system, producing a positive Babinski sign[1]. It is often associated with lesions, such as infarcts of internal capsule structures that give rise to hemiplegia.

Motor Cortices

Motor commands are generated by the motor cortices, also known as the upper motor neuron. There are three main cortical areas that contribute to the descending motor systems and provide motor commands, the primary motor area (M1) (Brodmann area 4, see Appendix A), SMA, and PMA (area 6) (SMA is also known as M2, and PMA is known as M3) (**Fig. 9.2**). Four divisions of the PMA are located on the medial wall of each hemisphere, which also includes the SMA that occupies a larger part of Brodmann area 6 (see Appendix A). These cortical areas are located on the frontal side of the central sulcus. Two premotor areas, the ventral premotor area (PMv) and the dorsal premotor area (PMd), are located on the lateral surface of the hemisphere. These premotor areas are extensive and occupy more than 60% of the cortical area in the frontal lobe that projects to the spinal cord (4). Three cingulate motor areas that occupy Brodmann areas 23 and 24 also contribute to motor control. Some cells in the somatosensory cortex (areas 1–3 located on the posterior side of the central sulcus) also contribute to descending motor pathways.

Each of these premotor areas has considerable direct projections to the spinal cord, and motor activity can be elicited by stimulation of these areas without involving the M1 area, but it should be noted that PMA and SMA also have abundant connections to M1. The motor cortices receive input from the prefrontal cortex and many other cortical areas.

Since neurons in these premotor areas project directly to the spinal cord, they can influence generation and control of movement independent of the primary motor cortex. This means that large parts of the corticospinal system originate from the premotor areas, either directly or through M1. This also means that M1 is not the only cortical region known as the "upper motoneuron" that provides central control of movement through the corticospinal system (the lateral system) (4).

There has been a substantial change in the understanding of the cortical motor areas. It is

---

[1]Babinski sign: extension of the great toe and abduction of the other toes instead of the normal flexion reflex to plantar stimulation, considered indicative of corticospinal tract involvement ("positive" Babinski). (Stedman's Electronic Medical Dictionary).

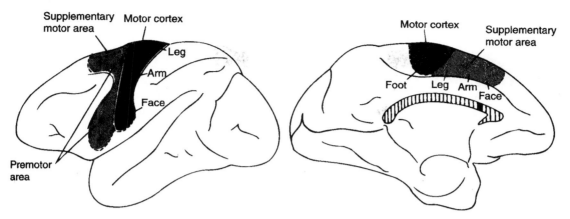

Figure 9.2: Motor, premotor, and supplementary motor cortical areas in the monkey. (Reprinted from (*3*) with the permission from Oxford University Press).

now clear that the frontal lobe of primates contains at least six premotor areas that project directly to the primary motor cortex (M1) (*5*). In addition to their connections to M1, these motor areas send axons to the basal ganglia, to the cranial nerve motor nuclei through the corticobulbar tract, and to alpha motoneurons in the spinal cord through the corticospinal tract. The basal ganglia returns processed motor information to the motor cortices via the thalamus (see page 175).

Anatomically, the main motor cortical areas are different from sensory cortices in that they lack layer 4, which is the main input layer of sensory cortices.

Many individuals who have congenital hemiparesis due to brain lesions acquired before, during, and immediately after birth have abnormalities in their corticospinal projections from the hemisphere that is opposite to the lesion. A study of individuals with such lesions indicates that PMd and M1 have possible roles in complex motor control even in individuals with congenital hemiparesis who control their paretic hands via crossed, corticospinal projections from the damaged hemisphere (*6*).

Somatotopic Organization. All motor cortical areas have their own somatotopic organization; the best-known cortical area is

that of M1 as described by Penfield and his co-workers (*7, 8*), and by Woolsey (*9*) (**Fig. 9.3**).

In general, the hands and face compose the largest parts of the M1, and they are located on the lateral and dorsal surfaces of the brain. Innervation of trunk muscles occupies a small part of the motor cortex, and the distal legs are represented by a region that is hidden between the two hemispheres.

The Organization of the Motor Cortices Is Dynamic. The organization of the motor cortex is dynamic, and its processing may change as a result of the activation of neural plasticity (*10*). Age-related changes may occur, and input from other parts of the brain may alter the function of primary motor cortices, which can affect cortical processing and excitability of cortical neurons. Use of specific muscles can extend their representation on the motor cortices (*11*).

Other Functions of Motor Cortices. While the motor areas of the cortex are mainly involved in control of muscles, it has become evident that electrical stimulation of some of these areas can have very different effects than simple muscle activation. One such effect is the control of severe, chronic pain (*12*). It has been shown that the effectiveness of such stimulation

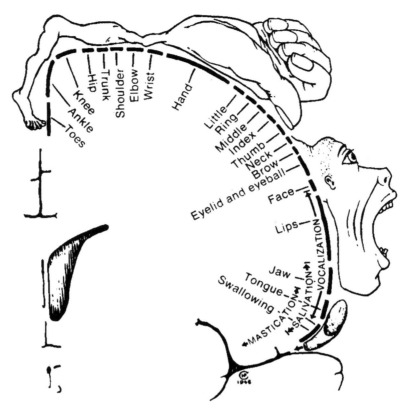

Figure 9.3: Illustration of the somatotopic organization of the primary motor cortex (M1). (Reprinted from: (*7*)).

is the greatest when it elicits a large D-wave that can be recorded from the corticospinal tract of the spinal cord.

Further information about the anatomical organization of the motor system can be found in Brodal, 2004 (*3*), and Kandel, Schwartz, and Jessel, 2008 (*13*).

BASAL GANGLIA

The basal ganglia receive input from cortical motor areas and relay the processed information to the thalamus, which then sends the information back to the motor cortex (**Fig. 9.4**). (The basal ganglia also process information from other parts of the cerebral cortex.)

The basal ganglia play an important role in movement control, and pathologies of the basal

ganglia seem to be involved in several important diseases, such Parkinson's and Huntington's diseases, and also some rare diseases such as Tourette's syndrome. The basal ganglia are important in intraoperative monitoring (or rather intraoperative neurophysiology) in that treatment using either lesions or implantation of stimulating electrodes (deep brain stimulation, DBS) benefits from the support of electrophysiologic recordings (known as intraoperative neurophysiology).

The fact that the basal ganglia receive input from the motor cortices and deliver their output back to the motor cortices through the thalamus (**Fig. 9.4**) means that descending motor pathways, such as the corticospinal tract, contain information that has been processed in the basal ganglia. The thalamus also provides some processing of the information it receives from the basal ganglia.

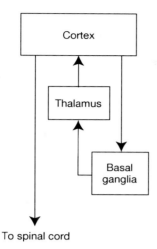

Figure 9.4: Connections among the basal ganglia, the thalamus, and the motor cortices. Reprinted from (*10*) with the permission from Cambridge University Press.

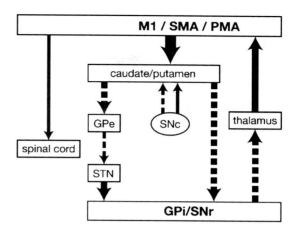

Figure 9.5: Simplified scheme of the connections among the cerebral motor cortices and some of the nuclei of the basal ganglia and the thalamus showing the indirect (*left*) and the direct pathway (*right*) from the caudate/putamen to the GPi/SNr. *Solid arrows* show excitation and segmented arrows show inhibition. The width of the arrows indicates the amount of excitation or inhibition one structure has on another. Modified from: (*10*).

Anatomical Organization of the Basal Ganglia

Traditionally, the term basal ganglia is used to describe specific nuclei collectively: the caudate nucleus, the putamen, and the globus pallidus. The terminology used by different authors regarding the basal ganglia varies, and different investigators have included different nuclei under the term basal ganglia. However, most authors include the substantia nigra (SN), the subthalamic nucleus (STN), and the claustrum (**Fig. 9.5**) because they are related functionally to the other parts of the basal ganglia (*3*). The caudate nucleus and the putamen, as the primary inputs to the basal ganglia, possess many similarities and are often referred to as the striatum or neostriatum. The putamen and the globus pallidus are known as the lentiform nucleus (because of their anatomical lens shape). Several previously unrecognized subdivisions of the nuclei of the basal ganglia are now known, and their functions are beginning to be understood. For example, the globus pallidus consists of an external segment (globus pallidus external part, GPe) and an internal segment (globus pallidus internal part, GPi). A part of the substantia nigra

is the pars reticulata (SNr), and another part is known as the substantia nigra pars compacta (SNc). These nuclei are of special interest in connection with movement disorders. **Fig. 9.5** shows the main connections between the different nuclei, and **Fig. 9.6** shows the anatomical relationship between the basal ganglia and adjacent structures.

The anatomical organization of the basal ganglia is shown in **Fig. 9.6A, B.**

It should be noted that all connections among the components of the basal ganglia are inhibitory with one exception, namely, the connections between the STN and the Gpi/SNr, which are excitatory (**Fig. 9.5**). The SNc has both inhibitory and excitatory inputs to the caudate/putamen.

The nuclei of the striatum send inhibitory input to the GPi and SNr via two separate routes: a direct route and an indirect route (**Fig. 9.5**). What is known as the "indirect" route projects from the striatum to the GPi/SNr via the GPe and the STN (**Fig. 9.5**). This means

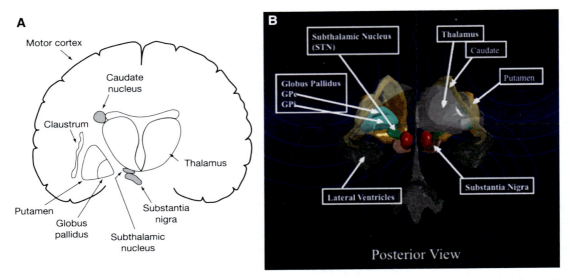

Figure 9.6: Anatomical organization of the basal ganglia and the motor thalamus. (**A**) Schematic drawing of the basal ganglia showing their relationship to other structures. (Reprinted from Møller AR (2006) Neural plasticity and disorders of the nervous system. 2006, by Aage Møller, Copyright © 2006 © A. Møller 2006. Reprinted with the permission of Cambridge University Press (*10*)). (**B**) A three-dimensional artist's rendition of the structures involved in surgery of the basal ganglia to treat movement disorders. (Modified from: (*14*), Reprinted from: (*15*) with permission from Elsevier).

that the GPi and SNr nuclei receive inhibitory input from the striatum that is interrupted in the GPe and STN, as well as input that is not interrupted by these structures (*16*). The output of GPi and SNr tonically inhibits thalamocortical neurons (*17*), but the direct dopaminergic nigrostriatal pathway from SNc may also modulate the activity in the two striato-pallidal pathways in two different ways: one of which facilitates transmission in the "direct" pathway, while the other inhibits transmission in the "indirect" pathway (*18*).

The input to the basal ganglia from the primary motor cortex converges on the striatum, which consists of the caudate nucleus and the putamen, the centromedian nucleus (CMN) of the thalamus, and the SNc. The putamen receives input from the M1, the SMA, and the PMA (**Fig. 9.5**), as well as from the primary somatosensory cortex (S1). The caudate nucleus primarily receives input from association cortices (*3*). (**Fig. 9.5** is a simplified drawing that omits some connections).

The STN connects to the GPe and the SNr in a reciprocal way, and to a lesser degree, the STN receives indirect input from the motor cortex (**Fig. 9.5**) and sends output to the GPi. The output from the basal ganglia to the thalamus primarily originates from the GPi and the SNr.

Dormant and Active Connections

Morphologic studies show connections from motor cortices to the striatum; several groups of thalamic nuclei; the red nucleus; pontine nuclei; the mesencephalic, pontine, and medullary parts of the reticular formation; dorsal column and trigeminal sensory nuclei; and the lateral reticular nucleus (*19*). It must, however, be pointed out that these connections that are often shown in diagrams in textbooks are based primarily on morphologic studies, and much less is known about the functional roles of these connections, and which of these connections are active at any given time.

The Role of the Basal Ganglia in Motor Control

Considerable neural processing occurs in the basal ganglia, the thalamus, and the motor cortex itself, which is evident in the descending activity that activates alpha motor nuclei. The role of the basal ganglia in control of motor activity is complex and several hypotheses about the role of these nuclei have been presented. It has been suggested that the basal ganglia are involved in the planning of movements (20), and this hypothesis is supported by the existence of connections to the PMA, the SMA, and to and from the prefrontal motor cortex (PFMC). More recently, the basal ganglia have been associated with nonmotor functions such as memory and learning (21).

THALAMUS

The motor portion of the thalamus is involved in processing movement information, and it links the output of the basal ganglia to the motor cortices (**Figs. 9.4** and **9.5**). Lesions made in specific nuclei of the thalamus have been shown to be effective in treating movement disorders, sensory disorders, and pain (see Chap. 15). Surgical lesions have now largely been replaced by implantation of electrodes for chronic electrical stimulation of specific nuclei (DBS).

CEREBELLUM

The cerebellum has so far been of less interest from an intraoperative neurophysiology and monitoring perspective than the basal ganglia and the thalamus. However, as the understanding of the many functions of the cerebellum increases, it may in the future be a target of similar interventions in the treatment of movement disorders we have seen to develop for the basal ganglia during the past two or three decades.

The cerebellum processes information from other CNS structures, but does not initiate movements. The cerebellum receives extensive input from sensory and (unconscious) proprioceptive sources such as receptors in the skin, joints, tendons, and muscle spindles through the spinocerebellar tract, and from the vestibular system. The cerebellum connects to the basal ganglia, the spinal cord, and neurons in the M1. As in many other motor and sensory systems, many of these connections are reciprocal, forming loops (**Fig. 9.6**).

The cerebellar hemispheres receive input from many sources such as the superior colliculus, pretectal nuclei, and the red nucleus through the inferior olive in the medulla (3) (**Fig. 9.7**). The cerebellum has been divided into the spinocerebellum, the cerebrocerebellum, and the intermediate zone. The spinocerebellum receives proprioceptive input from muscle spindles, tendon organs, and low-threshold receptors in the skin.

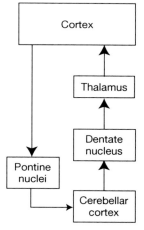

Figure 9.7: Schematic diagram showing some important connections from the cerebral cortex to the cerebellum and illustrating reciprocal connections. The cerebellum receives information from the primary motor cortex via pontine nuclei and communicates back to the primary motor cortex via the dentate nucleus of the cerebellum and the thalamus. (Reprinted from (10) with the permission from Cambridge University Press).

The intermediate zone receives connections from both the cerebral cortex (mainly M1) and the spinal cord. These neurons may compare motor commands sent from the cerebral cortex with information from the periphery about the actual movement.

The spinocerebellum also receives input from spinal interneurons and monitors the level of activity in these neurons, thus providing the cerebellum with information about the commands issued to motoneurons and the movements produced.

The cerebrocerebellum receives input from cerebral motor cortices (M1, SMA, and PMA) via nuclei in the pons and sensory cortices, and it sends the information back to the cerebral cortices via the dentate nucleus and the ventrolateral thalamic nucleus. This part of the cerebellum is supposed to receive information about planned movements and about the motor commands that are sent out by the cerebral cortices. On the basis of the received information, the cerebellum can modify the activity in the cerebral motor cortices. The pontine nuclei also receive visual input and that may provide information about moving objects.

Anatomical studies have shown that the output of the cerebellum targets not only motor circuits in the brain and the spinal cord, but also many nonmotor areas in the prefrontal and posterior parietal cortex (22). This explains why the cerebellum has many other functions than motor functions, including cognitive and memory functions. The loops of the connections between the cerebral cortices and the cerebellum, thus, provide control not only of motor functions, but also of cognitive functions, the latter being largely ignored until recently. Neuroimaging has provided support for this wide range of influence from the cerebellum. The range of tasks associated with activation of neural circuits in the cerebellum includes attention, language, working memory, learning, pain, emotion, and addiction (22). Cerebellar areas around the vermis are activated during mental recall of emotional, personal episodes.

The effects of lesions in the cerebellum also support the notion that the cerebellum has nonmotor functions. For example, individuals who have had a cerebellar stroke may fail to show overt emotional changes (23).

DESCENDING MOTOR PATHWAYS

As mentioned above, there are two main descending motor pathways, the lateral system and the medial system, according to Kuypers' definition (2). The lateral system, also known as the specific or the pyramidal system, is phylogenetically younger than the medial system.

The lateral system (also known as the dorsolateral system) comprises two pathways, the corticospinal and rubrospinal pathways (**Fig. 9.8**). Of these two systems, the

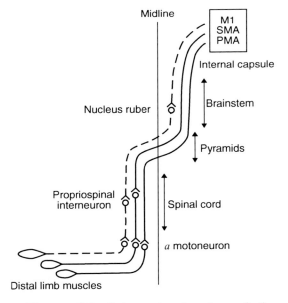

Figure 9.8: Schematic drawing of the crossed lateral corticospinal tract and the rubrospinal tract. The dashed line indicates that the rubrospinal tract is small and less influential in humans compared to that in other mammals.

corticospinal system is the more developed in primates (*24*), which makes the results of studies of the motor system in other mammals less representative for humans. The axons of the corticospinal tract originate in cells of M1, PMA, SMA, and S1 cortices (M1 occupies Brodmann area 4, PMA, and SMA area 6 and S1, areas 1–3) (see **Fig. 9.2**).

The contributions from areas other than M1 to major descending motor pathways are not always recognized and many descriptions of the "motor cortex" do not specify whether only the M1 area is concerned or whether the other cortical motor areas that contribute to the corticospinal tract are included in the description. Almost all fibers of the lateral system travel in the lateral part of the spinal cord and they cross the midline at the level of the pyramids. A small and somewhat variable part of the corticospinal system travels in an anterior (ventral) part of the spinal cord near the midline (median fissure of the spinal cord). The axons of this part of the corticospinal tract (approximately 10%) are assumed to travel uncrossed to the spinal cord and terminate bilaterally in the ventral horn of the spinal cord. The importance of this anterior (or ventral) corticospinal tract is poorly known. The lateral system, mainly evolved in primates, is very small in animals such as the cat, which has been used in many studies of the motor system.

Many aspects of the corticospinal system in humans are incompletely known because of the limited number of studies of primates and the possibilities of differences between humans and other primates. The rubrospinal tract in humans is small; the exact size not known. For monitoring purposes, it does not play any important role.

The medial system is also known as the non-specific system, and it innervates proximal limbs and trunk muscles.

Some fiber tracts from the motor cortices innervate nuclei in the brainstem that send their axons down the spinal cord, forming the medial system. The axons of the cells in these nuclei, in turn, descend in the spinal cord as the vestibulospinal, the reticulospinal, and tectospinal

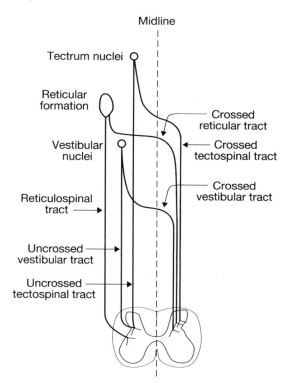

Figure 9.9: Simplified schematic diagram of medial descending motor pathways showing the vestibular, tectospinal, and reticulospinal tracts.

tracts. These tracts are to a great extent bilateral (**Fig. 9.9**).

In addition to these two main descending tracts, often known as the direct and the indirect pathways, there is a small, uncrossed corticospinal pathway, the ventral corticospinal tract, that originates in the neurons in the SMA and the PMA (Brodmann area 6).

Origin of the Descending Pathways from the Motor Cortices

The descending corticospinal pathways (**Fig. 9.8**) originate in motor cortices (**Fig. 9.2**). Layer 5 in the primary motor cortex (M1, Brodmann area 4, see Appendix A) contains giant pyramidal (Betz) cells, the axons of which travel in the corticospinal tract. These cells, however, are few compared with the total number of corticospinal fibers (about 1 million), which means that other central regions must contribute to the corticospinal tract. The proportion of axons that these other sources contribute to the corticospinal tract in humans is not known exactly, and different investigators have reported different values. One study states that all cells in layer 5 of the M1 cortex contribute to the corticospinal tract and that M1 provides about half of all fibers in the corticospinal tract in humans. Most of the remaining fibers come from the SMA (Brodmann's area 6, see Appendix A) and a smaller part from the lateral PMA (area 6) and from the somatosensory cortex (areas 1–3). Neurons in areas 23 and 24 in the cingulated cortex also contribute. Other sources state that only one-third of the fibers come from M1, one-third from SMA and PMA, and the remaining third comes from the primary somatosensory cortex. The corticospinal tract also receives input from motor areas in the frontal lobe.

As shown above, the primary motor cortex receives input from higher order cortical motor regions such as motor regions of the prefrontal cortices (PFC) (**Fig. 9.2**). The motor cortex also receives input from the somatosensory cortical areas such as S1, mostly from area 3a, which is close to area 4 (see Chap. 5, **Fig. 5.5**).

Corticospinal Tract

The corticospinal tracts are the main part of the lateral system, along with the axons of the corticobulbar tract that also originate in motor cortices and innervate cranial motor nuclei. The rubrospinal tract, which is small and of little importance in humans, is also usually regarded as a part of the lateral system.

Most of the fibers of the corticospinal tract (from M1, SMA, and PMA) cross the midline at the level of the medulla (Pyramidal decussation, **Fig. 9.8**), but a small number of fibers continue uncrossed in the ventral corticospinal tract down the spinal cord.

The corticospinal tract alone passes through the pyramids, while other descending pathways pass through other parts of the medulla. This is why the corticospinal tract has been known as the pyramidal tract and the other tracts were

known as the extrapyramidal tracts – a distinction that is no longer valid. The corticospinal tract innervates distal limbs and provides fine control of muscles, especially those that control the fingers.

The corticospinal tract connects cortical motor neurons with alpha motoneurons in the spinal cord, either directly synapsing with alpha motoneurons or indirectly via propriospinal interneurons. Most of the approximately two million fibers of the corticospinal tract are fast conducting fibers, but only a small percentage connects directly (monosynaptical) to alpha motoneurons; most remaining fibers terminate on propriospinal interneurons that connect to alpha motoneurons.

The rubrospinal tract originates in the nucleus ruber, which receives indirect input from the motor cortex. Because this pathway has very few fibers in humans (estimated to be one percent of the number of the corticospinal tract fibers in primates (3)), the functional importance of the rubrospinal tract in humans has been questioned, and it is of little importance for monitoring purposes.

The main parts of the lateral system cross the midline at the level of the lower medulla (lateral corticospinal tract and the rubrospinal tract), but it has been stated that approximately 10% of the corticospinal fibers in humans do not cross the midline and form the ventral corticospinal tract; there are large individual variations (3). The corticospinal tract is asymmetric in about 75% of the population (3), the right side often being larger than the left side (3).

Most of the connections from cells in the motor cortices reach cells in the contralateral ventral horn of the spinal cord, but some cells in the middle portion of the spinal horn receive input from the S1 (**Fig. 9.10**). Cells in the dorsal horn indirectly connect to cells in the somatosensory cortices.

The anatomy of the projections from motor areas described above is representative for most individuals, but large deviations from that can be found. Such variations have been especially noted in individuals with scoliosis and other disorders, such as congenital hemiparesis,

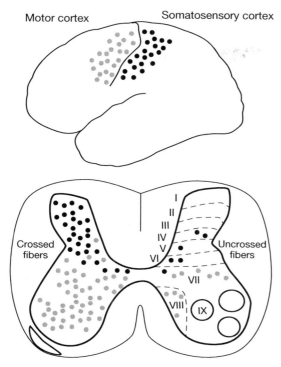

Figure 9.10: Termination of the corticospinal tract in the spinal cord based on studies in monkeys, using histological methods for tracing axons from the motor somatosensory cortices. **(A)** Fibers of the corticospinal tract from M1 terminate in the ventral part of the spinal horns, and those originating in the S1 terminate in the dorsal horn. **(B)** Most fibers cross to the opposite side, and a few uncrossed fibers terminate in the middle part of the ipsilateral spinal horns. Reprinted from (*10*) with the permission from Cambridge University Press.

where large abnormalities in motor pathways in the spinal cord may be present (see page 220).

There are reports that the left and right corticospinal tracts are different and most often the right side is larger than the left side. It has been reported that the corticospinal tracts proceed

uncrossed in a few individuals such as in Joubert syndrome[2] (*26*). It is also known that there are anatomical abnormalities in many individuals with scoliosis (*26, 27*) where the corticospinal pathways may be mainly uncrossed in some individuals.

Medial System

Axons of the pontine motor nuclei form the medial spinal motor tracts (**Fig. 9.9**) of the medial system. There are two kinds of nuclei in the brainstem that receive axons from motor cortices. One kind is the cranial nerve motonuclei that control muscles in the face, mouth, and throat. The other kind is the nuclei of the medial system that control trunk muscles and muscles on the proximal limbs (pontine motonuclei). These nuclei were parts of what was known as the extrapyramidal system, now known as the medial system.

Pontine Motonuclei. The medial tract mainly consists of three parts: the vestibulospinal, the reticulospinal, and the tectospinal tracts that originate in the vestibular nucleus, the superior colliculus, and the pontine reticular formation (**Fig. 9.9**). It is believed that the vestibular nucleus receives its main input from the vestibular system and little, if anything, from the motor cortices, whereas the other two nuclei receive input from motor cortices (**Fig. 9.9**). The nuclei of the medial system give rise to both crossed and uncrossed descending tracts and thus, control muscles on both sides of the body.

The tracts of the medial system are less direct motor pathways than those of the lateral system, and the medial system comprises pathways with different origins. From a phylogenetic perspective, the tracts of the medial system are the oldest motor pathways. The medial system controls muscles in the proximal limbs and especially trunk muscles, including "antigravity" muscles. This tract is important

---

[2]Joubert syndrome: agenesis of the cerebellar vermis, characterized clinically by attacks of tachypnea or prolonged apnea, abnormal eye movements, ataxia, and mental retardation. (Stedman's Electronic Medical Dictionary).

for control of posture and for providing necessary facilitation of alpha motoneurons.

The anatomy of the motor tracts that belong to the medial system is generally poorly understood. Some investigators have found that, normally, these pathways have both crossed and uncrossed tracts (some sources state that only the tectospinal tract is bilateral and that this tract only extends to the cervical part of the spinal cord).

Other investigators found that the tectospinal and vestibulospinal fibers are mainly crossed, (28) (**Fig. 9.9**) but have small, uncrossed parts. The reticulospinal pathways are bilateral.

Origin of the Tracts of the Medial System. The tectospinal tracts have their origin in the neurons of the superior colliculus, which receive input not only from the visual system, but also from other sensory systems, such as the auditory system and the somatosensory system, and from motor cortices.

The vestibulospinal pathway receives its main input from the vestibular nuclei, which in turn receive input from the balance organs in the inner ears. The vestibulospinal tracts have two parts: the lateral vestibulospinal tract, which reaches all parts of the spinal cord, and the much smaller medial vestibulospinal tract, which reaches only the cervical and upper thoracic parts of the spinal cord. The fibers of the vestibulospinal tracts terminate on neurons in the medial part of the spinal horn and provide excitatory influence on both alpha and gamma neurons.

The vestibular nuclei have little input from the cerebral cortex and, therefore, mainly mediate automatic reflex movements and adjustments of muscle tonus. Most of the functions of the vestibulospinal system are regained after loss of input from the balance organ in the inner ear, which is an indication that the system receives connections from other parts of the CNS through synapses that normally are dormant, but which can be unmasked when their normal input is lost. The reticulospinal system may also be able to take over such functions from the vestibulospinal system when the balance organ is damaged.

The reticulospinal pathway originates in cells in the reticular formation of the brainstem, mainly the pons and the medulla. These neurons receive input from many other nuclei and from the cerebral cortex through corticoreticular fibers. Thus, this is one way the motor cortices can influence motoneurons in the spinal cord. The reticulospinal pathway is important for posture and for movements related to orientation of the body (thus, some similarities with the vestibulospinal system). The reticulospinal system can also provide crude voluntary movements through the corticoreticular connections from the motor cortices along with contributions from the tectum (superior colliculus) and the cerebellum.

The fibers of the reticulospinal tract that originate in the pontine reticular formation travel in the ventral funiculus, while fibers from the medullary portion travel in the ventral part of the lateral funiculus (**Fig. 9.9**) (*3*).

Because of its role in facilitating alpha motoneurons, the reticulospinal tract has some importance for intraoperative monitoring. However, many forms of anesthesia suppress the reticular formation, and thus, decrease the activity in the reticulospinal tracts and render monitoring of the tract ineffective because of lack of facilitatory input to alpha motoneurons.

Nonspecific Descending Systems

The NA–serotonin pathways belong to a nonspecific system originating in the raphe nuclei (*3*) (see (*10*)), which project to the spinal cord. Neurons in the locus coeruleus also project to the spinal cord where they can affect the excitability of spinal neurons that are part of the motor system. In addition, the neurons of these nuclei connect to many regions of the brain (*3*).

The fibers of the NA–serotonin pathways terminate throughout the gray matter in the spinal cord, where they can modulate neural activity in neurons that are part of the motor system, including alpha motoneurons. The NA–serotonin system generally increases the excitability of alpha motoneurons (*29*) (for an overview, see (*30*)). One important function of these descending pathways is adjusting muscle tone, such as suppressing skeletal muscle activity, which occurs, for example, during rapid eye movement (REM) sleep (3). These facilitatory systems are sensitive to anesthetic agents, and the reduction in the activity of these systems, caused by anesthetics, is likely to contribute to the decreased excitability of motor systems that is observed during surgical operations.

THE SPINAL CORD

The spinal cord is comprised of white matter and gray matter areas, also known as the spinal horns, because of the way the areas appear anatomically (**Fig. 9.11**). The white matter consists of nerve axons grouped together in descending motor fiber tracts and ascending sensory tracts. The gray matter consists of nerve cell bodies and glia cells. This complex network of nerve cells performs complex processing of motor and sensory information. The neurons in the dorsal horns are involved in sensory processing of information that arrives in dorsal roots. The ventral horns contain the lower motor neurons including the alpha motoneurons that serve as the final common pathways for motor commands that activate somatic muscles. Cells in the ventral horns process motor commands that arrive in descending motors tracts that terminate on nerve cells in the ventral horn. The functions of the dorsal horn were discussed in Chap. 5, and in this chapter, the anatomy and function of the ventral horn will be discussed.

Descending activity in the lateral spinal system (2) (corticospinal and rubrospinal tracts) from the M1, SMA, and PMA provides input to neurons in the ventral spinal cord that can control reflexes and activate alpha motoneurons. Input from the somatosensory system (S1) can also reach neurons in the ventral spinal cord (including the alpha motoneurons) indirectly.

Corticospinal axons from the premotor areas terminate in cells in the intermediate zone of the spinal cord, but some also terminate in the ventral horn around motoneurons. This means that the projection of neurons in the premotor areas to the spinal cord is similar to that of neurons from M1.

Some axons from cells in the PMA also appear to have direct connections with spinal motoneurons, particularly those innervating hand muscles, as indicated by the finding that low current stimulations of the premotor areas can evoke movements of the distal and proximal forelimb. Hence, the premotor areas can influence movement directly at the level of the spinal cord. Because of this observed influence, Dum and co-workers have suggested that the premotor areas may operate at a hierarchical level comparable to M1, and that each premotor area is a functionally distinct system that generates and/or controls specific aspects of motor behavior (5). The corticospinal projections to cervical segments of the spinal cord originate from M1 and the six PMAs in the frontal lobe (4).

The main descending pathways from the motor cortices terminate in interneurons in different segments of the spinal cord. It is also important to point out that each alpha motoneuron receives input from a large territory of M1 and that the territory supplying input to a given muscle overlaps extensively with that providing input to other muscles in the same part of the body (31). The degree of overlap can be changed by activation of neural plasticity (10) that may be controlled by the use of the different muscles.

The axons of the medial system terminate on neurons in the ventromedial zone of the spinal horn. These pathways mostly innervate propriospinal interneurons whose axons terminate on the alpha motoneurons that control muscles of the trunk and girdle, as well as proximal limb muscles.

The Importance of Synaptic Efficacy

There is no doubt that activity in many of the fibers in these fiber tracts terminates in synapses that do not normally conduct. The existence of such dormant connections

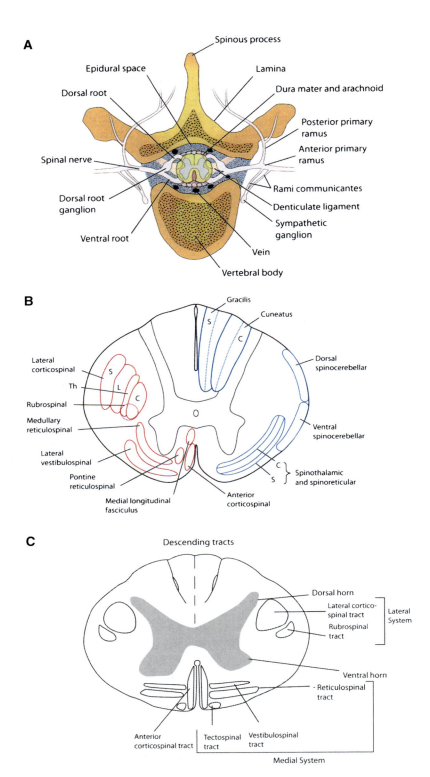

Figure 9.11: Spinal motor systems: Cross section of the spinal cord. (**A**) Bone structures and the spinal cord. (Reprinted from (*42*) with permission from Mayo Foundation). (**B**) Schematic drawing of the anatomical location of ascending sensory pathways in the spinal cord. (**C**) Schematic drawing of the anatomical location of descending motor pathways in the spinal cord. Figures A and B from (*42*) reprinted with the permission from the Mayo Foundation, Rochester, Minnesota).

represents redundancy that may be activated through expression of neural plasticity (see (*10*)). Many phenomena can cause expression of neural plasticity, such as injuries or changes in demand. More important for intraoperative monitoring is perhaps the fact that connections that normally are conducting nerve impulses may cease to do so because of the effect of anesthetics. This adverse effect is probably most apparent when it results in reduced facilitatory input to motoneurons.

LOWER SPINAL MOTONEURON

Lower motor neurons are alpha and gamma motoneurons and interneurons located in the ventral part of the spinal horn. All spinal motor activity must pass through the alpha motoneuron from which the motor nerves emerge (the "common final pathway"). The motor portion of peripheral nerves also contains the axons of gamma neurons that innervate the (intrafusal) muscles of muscle spindles (see page 171).

Segmental Pathways

At first glance, the corticospinal tract appears as a rather simple pathway that connects neurons in the primary motor cortex to alpha motoneurons in the spinal cord. However, it is a pathway that activates complex circuitry in the spinal cord. Most fibers from the cortices terminate on interneurons, and only a few fibers terminate directly on alpha motoneurons. It is not only the M1 cortex that contributes to the corticospinal tract, but the SMA, PMA, and some cells in the S1 also send axons to the spinal cord in the corticospinal tract. The processing of motor commands in the spinal cord is extensive. In fact, most input to cells in the ventral spinal horn originates in other cells in the gray matter of the spinal cord, and there is a complex network of connections among neurons in the spinal cord that provides extensive intra- and inter-segmental processing. Corticospinal fibers make complex collateral connections with neurons in many parts of the spinal cord (*2, 28, 32*), and they reach neurons in several different areas of the spinal cord and extend over many spinal

cord segments. The lateral system of descending pathways (corticospinal and rubrospinal systems) provides disynaptic and polysynaptic input to spinal motoneurons from different parts of the cerebral motor areas and from other sources in the brain.

The neural networks in the spinal cord perform extensive integration of somatosensory and proprioceptive information with motor commands from the brain. Spinal cord processing involves multiple feedback loops (including reflexes), and the gain of these multiple feedback loops is affected by several sources of input from the brain and by proprioceptive input. This means that the spinal cord has wide ranges of computational capabilities. Processing in the spinal cord is important not only for the normal function of the motor system, but also for assessing changes in function, such as in diagnosis of movement disorders and in intraoperative monitoring of motor systems.

The interneurons in the spinal cord provide local processing of the input from sources in the brain and in the spinal cord, which can be extensive, before the motor commands reach the alpha motoneurons. Propriospinal interneurons that receive their input from corticospinal fibers also receive excitatory and inhibitory inputs from other pathways and from many segmental sources in the spinal cord. This makes it possible to modulate the commands from the motor cortices before they reach the alpha motoneurons (*33–36*).

Studies, in which a specific site on the cortex was micro-stimulated, showed that activity in small groups of cortical neurons can cause descending activity in many different tracts and evoke contraction of many different muscles (*28*).

Local spinal circuits can generate complex commands on their own without input from the brain. For example, the CPG in the spinal cord can generate the rhythmic movements of walking. This means that walking may be possible without signals from the brain, and thus, in individuals with spinal cord injuries, but the CPG itself must receive initial input from commands from the brain. Neural circuits in the spinal cord can also generate motor functions necessary for breathing without supraspinal input, but descending activity from structures of the brain can modulate these functions.

Alpha Motoneurons

As mentioned above, alpha motoneurons, located in layer IX of the ventral horn of the spinal cord, are the targets of the descending motor tracts. These neurons are the "final common pathway" for motor control through which all motor commands must pass. Their axons form the ventral spinal roots and the motor portions of spinal nerves that innervate skeletal (extrafusal) muscles. Gamma motor neurons that innervate the fibers of muscles spindles (intrafusal) are also located in the ventral horns of the spinal cord. These fibers control the length of muscle spindles and, thereby, adjust the working range of the muscle spindles that measure the length of muscles and report back to the CNS (mostly the cerebellum) as a feedback loop of muscle contractions.

Each alpha motoneuron has many synapses (estimated to be somewhere between 10,000 and 50,000 for each individual alpha motoneuron) that connect input from different sources. Alpha motoneurons receive some direct input from corticospinal fibers, but most corticospinal fibers activate alpha motoneurons through propriospinal interneurons and other local (excitatory and inhibitory) segmental interneurons. These spinal interneurons receive some of their input from sources in the brain through long descending pathways (corticospinal, rubrospinal, tectospinal, vestibulospinal, and reticulospinal tracts), but most of the input to neurons in the spinal cord comes from other neurons in the spinal cord that create local spinal circuits (28, 31). Some of the inputs from descending motor pathways, such as the reticulospinal tract, serve to facilitate activation of the motoneurons and, thereby, influence the ability to evoke motor responses by stimulation of

the motor cortex. Some of the activity in the corticospinal pathways, such as the activity represented by I waves, also provide facilitatory input to alpha motoneurons.

There are, thus, several anatomical means in the spinal cord for extensive modulation of the motor commands from the brain.

SPINAL REFLEXES

The fibers of all descending pathways give off many collateral fibers to neurons that are involved in spinal reflexes. Spinal reflexes are important for many types of movements, and to a great extent, descending motor pathways control spinal reflexes as a way to induce normal motor activity.

Some reflexes, such as the monosynaptic stretch reflex, are relatively simple, and other reflexes are complex and involve circuits in the brain. However, all spinal reflexes can be modulated by descending input from the brain and from input from neurons in the same and other spinal segments. The input to spinal reflexes from descending pathways, such as the corticospinal tract and those of the medial system, plays an important role in execution of motor commands. One of the simplest of spinal reflexes is the Renshaw reflex, which feeds information that travels in the motor nerves back to the alpha motoneurons as inhibition. This information acts as a negative feedback that stabilizes the movement. Even though this reflex appears as a simple one-synapse feedback system, its action can be modulated by input from neurons in the spinal cord and from sources in the brain (**Fig. 9.12A**). The same is the case for other spinal reflexes. In a similar fashion, the "simple" monosynaptic stretch reflex can be modulated by input from the brain and input from other segments of the spinal cord (**Fig. 9.13B**).

Neurologists often test the monosynaptic stretch reflex clinically by tapping on the patella tendon with a small hammer. More quantitative tests of the monosynaptic stretch reflex are made by electrical stimulation of a

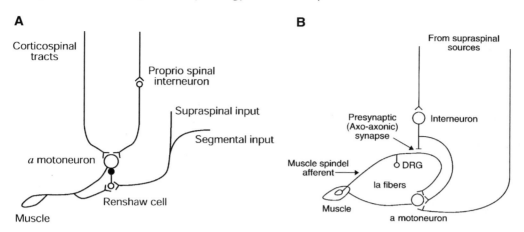

Figure 9.12: (A) Input from corticospinal tracts to alpha motoneurons, showing Renshaw inhibition and modulation of that input. Reprinted from: Møller AR (2006) Neural plasticity and disorders of the nervous system. 2006, by Aage Møller, Copyright © 2006 © A. Møller 2006. Reprinted with the permission of Cambridge University Press (*10*). (B) Monosynaptic stretch reflex. Simplified diagram of the monosynaptic stretch reflex, showing the modulatory input from sources in the brain and spinal sources via an interneuron. (Reprinted from (*10*) with the permission of Cambridge University Press).

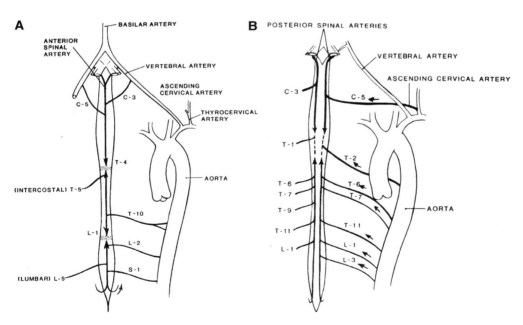

Figure 9.13: General principles for blood supply to the spinal cord. (A) Schematic drawing of the spinal cord with the single anterior spinal artery (ASA), and three radicular arteries from the aorta as C-3, C-5, T-4, T-10, L-1, L-2, and S-1. (B) Posterior spinal arteries (PSA). Seven radicular arteries are shown here as C-5, T-2, T-6, T-7, T-11, L-1, and L-3. *Stippled areas* indicate zones of marginal blood supply. (Reprinted from: (*42*) with permission from the Mayo Foundation).

peripheral (mixed) nerve while recording electromyographic (EMG) potentials from the related muscle (known as the Hoffman reflex). The Hoffman reflex is beginning to come into use for intraoperative monitoring.

In spinal cord injuries, spinal reflexes are present below the location of the injuries. Spinal reflexes can be elicited independent of input from the brain as shown by the fact that electrical stimulation through epidural electrodes of the lumbosacral spinal cord in individuals with complete spinal cord injury can elicit responses from spinal cord reflexes. Low-frequency (2.1 Hz) stimulation has been shown to produce twitches in muscles in paralyzed lower limbs (37), while high frequency (25–50 Hz) stimulation has caused stepping-like movements (38) in individuals with long-standing paralysis, and thus, electrical stimulation can initiate complex movements that are programmed in the spinal cord.

Reflexes are depressed below the site of injury immediately after spinal cord injuries because the absence of input from the brain affects the normal modulation of reflexes. Over time, this absence produces plastic changes in spinal cord circuits that are involved in producing spasticity and results in exaggerated reflexes. These changes in reflexes may be the consequence of synaptic efficacy changes that cause depression of inhibition in spinal cord neural circuits – less inhibition results in greater exaggeration. Spasticity[3] is one such sign that often appears months after spinal injuries (39) and can be treated by medicine such as baclofen, but spasticity can also be treated by severing a few fascicles of dorsal roots (see Chap. 15) (40) or by other microsurgical procedures regarding spinal nerve roots (41). In order to perform these types of procedures effectively, intraoperative neurophysiology is important.

BLOOD SUPPLY TO THE SPINAL CORD

Bleeding or compromise to the blood supply and the venous drainage of the spinal cord are common causes of spinal cord trauma that may occur during surgical operations on the spine (bone) and on the spinal cord itself. Intraoperative monitoring is important in such operations, and it can reduce the risk of permanent deficits considerably. It is, therefore, important to understand the blood supply to the spinal cord and the venous drainage, which are complex and vary from individual to individual. Since the blood supply to the spinal cord is variable, a description of the blood supply given here will not apply to all individuals.

The fact that two parts of the spinal cord, the dorsal and the ventral, receive blood from different sources implies that these two parts of the spinal cord can be injured separately if the blood supply is impaired. Monitoring of both the dorsal and the ventral parts of the spinal cord is, therefore, necessary to optimally reduce the risks of injuries from ischemia that is caused by insufficient blood supply as might occur during operations that involve the spine. Monitoring somatosensory evoked potentials (SSEP) mainly tests the function of the sensory parts of the dorsal spinal cord. In the same way, monitoring only motor evoked responses mainly covers the ventral part of the spinal cord.

Recording of SSEP was the earliest method used to monitor the function of the spinal cord intraoperatively, as described in Chap. 6. Since the sensory pathways that are monitored by recording SSEP occupy the dorsal and lateral portions of the spinal cord, while the motor pathways occupy mainly the ventral portion, the effect of ischemia and other insults to the ventral portion of the spinal cord does not cause direct changes in the SSEP. If only SSEP

---

[3]Spasticity: One type of increase in muscle tone at rest, characterized by increased resistance to passive stretch, velocity dependent, and asymmetric about joints (i.e., greater in the flexor muscles at the elbow and the extensor muscles at the knee). Exaggerated deep tendon reflexes and clonus are additional manifestations. (Stedman's Electronic Medical Dictionary).

are monitored, changes in the function of the ventral part of the spinal cord can, therefore, proceed unnoticed.

Such selective damage to the spinal cord can occur because the dorsal and the ventral potions have different blood supplies. Because the motor (ventral) portion of the spinal cord, in general, has a different blood supply than the sensory portion of the spinal cord (**Fig. 9.16**), compromises of the blood supply to the ventral portion of the spinal cord may occur without the dorsal part of the spinal cord being affected, and thus, go unnoticed if only SSEP are monitored. Monitoring the function of both the dorsal and the ventral portions of the spinal cord is important during operations in which there is risk of ischemia of the spinal cord.

Technical difficulties, mainly related to producing a satisfactory activation of the motor systems of the spinal cord in an anesthetized patient, delayed the introduction of such monitoring for general use. Techniques for extracranial stimulation of the motor cortex by activating descending motor tracts in the spinal cord are now available, and the use of such techniques is increasing (Chap. 10). Development of a suitable anesthesia regimen has contributed to the success of monitoring of motor systems (see Chap. 16).

Arteries

The general outline of the arterial blood supply to the spinal cord is shown in **Fig. 9.13**. The two main sources of blood supply to the spinal cord are the anterior spinal artery (ASA) and the posterior spinal artery (PSA). The ASA branches off from the vertebral artery just after its bifurcation (**Fig. 9.13A**). The PSA (**Fig. 9.13B**) branches off the vertebral artery a little more distally.

There are two PSAs, one on each side of the spinal cord, located just medial to the dorsal roots (**Fig. 9.13**). They normally originate from the vertebral arteries, but they may also originate from the posterior inferior cerebellar arteries (PICA). The PSAs travel all the way along the spinal cord, not as two independent arteries, but rather as an arterial plexus. Occasionally they become very small and are occasionally

interrupted for a short distance on their path along the spinal cord.

The ASA travels caudally as a single artery in the middle of the anterior (ventral) spinal cord. The ASA is a continuation of paired vessels, each one originating from the two vertebral arteries. The two arteries travel a short distance ventromedially before uniting into the ASA at the level of the foramen magnum. The ASA travels along the entire length of the spinal cord in the sulcus of the anterior median fissure.

There are 31 pairs of segmental arteries along the spinal cord (**Fig. 9.14**).

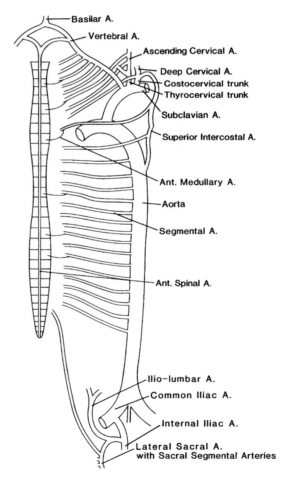

Figure 9.14: The segmental arteries of the spinal cord. (Reprinted from: (*43*) with permission from Elsevier).

The segmental arteries arise from several sources, the most rostral originates from the vertebral arteries, and only a few supply blood to the spinal cord. The sixth and seventh cervical segmental arteries arise from ascending cervical arteries; the eighth cervical segmental arteries arise from deep cervical arteries. The remainder of the thoracic segmental arteries originates from the aorta (**Fig. 9.14**). Four pairs of lumbar segmental arteries also arise from the aorta; the sacral segmental arteries are branches of the lateral sacral arteries (*43*).

The number of vessels from the spinal arteries that contribute to the blood supply of the spinal cord varies. Different authors have referred to these vessels with different names, such as radical, radicular, radiculomedullary, or medullary arteries. These arteries travel either anteriorly or

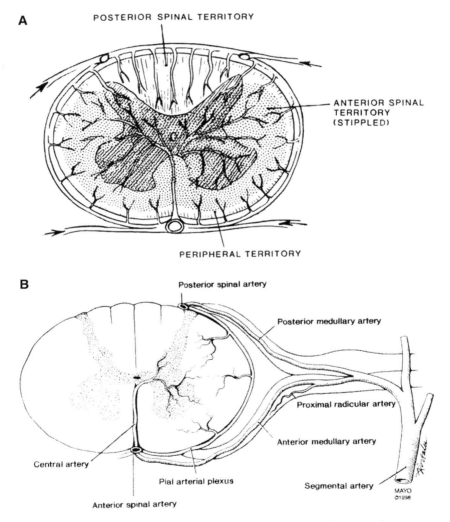

Figure 9.15: (**A**) Schematic drawing of the blood supply to the dorsal and ventral parts of spinal cord. (Reprinted from: (*42*) with permission from the Mayo Foundation). (**B**) Arterial blood flows in a single segment of the spinal cord, showing both anterior and posterior branches of a segmental artery. (Reprinted from: (*44*) with permission from Elsevier).

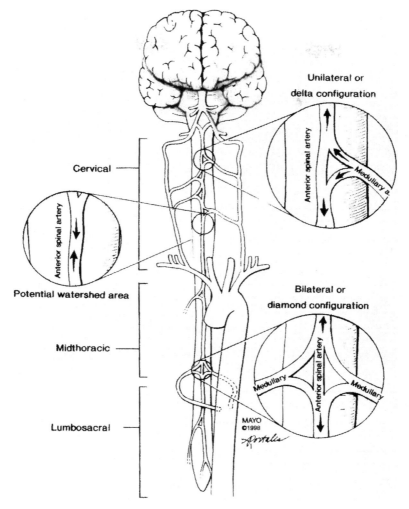

Figure 9.16: Because of the configuration of the anterior spinal artery, medullary artery anastomosis blood can flow in both directions. This is an area of potential risk of ischemia. (Reprinted from: (*44*) with permission from Elsevier).

posteriorly and supply blood to the ASA and the PSA, which in turn supply the spinal cord with blood. There are between 2 and 17 (10 as average) anterior medullary arteries and between 10 and 23 (smaller) posterior arteries (*43*).

Fig. 9.15A shows how the dorsal and the ventral parts of the spinal cord are supplied by different arteries. Each of the segmental arteries typically divides into an anterior (ventral) and a posterior (dorsal) branch (**Fig. 9.16**). The posterior branch bifurcates into an anterior and a posterior radicular artery that supplies the ventral and dorsal nerve roots and dorsal root ganglia (DRG).

In general, the ASA supplies the larger part of the spinal cord, and the PSA supplies dorsal tracts and dorsal horns, as shown in a cross section of the spinal cord in (**Fig. 9.17**). There may be extensive overlap of perfusion in the posteriolateral spinal cord. Again, this description must be taken only as a guide; the exact territories of the dorsal and ventral blood supply to the spinal cord vary among individuals.

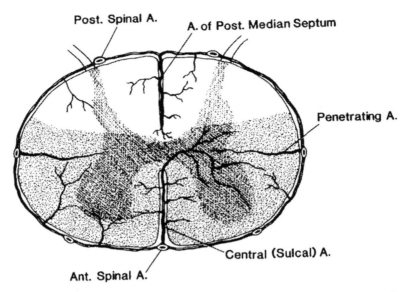

Figure 9.17: Intrinsic arteries of the spinal cord, illustrated for a single segment. The dark areas are the territories of the ASA and its branches. (Reprinted from: (*43*) with permission from Elsevier). A more detailed drawing of the blood supply to a segment of the spinal cord is shown in **Figure 9.18**.

The ASA and PSA give rise to surface vessels that form a ring (vasa corona) around the spinal cord. Vessels from this ring penetrate the spinal cord, but the ASA and PSA send penetrating vessels into the interior of the spinal cord as well (**Fig. 9.18**).

The largest penetrating vessels are the central arteries that are branches of the ASA. These enter the spinal cord through the anterior median fissure, and they also give off longitudinal branches. There are reported to be 200–240 central arteries, 45–60 in the cervical area, 50–80 in the thoracic area, 35 or more in the lumbar region, and approximately 28 in the sacral region (for a review, see Sliwa J and I Maclean (1992) (*43*)).

Spinal Perfusion Varies Along the Spinal Cord. The blood supply to the spinal cord from the anterior medullary arteries varies along the spinal cord. To describe this variation, the spinal cord has been divided into three different regions (*45*):

1. The cervicodorsal area, caudally from T_2 or T_3. This area is richly supplied with blood from three to five medullary arteries.

2. The intermediate zone from T_4 to T_7 or T_8. This area is poorly vascularized with only one medullary artery, or occasionally none.

3. The dorsolumbar region of the spinal cord is the part that is caudal to T8. A large artery, the Great Artery of Adamkiewicz, the arteria radicularis magna (ARM), is the main supply of blood to this area, although as many as three other vessels can reach the area. The ARM is the largest vessel to reach the spinal cord, and it supplies one-fourth of the cord in 50% of individuals (for a review, see (*43*)).

Spinal perfusion includes not only discrete arteries, but also an arterial plexus (*46*). In addition, a capillary system supplies nerve fibers and ganglion cells in the gray and white matter of the spinal cord.

Spinal blood supply resembles that of a plexus. The demand for spinal cord perfusion varies along the spinal cord, and the perfusion depends on the degree of collateral flow. Centrifugal perfusion is more directed toward the anterior gray cell column and less posterior. At the thoracic level of the spinal cord, centrifugal perfusion projects further posterior, while centrifugal perfusion at the cervical and

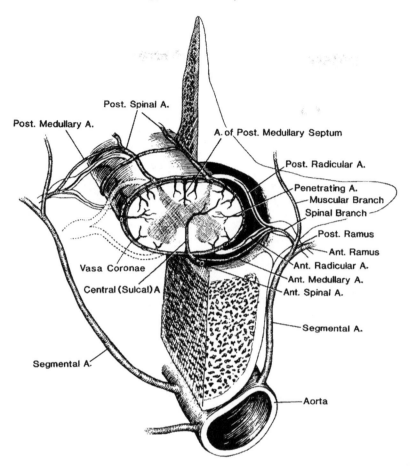

Figure 9.18: A more detailed illustration of the arterial supply to the spinal cord. (Reprinted from: (*43*) with permission from Elsevier).

lumbar levels is more directed toward anterior gray cell column and less posterior. The blood supply to the corticospinal tract is more vulnerable at thoracic levels because blood is not directed anteriorly.

Individual Variations. Anterior and posterior medullary arteries show great variability, and the number of each and the volume of blood they supply to the spinal cord may not be equal. The degeneration that occurs after specific lesions of vessels that supply blood to the spinal cord varies. It is not possible to provide all individual variations that are known, but two examples are shown below in **Fig. 9.20**.

Examples of variations that may have been caused at least partly by individual variations in the specimens that were studied by different investigators are illustrated in **Fig. 9.19**. There are also age-related changes in the blood supply such as the decrease in the number of collateral vessels, which can limit the extent to which blood vessels can be scarified without causing damage (ischemia).

The centrifugal arterial system that is composed of branches of the sulcal arteries (SA) supplies the central areas of the spinal cord. The peripheral white matter is supplied by the PSAs and the pial arteries (PA) (*46*). The shaded areas in **Fig. 9.19** show the overlap or "watershed zone" between the centrifugal and centripetal

Turnbull

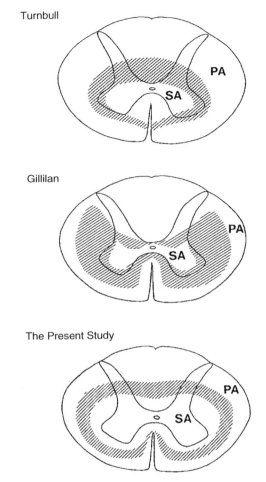

Gillilan

The Present Study

Figure 9.19: Illustrations of how the descriptions of the patterns of arterial supply vary as described by different authors who studied degenerations that followed vascular lesions of the spinal cord. The *shaded areas* show the extent of degeneration that occurs after vascular lesions to the spinal cord. (Reprinted from: (*46*) with permission from the Journal of Neurosurgery).

arterial systems. The three figures are from three different studies, and the difference in the results regarding the pattern of arterial supply between different authors is apparent.

Veins

In connection with operations upon the spine and the spinal cord, veins are important for two reasons: they bleed easily, and obstruction of veins causing venous congestion and swelling of the spinal cord is a serious threat to the spinal cord. Anatomically, veins do not follow arteries in the spinal cord as is common in other places of the body, and this fact is another important difference between blood circulation in the spinal cord and that in many other places of the body.

While the arterial supply to the spinal cord is delivered through three vessels, there are only two unpaired veins: the anterior central veins and the posterior central veins (*43*), which together drain the interior of the spinal cord.

The anterior central veins are twice as numerous as the anterior central arteries and, together with intrinsic veins, drain blood from the spinal cord. The anterior system provides the main drainage from the spinal cord, but it is not capable to drain all blood from the spinal cord.

The posterior central veins drain structures that are located adjacent to the median septum. The posterior vein is the largest of the posterior central veins, and it communicates with the radicular veins at the neck and ends where the spinal cord ends. Radicular veins that are present at only certain segments of the spinal cord connect together these veins that lie within the pia.

The intrinsic peripheral venous system drains the remaining areas of the spinal cord (*43*) (**Fig. 9.20**). However, there are considerable individual variations of the venous drainage.

Blood from the spinal cord drains into the superior vena cava; blood from the intercostal veins drain into the superior vena cava via the unpaired and hemiazygos[4] system. Veins are different for the different segments (**Fig. 9.20**).

It is again worth pointing out that the blood vessels, and especially veins of the spinal cord, have large individual variations. There are likely to be surprises regarding which arteries can be

---

[4]Hemiazygos vein: formed by the merger of the left ascending lumbar vein with the left subcostal vein or a communication from the inferior vena cava, it pierces the left crus of the diaphragm, ascends along the left side of the bodies of the lower thoracic vertebrae, opposite the eighth vertebra, crosses the midline posterior to the aorta, thoracic duct, and esophagus and empties into the azygos vein, sometimes in common with the accessory hemiazygos vein.

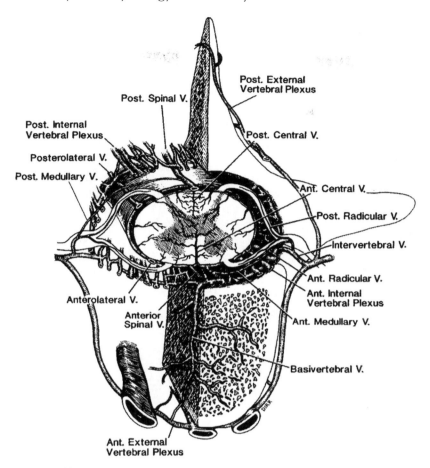

Post. Spinal V.

Post. External
Vertebral Plexus

Post. Internal
Vertebral Plexus

Post. Central V.

Posterolateral V.

Post. Medullary V.

Ant. Central V.

Post. Radicular V.

Intervertebral V.

Anterolateral V.

Ant. Radicular V.

Ant. Internal
Vertebral Plexus

Anterior
Spinal V.

Ant. Medullary V.

Basivertebral V.

Ant. External
Vertebral Plexus

Figure 9.20: Detailed picture of the veins that drain a segment of the spinal cord. (Reprinted from (*43*) with the permission from Elsevier).

clamped without risk of damage to the spine during operation on the spine. In particular, operating upon the spinal cord and obstructing or sacrificing a vein can cause dangerous venous congestion in the spinal cord. These variations are seldom known before the operations.

PHYSIOLOGY OF THE SPINAL MOTOR SYSTEM

The physiology of the lateral system is better known than that of the medial system. However, an obstacle to understanding the physiology of the lateral system is that this system is different in the animal species, from which much of our knowledge originates. Studies in humans made during surgical operations have contributed to our understanding of the physiology of these systems, and further use of neurophysiologic methods in connection with operations on the spinal cord can provide crucial information about the function of the spinal motor system.

DESCENDING ACTIVITY OF THE CORTICOSPINAL SYSTEM

Recording from the Spinal Cord

D and I Waves. Transcranial magnetic and electrical stimulation of the motor cortex can elicit responses in descending motor tracts that can be recorded from the surface of the spinal cord. Such recordings are useful in monitoring of the spinal cord. The responses to transcranial electrical and magnetic stimulation of the primary motor cortex, or direct stimulation of the cerebral cortex, consist of a series of distinct (negative) waves (*47–51*) that are often labeled D and I waves (**Fig. 9.21**). The "D" wave (direct wave) is generated by direct activation of descending pathways from the primary motor cortex. Studies in the monkey (**Fig. 9.2**) show that the I waves, or indirect waves, are assumed to be generated by successive activation of cortical neurons in deeper and deeper layers of the primary motor cortex. The D and I waves are

similar when elicited by transcranial electrical or magnetic stimulation, or when elicited by direct stimulation of the exposed motor cortex.

It has been hypothesized that (transcranially applied) electrical current impulses activate vertical fibers in the M1 cortex and generate D waves, while the subsequent activation of cells transynaptically in succession produces the I waves. The interval between I waves of approximately 1.5 ms can be explained by synaptic delay and conduction delay in the associated axons. The fact that frontally oriented electrode placement for transcranial stimulation (**Fig. 9.24**, anode at C_z-, cathode 6 cm frontal to C_z) favors generation of I waves has been explained by

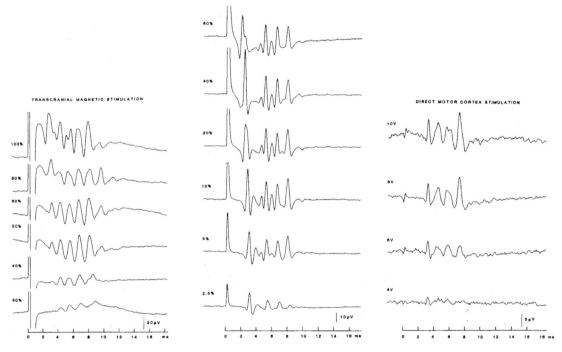

Figure 9.21: Effect of stimulus intensity on the response from the surface of the exposed spinal cord in a monkey to different forms of cortical stimulation. *Left hand column*: transcranial magnetic stimulation. *Middle hand column*: transcranial electrical stimulation. *Right hand column*: direct electrical stimulation of the exposed motor cortex. The responses were recorded from the spinal epidural space by a monopolar electrode placed on the dorsal surface of the dura at the T_{11} level. Negativity is shown as an upward deflection. (Reprinted from (*49*) with permission from Elsevier).

assuming that such orientation of the stimulating electrical field activates cortico-cortical projections of vertically oriented interneurons (*52*) (**Fig. 9.22**).

The effect of anesthesia on D and I waves differs. The primary response recorded from the corticospinal tract of the spinal cord (the "D" wave) in response to transcranial electrical or magnetic stimulation (*51*) is insensitive to common anesthetics, while anesthesia decreases the number of identifiable I waves (*54*), which supports the hypothesis that the I waves depend on synaptic transmission in cortical interneurons. The effect of anesthesia on the I waves can thus be explained by a change in synaptic efficacy. In deeply anesthetized animals or humans, the synaptic transmission in these vertically oriented axons to the cell bodies is abolished, and therefore, only the D waves are present in recordings from the spinal cord (see (*55, 56*)).

Several studies show that D waves are slightly affected by anesthesia, which is contrary to the hypothesis that the D waves are generated by stimulation of descending axons. Some investigators have reported that D waves are affected by anesthesia in a similar way as a decrease in stimulus intensity affects the amplitude of the D waves (54).

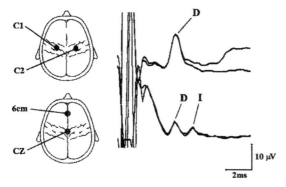

Figure 9.22: Effect of orientation of TES on D and I waves recorded from the upper thoracic spinal cord in an operation for a spinal tumor. C_1 and C_z were anodes. (Based on: (*50*) after (*53*). Reprinted with permission from Elsevier).

Another mechanism offered as to the effect of anesthesia on the D waves is that the effect is due to a change in the fluid space in the cortex rather than a change in synaptic efficacy. Deletis (57) has presented evidence that the effect of anesthesia on D waves is caused by vasodilatation that changes the electrical properties of the surroundings of the areas of the cerebral cortex that generate the D waves.

When electrical stimulation is applied to the exposed surface of the cortex, there is no noticeable effect of anesthesia on the D waves, which is in good agreement with the assumption that the D waves that are elicited by electrical stimulation of the motor cortex are in fact a result of stimulation of the axons that leave the cerebral cortex and begin the corticospinal tract. Electrical stimulation of axons is normally unaffected by anesthesia.

Responses recorded in conscious humans who had epidural electrodes placed at the C_1–C_2 spinal levels (*58*) or in operations for scoliosis in response to transcranial magnetic and electrical stimulation are similar (*50*). The direction of the induced current in the cortex (and thus, the position of the stimulating coil) affects the waveform of the recorded potentials (*52*). An example of recordings of D and I waves to TES in a patient operated upon for scoliosis is shown in **Fig. 9.23**.

Response from Muscles

Reduced facilitatory input to the spinal cord from sources in the brain is one of the reasons why it is necessary to use trains of impulses to elicit muscle responses from cortical stimulation in anesthetized individuals (see page 171) (*10*).

Stimulating the primary motor cortex with a single impulse in a conscious individual evokes activity in descending motor pathways that generate excitatory postsynaptic potentials (EPSP) that are sufficient to reach the threshold of alpha motoneurons. Single-pulse transcranial stimulation can, thus, elicit contractions of skeletal muscles in conscious individuals, but its effectiveness is diminished in patients under general (surgical)

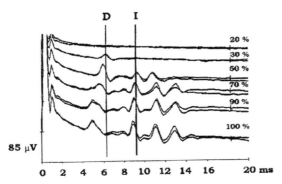

Figure 9.23: D and I waves recorded from the spinal cord in a 14-year-old child with idiopathic scoliosis. The stimuli were applied through electrodes placed at C_z and 6 cm anterior. 100% = 750 V (Reprinted from (*50*) after (*57*) with permission from Elsevier).

anesthesia (*55, 56, 59*). In the anesthetized (unconscious) individual, it is not possible to elicit a muscle contraction by a single magnetic impulse through transcranial magnetic stimulation (TMS) (*55*). The reason is assumed to be that the facilitation of alpha motoneurons that is normally present and necessary for activation of alpha motoneurons from the cerebral cortex and the spinal cord is suppressed by the agents used for the anesthesia.

In the conscious individual, facilitation of motoneurons is provided by descending pathways, such as the reticulospinal tract, that originate in the reticular formation of the brainstem and influence the excitability of spinal interneurons (see page 171). The NA–serotonin pathways also have facilitatory influence on alpha motoneurons.

The activity in these nonspecific pathways is sensitive to anesthetics because the pathways originate in structures in the brain that have long chains of neurons. The activity that produces the I waves probably also has facilitatory influence on alpha motoneurons. The I waves are also depressed by anesthetics (*55, 56*). In the anesthetized individual, the EPSP elicited by a single impulse are, therefore, not sufficient to reach the threshold of alpha motoneurons because of a lack of such facilitation, but a lack

of normal facilitation can be compensated for by delivering several successive stimuli. The EPSP elicited by trains of stimuli can reach the threshold of alpha motoneurons through temporal summation despite the lack of normal facilitatory input to the neurons. Trains of stimuli are easier to generate by electrical transcranial stimulation than by magnetic stimulation (see Chap. 18).

Common anesthetics do not affect the function of muscle endplates noticeably. Therefore, it is not assumed that common anesthetics contribute to the depression of muscle responses as is evident from the fact that muscle contractions (and EMG responses) can be elicited by electrical stimulation of motor nerves in surgically anesthetized (but not paralyzed) patients.

BRAINSTEM CONTROL OF MOTOR ACTIVITY

The importance of facilitatory input to the alpha motoneurons has been discussed in other places of this chapter. The reticular formation of the brainstem plays a central role in controlling muscle tone and exciting spinal motoneurons and the alpha motoneurons. This influence is mainly mediated in the spinal cord through the reticulospinal tract, which originates in the brainstem. This system enables brainstem structure to control the excitability of spinal motoneurons and interneurons. While too much activity from the reticular activating system in the conscious individual causes hyper-excitability and hyperactivity, too little activation results in difficulties in eliciting muscle responses from the cerebral motor cortices such as is experienced in the anesthetized individuals (see page 182).

Central Control of Muscle Tone and Excitability

The effect of normal facilitation from high brain centers on the excitability of motor systems can be demonstrated in the conscious individual. The response to single stimuli of the motor cortices using TMS can be modulated by an individual's

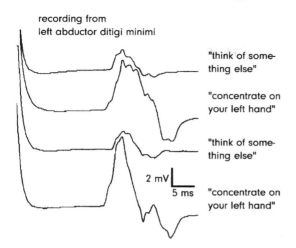

recording from
left abductor ditigi minimi

"think of some-
thing else"

"concentrate on
your left hand"

"think of some-
thing else"

2 mV

5 ms   "concentrate on
your left hand"

Figure 9.24: Illustration of facilitatory and inhibitory influence from the conscious brain on the response of a muscle in the hand of a conscious human individual to transcranial magnetic stimulation of the motor cortex showing EMG recordings from muscles in the hand. (Reprinted from: (*60*) with permission from the American Physiological Society).

attention to the muscles that are activated (*60*) (**Fig. 9.24**). The amplitude of the recorded EMG response increases when the subject "thinks of the hand," while the amplitude decreases when the subject "thinks of something else."

Activation of the corticospinal system by stimulation of the motor cortex does not involve processing in the cortex. The observed, increased excitability must, therefore, be caused by increased excitability of the alpha motoneurons. This study, thus, shows that the excitability of the alpha motoneurons is affected by descending signals from high CNS centers.

Spinal Control of Muscle Excitability

The observed effect, changing the attention can change the muscle response elicited by

cortical stimulation (**Fig. 9.24**), demonstrates clearly how activity from high CNS structures (including mental activity) can modulate the excitability of motor systems. A somewhat different example of facilitation of spinal motor activity is the familiar "Jendrassik maneuver"[5] where a spinal reflex (monosynaptic stretch reflex) is modulated (enhanced) by voluntary contraction of muscles that are innervated from different spinal segments. This is an example of how activity in one segment of the spinal cord can affect the function of different and distant spinal segments. That the facilitation is accomplished in the spinal cord and not the brain is evident from the finding that the D wave recorded from the surface of the spinal cord is not affected from the activation of the muscles by CNS structures that provide facilitation. On the contrary, the brain is involved in fatigue that causes reduced muscle contraction strength as indicated by the finding that the D wave is reduced as are EMG and I waves.

It has, thus, been clearly demonstrated in different kinds of experiments that a multitude of factors can influence the excitability of alpha motoneurons (*34, 61, 62*).

THE VALUE OF ANIMAL STUDIES

A large part of our knowledge about the function of the spinal motor systems and the processing that occurs in the spinal cord is based on studies in animals such as the cat. The cat, however, has only a few corticospinal fibers, mostly located in the neck. The results of some of these studies performed in cats are, therefore, not representative for humans. Intraoperative recordings that can be performed together with monitoring are important for increasing our understanding of the function of these systems in humans. Early work by

---

[5] The Jendrassik maneuver is used clinically to increase the excitability of lower extremity stretch reflexes. Practically, the patient is asked to hook the hands together by the flexed fingers and strongly pull against them while the monosynaptic stretch reflex is activated by tapping on the patella tendon or by stimulating a peripheral nerve to elicit the H-reflex.

Penfield (*1, 7*) has paved the way for such studies.

DISORDERS AND ABNORMALITIES IN MOTOR SYSTEMS

Lesions in the adult motor nervous system (like that in any other part of the central nervous system) can cause changes in the function in many other structures either directly through anatomical connections, or indirectly through activation of neural plasticity (*10*). The PMA and SMA share many connections with M1 and project to the spinal cord through the corticospinal pathways, and they play an important role in recovery from lesions that affect the M1 and its corticospinal projections. Premotor areas have a potential to take over functions normally carried out by M1 (*63*). While activation of neural plasticity mainly serves beneficial roles, it can also cause explicit maladaptive processes (*10*). An example is spasticity (see page 281) that often develops after spinal cord injuries and is regarded as a result of activation of neural plasticity by the decreased activity in injured structures.

Trauma to the spinal cord is a common cause of disorders of motor systems. Traumatic injury to the brain and stokes are additional common causes of problems related to the motor system, in the form of pareses, paralysis, and spasm.

Malformations of the spinal motor nervous system, such as abnormal organization of descending pathways, have also been reported (*27*).

Disorders Related to the Basal Ganglia and Their Treatment

The basal ganglia are associated with movement disorders such as Parkinson's disease, Huntington's disease, Gilles de la Tourette's Syndrome (*64, 65*), and probably several other disorders such as blepharospasm. Parkinson's disease was the first disease where the treatment was directed to the basal ganglia, first by surgically made lesions, then by medications such as l-dopa, and now by electrical stimulation by implanted electrode. While it is true that medications at one time supplanted the lesioning treatment for the disease, it was found that these medications lost their effectiveness after continued use, and surgical methods in the form of lesions in specific parts of the basal ganglia again came into use. Technology had advanced since lesioning was first introduced, and by this time, stereotactic techniques that could be used to place the lesions more exactly had been developed. Later, lesions were replaced by electrical stimulation applied through implanted electrodes, and this method became the most common way of surgical treatment of Parkinson's disease in patients who no longer received a beneficial effect from medications. The technique is known as DBS, and it is now in routine use for treatment of not only patients with Parkinson's disease, but also patients with other movement disorders such as Tourette's syndrome. Using appropriate stimulus parameters, the technique of electrical stimulation can produce a similar effect as making lesions.

While lesions or implantation of electrodes for DBS can be made using stereotactic techniques alone, it is advantageous to use electrophysiologic guidance (intraoperative neurophysiology) for placement of the electrodes (see Chap. 15).

Pathologies of the Basal Ganglia

Degeneration of dopamine-producing cells in the SNc has for a long time been assumed to play the major role in producing the typical symptoms of Parkinson's disease (Fig. 9.25). The subsequent re-routing of information in the basal ganglia is assumed to cause the bradykinesia (slow movements), tremor, and postural instability that are the classical signs of Parkinson's disease. Patients with Parkinson's disease have other, more complex symptoms, such as "freezing," and some have cognitive deficits, which indicates that the pathology localized to the basal ganglia cannot explain all the symptoms of the disease and that different individuals have different symptoms.

There is evidence that many factors are involved in the pathogenesis of Parkinson's disease.

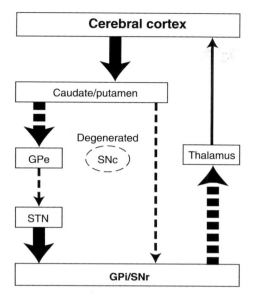

Figure 9.25: Basal ganglia in Parkinson's disease (Reprinted from (*10*) with the permission of Cambridge University Press).

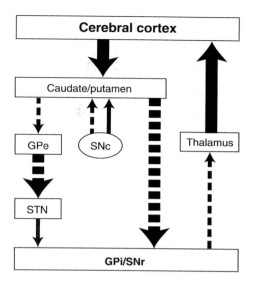

Figure 9.26: Basal ganglia in Huntington's chorea. (Reprinted from (*10*) with permission from Cambridge University Press).

Hereditary factors and oxidative stress are probably implicated. Neurotoxicity by the neurotransmitter glutamate also likely contributes to the development of the disease (66). Age is the major risk factor for Parkinson's disease, and patients with Parkinson's disease often have other typical age-related neurological disorders (67). The involvement of neural plasticity (10) has, however, been mostly ignored in forming hypotheses about the pathologies of Parkinson's disease. The fact that training of various kinds has now been found to be beneficial (68) in reducing the symptoms and signs of Parkinson's disease supports the hypothesis that expression of neural plasticity is involved in creating the symptoms and signs of Parkinson's disease, and that brain chemicals other than dopamine may be involved. For example, the beneficial effect of physical exercise may be achieved because of the increase in the brain-derived neurotrophic factor BDNF (69).

Huntington's disease is a progressive, neurodegenerative disorder clinically characterized by chorea, cognitive decline, and a poor prognosis. Anatomically, the abnormalities primarily affect the caudate nucleus and the putamen (Fig. 9.26). Although individuals with Huntington's disease have massive degeneration in these nuclei, the substantia nigra does not seem to be affected, and this explains why the clinical manifestations of these two disorders (Huntington's disease and Parkinson's disease) of the basal ganglia are substantially different. The excitatory input from the thalamus to the cortex, which is decreased in Parkinson's disease, is increased in Huntington's disease (66). The globus pallidus is often affected in Huntington's disease, but not in Parkinson's disease.

Studies have shown that the input to the striatum from the SNc is unaffected in Huntington's disease, but that inhibition from the striatum on the GPe is decreased because the indirect pathway degenerates, and inhibition on the STN from GPe is increased, at least in the early stages of the disease. The excitation from both the STN to SNr and to the medial segment of the GPi (MGP) is decreased, while it is increased in Parkinson's disease. In Huntington's disease, inhibition on the thalamus from the MGP and SNr is decreased, while it is increased in Parkinson's disease.

In later stages, neurons in the striatum that project to the GPi also degenerate as do many other cells in the brain. Other areas of the CNS become affected as the disease progresses and neuronal loss occurs in the cerebral cortex, mainly affecting layers III, V, and VI, confirming that Huntington's disease is a more general neurodegenerative disease than if it were produced by changes in the basal ganglia only. Increase in thalamic excitation of the cortex is assumed to be the cause of the increased, and often inappropriate, motor activities that are characteristic for patients with Huntington's disease (70).

Much less is known about the pathophysiology of Gilles de la Tourette's syndrome (64, 65), which is a movement disorder (often classified as a neuropsychiatric disorder) that is characterized by sudden, rapid, and recurrent movements (tics). Individuals with this disorder also have other symptoms such as uttering of odd and inappropriate sounds (coprolalia). It is believed that abnormalities within the cortico-striato-palido-thalamic circuit contribute to these symptoms.

Recently, some patients with Tourette's syndrome have been treated successfully using DBS (bilateral thalamic stimulation), which reversed the symptoms (71).

The increased interest in treatments that involve surgical interventions of specific parts of nuclei of the basal ganglia and the thalamus has resulted in a need to better understand the function of the basal ganglia and their anatomy. The use of electrophysiologic methods in connection with placement of stimulating electrodes for DBS has provided many research opportunities, and in fact, much of our current understanding of the role of the basal ganglia in motor control has been gained from studies in patients with Parkinson's disease and other motor disorders, who were treated either by making lesions in the basal ganglia or by implantation of electrodes in specific parts of these nuclei using DBS (see for example work by Fred Lenz and co-workers (72) and by T. Hashimoto (73)). Such research has also led to a more differentiated view of the role of these ganglia in movement control and movement disorders.

Stimulation of Structures Other Than the Basal Ganglia for Motor Diseases

Although it is established knowledge that the basal ganglia are involved in generation of symptoms and signs of motor disorders such as

Parkinson's disease, Tourette's syndrome, and Huntington's chorea, it has recently become evident that electrical stimulation of structures other than the basal ganglia can alleviate symptoms from disorders in which the pathology is assumed to be located near the basal ganglia. For example, it has been shown that electrical stimulation of the motor cortex can alleviate some of the symptoms of Parkinson's disease (74–76), and animal experiments have shown indications that epidural spinal stimulation of the dorsal column of the spinal cord can alleviate some symptoms in dopamine-depleted mice, thus a model of Parkinson's disease (77).

ORGANIZATION OF CRANIAL MOTOR NERVE SYSTEMS

Cranial Motonuclei

Cranial nerves III, IV, V, VI, VII, XI, and XII have large motor parts, and CN IX sends a minor motor part to innervate a muscle involved in swallowing, the stylopharyngeus muscle of the head. Cranial nerves X and XI also innervate muscles in the neck and the upper body.

The motor cortices send information to the brainstem motonuclei through the corticobulbar tract (also known as the corticonuclear fibers (78)). The corticobulbar tract branches from the corticospinal tract (also earlier known as the pyramidal tract). In this way, cranial nerve nuclei in the pons of the brainstem receive information from the motor cortices (M1, SMA, and PMA) and sensory cortices.

Unlike skeletal muscles innervated by the spinal cord, the nuclei that innervate the mastication muscles (CN V) have bilateral cortical innervation, and that is also the case for the part of CN VII that innervates the forehead. The part of the nucleus of CN VIII that innervates the mimic muscles of the middle and lower face and the tongue receives crossed fibers from the motor cortices. CN VI and CN XII also receive only contralateral (crossed) innervation from motor cortices. The part of CN XI that innervates the sternocleidomastoid muscle receives ipsilateral cortical innervation only. The motor nuclei of the tectum (CN III and CN IV) do not receive direct input from the motor cortices, but receive their cortical signal via the abducens (CN VI) nucleus (*78*).

REFERENCES

1. Penfield W and E Boldrey (1937) Somatic motor and sensory representation in the cerebral cortex of man as studied by electrical stimulation. Brain 60:389–443.
2. Kuypers HGJM (1981) Anatomy of the descending pathways, in *Handbook of physiology-the nervous system*, JM Brookhart and VB Mountcastle, Editors. American Physiological Society: Bethesda, MD. 597–666.
3. Brodal P (2004) The Central Nervous System Third Edition. 2004, New York: Oxford University Press.
4. Dum R and P Strick (1991) The origin of corticospinal projections from the premotor areas in the frontal lobe. J Neurosci 11:667–89.
5. Dum R and P Strick (2002) Motor areas in the frontal lobe of the primate. Physiol Behav 77:677–82.
6. Lotze M, P Sauseng and M Staudt (2009) Functional relevance of ipsilateral motor activation in congenital hemiparesis as tested by fMRI-navigated TMS. Exp Neurol 217:440–3.
7. Penfield W and T Rasmussen (1950) The cerebral cortex of man: a clinical study of localization of function. New York: Macmillan.
8. Penfield W and K Welch (1951) The supplementary motor area of the cerebral cortex. Arch Neurol Psychiatry 66:289–316.
9. Woolsey CN, PH Settlage, DR Meyer et al (1951) Patterns of localization in precentral and "supplementary" motor areas and their relation to the concept of a premotor area. Res Pub Assoc Res Nerv Ment Dis 30:238–64.
10. Møller AR (2006) Neural plasticity and disorders of the nervous system. 2006, Cambridge: Cambridge University Press.
11. Elbert T, C Pantev, C Wienbruch et al (1995) Increased cortical representation of the fingers of the left hand in string players. Science 270:305–7.
12. Meyerson BA, U Lindblom, B Linderoth et al (1993) Motor cortex stimulation as treatment of trigeminal neuropathic pain. Acta Neurochir Suppl 58:105–3.
13. Kandel ER, JH Schwartz and TM Jessell (2008) Principles of Neural Science. New York: Oxford University Press.
14. Kretchmann HJ and W Weinrich (1999) Neurofunctional Systems. Thieme: New York.
15. Shils JL, M Tagliati and RL Alterman, (2002) Neurophysiological monitoring during neurosurgery for movement disorders, in *Neurophysiology in Neurosurgery*, V Deletis and JL Shils, Editors. Academic Press: Amsterdam. 405–48.
16. Alexander GE, MD Crutcher and MR DeLong (1990) Basal ganglia-thalamocortical circuits: parallel substrates for motor, oculomotor, "prefrontal" and "limbic" functions. Progr Brain Res 85:119–46.
17. Yoshida M, A Rabin and A Anderson (1972) Monosynaptic inhibition of pallidal neurons by axon collaterals of caudatonigral fibers. Exp Brain Res 15:33–347.
18. Albin RL, AB Young and JB Penney (1989) The functional anatomy of basal ganglia origin. Trends Neurosci 12:366–75.
19. Wiesendanger M, (1981) The pyramidal tract. its structure and function., in *Handbook of behavioral neurobiology*, AL Towe and ES Luschei, Editors. Plenum: New York. 401–90.
20. Alexander GE and MD Crutcher (1990) Functional architecture of basal ganglia circuits: neural substrate of parallel processing. Trends Neurosci 13:266–71.
21. Pennartz C, B JD, G AM et al (2009) Corticostriatal interactions during learning, memory processing, and decision making. J Neurosci 29:12831–8.
22. Strick P, R Dum and J Fiez (2009) Cerebellum and nonmotor function. Annu Rev Neurosci 32:413–34.
23. Sacchetti B, B Scelfo and P Strata (2009) Cerebellum and emotional behavior. Neuroscience 162:756–62.
24. Schieber MH (2007) Comparative anatomy and physiology of the corticospinal system. Handb Clin Neurol 82:15–37.
25. Ralston DD and HJr Ralston (1985) The terminations of corticospinal tract axons in the macaque monkey. J Comp Neurol 242:325–37.
26. Spampinato M, J Kraas, B Maria et al (2008) Absence of decussation of the superior cerebellar peduncles in patients with Joubert syndrome. Am J Med Genet A 146:1389–94.

27. MacDonald D, L Streletz, Z Al-Zayed et al (2004) Intraoperative neurophysiologic discovery of uncrossed sensory and motor pathways in a patient with horizontal gaze palsy and scoliosis. Clin Neurophysiol 115:576–82.

28. Porter R and R Lemon (1993) Cortical function and voluntary movement. Oxford: Clarendon Press.

29. White SR and RS Neuman (1980) Facilitation of spinal motoneuron by 5-hydroxytryptamine and noradrenaline. Brain Res 185:1–9.

30. Davis M (1992) The role of the amygdala in fear and anxiety. Ann Rev Neurosci 15:353–75.

31. Andersen P, PJ Hagan, CG Phillips et al (1975) Mapping by microstimulation of overlapping projections from area 4 to motor units of the baboon's hand. Proc R Soc London ser B 188:31–60.

32. Humphrey DR and WS Corrie (1978) Properties of pyramidal tract neuron system within functionally defined subregion of primate motor cortex. J Neurophys 41:216–43.

33. Brodal P (1998) The central nervous system. New York: Oxford Press.

34. Burke D (1988) Spasticity as an adaptation to pyramidal tract injury, in *Functional Recovery in Neurological Disease*, SG Waxman, Editor. Raven Press: New York.

35. Pierrot-Deseilligny E (2002) Propriospinal transmission of part of the corticospinal excitation in humans. Muscle & Nerve 26:155–72.

36. Nicolas G, V Marchand-Pauvert, D Burke et al (2001) Corticospinal excitation of presumed cervical propriospinal neurons and its reversal to inhibition in humans. J Physiol 533:903–19.

37. Murg M, H Binder and M Dimitrijevic (2000) Epidural electric stimulation of posterior structures of the human lumbar spinal cord: 1. Muscle twitches – a functional method to define the site of stimulation. Spinal Cord 38:394–402.

38. Minassian K, I Persy, F Rattay et al (2007) Human lumbar cord circuitries can be activated by extrinsic tonic input to generate locomotor-like activity. Hum Mov Sci 26:275–95.

39. Frigon A and S Rossignol (2006) Functional plasticity following spinal cord lesions. Prog Brain Res 157:231–60.

40. Sindou M and P Mertens (2002) Selective spinal cord procedures for spasticity and pain, in *Neurophysiology in Neurosurgery*, V Deletis and JL Shils, Editors. Academic Press: Amsterdam. 93–117.

41. Sindou M and D Jeanmonod (1989) Microsurgical-DREZ-otomy for treatment of spasticity and pain in the lower limbs. Neurosurgery 24:655–70.

42. Benarroch EE, JR Daube, KD Flemming et al (2008) Mayo Clinic Medical Neurosciences, 5th edn, Mayo Foundation, Rochester, Minnesota.

43. Sliwa J and I Maclean (1992) Ischemic myelopathy: a review of spinal vasculature and related clinical syndromes. Arch Phys Med Rehabil 73:365–72.

44. Krauss WE (1999) Vascular anatomy of the spinal cord. Neurosurg Clin N Am 10:9–15.

45. Garland H, J Greenberg and D Harriman (1966) Infarction of the spinal cord. Brain 89:645–62.

46. Tator C and I Koyanagi (1997) Vascular mechanisms in the pathophysiology of human spinal cord injury. J Neurosurg 86:483–92.

47. Edgeley SA, JA Eyre, R Lemon et al (1990) Excitation of the corticospinal tract by electromagnetic and electrical stimulation of the scalp in the macaque monkey. J Physiol 425:301–20.

48. Amassian VE, GJ Quirk and M Stewart (1990) A comparison of corticospinal activation by magnetic coil and electrical stimulation of monkey motor cortex. Electroenceph Clin Neurophys 77:390–401.

49. Kitagawa H and AR Møller (1994) Conduction pathways and generators of magnetic evoked spinal cord potentials: a study in monkeys. Electroenceph Clin Neurophys 93:57–67.

50. Deletis V (2002) Intraoperative neurophysiology and methodologies used to monitor the functional integrity of the motor system, in *Neurophysiology in Neurosurgery*, V Deletis and JL Shils, Editors. Academic Press: Amsterdam. 25–51.

51. Amassian VE, (2002) Animal and human motor system neurophysiology related to intraoperative monitoring, in *Neurophysiology in Neurosurgery*, V Deletis and JL Shils, Editors. Academic Press: Amsterdam. 3–23.

52. Kaneko K, S Kawai, Y Fuchigami et al (1966) The effect of current direction induced by transcranial magnetic stimulation on corticospinal excitability in human brain. Electroenceph Clin Neurophys 101:478–82.

53. Maccabee PJ, VE Amassian, P Zimann et al, (1999) Emerging application in neuromagnetic stimualtion, in *Comprehensive clinical neurophsysiology*, K Levin and H Luders, Editors. W.B. Saunders: Philadelphia. 325–47.

54. Hicks R, D Burke, J Stephen et al (1992) Corticospinal volleys evoked by electrical

stimulation of human motor cortex after withdrawal of volatile anaesthetics. J Physiol 456:293–404.

55. Sloan T (2002) Anesthesia and motor evoked potential monitoring, in *Neurophysiology in Neurosurgery*, V Deletis and JL Shils, Editors. Elsevier Science: Amsterdam. 451–74.

56. Sloan TB and EJ Heyer (2002) Anesthesia for intraoperative neurophysiologic monitoring of the spinal cord. J Clin Neurophysiol 19:430–43.

57. Deletis V (1993) Intraoperative monitoring of the functional integrety of the motor pathways, in *Advances in neurology: Electrical and magnetic stimulation of the brain*, O Devinsky, A Beric and M Dogali, Editors. Raven Press: New York. 201–14.

58. Lazzaro Di V, A Oliviero, F Pilato et al (2003) Corticospinal volleys evoked by transcranial stimulation of the brain in concious humans. Neurol Res 25:143–50.

59. Barker AT, R Jalinous and IL Freeston (1985) Non-invasive magnetic stimulation of the human motor cortex. Lancet 1:1106–7.

60. Rösler KM (2001) Transcranial magnetic brain stimulation: a tool to investigate central motor pathways. News Physiol Sci 16:297–302.

61. Jankowska E and A Lundberg (1981) Interneurons in the spinal cord. Trends Neurosci 4:230–3.

62. Wolpaw JR and JA O'Keefe (1984) Adaptive plasticity in the primate spinal stretch reflex: evidence of a two-phase process. J Neuro Sci 4:2718–24.

63. Dancause N (2006) Vicarious function of remote cortex following stroke: recent evidence from human and animal studies. Neuroscientist 12:489–99.

64. Ackermans L, Y Temel and V Visser-Vandewalle (2008) Deep brain stimulation in Tourette's Syndrome. Neurotherapeutics 5:339–44.

65. Jankovic J (1993) Tics in other neurological disorders, in *Handbook of Tourette's Syndrome and Related Tic and Behavioral Disorders*, R Kurlan, Editor. Marcel Dekker: New York. 167–82.

66. Blandini F, C Tassorelli and JT Greenamyre, (1997) Movement disorders, in *Principle of Neural Aging*, SU Dani, A Hori and GF Walter, Editors. Elsevier: Amsterdam.

67. Bennett DA, LA Beckett, AM Murray et al (1996) Prevalence of parkinsonian signs and associated mortality in a community population of older people. N Engl J Med 334:71–6.

68. Hirsch MA and BG Farley (2009) Exercise and neuroplasticity in persons living with Parkinson's disease. Eur J Phys Rehabil Med 45:215–29.

69. Gómez-Pinilla F, Z Ying, RR Roy et al (2002) Voluntary exercise induces a BDNF-mediated mechanism that promotes neuroplasticity. J Neurophysiol 88:2187–95.

70. DeLong MR (1990) Primate models of movement disorders of basal ganglia origin. Trends Neurosci 13:281–85.

71. Temel Y and V Visser-Vandewalle (2004) Surgery in Tourette syndrome. Mov Disord 19:3–14.

72. Hua S, SG Reich, AT Zirh et al (1998) The role of the thalamus and basal ganglia in parkinsonian tremor. Mov Disord 13:40–2.

73. Hashimoto T (2000) Neuronal activity in the globus pallidus in primary dystonia and off-period dystonia. J Neurol 247 Suppl 5:V49–52.

74. Lefaucheur JP (2009) Treatment of Parkinson's disease by cortical stimulation. Expert Rev Neurother 9:1755–71.

75. Arle J, D Apetauerova, J Zani et al (2008) Motor cortex stimulation in patients with Parkinson disease: 12-month follow-up in 4 patients. J Neurosurg 109:133–9.

76. Cioni B, M Meglio, V Perotti et al (2007) Neurophysiological aspects of chronic motor cortex stimulation. Neurophysiol Clin 37(6):441–7.

77. Fuentes R, P Petersson, W Siesser et al (2009) Spinal cord stimulation restores locomotion in animal models of Parkinson's disease. Science 323:1578–82.

78. Schuenke M, E Schulte and U Schumacher (2007) Thieme atlas of anatomy. head and neuroanatomy, in LM Ross, ED Lamperti and E Taub Editors. Stuttgart, New York: Thieme.

10

Practical Aspects of Monitoring Spinal Motor Systems

From: *Intraoperative Neurophysiological Monitoring: Third Edition*
By A.R. Møller, DOI 10.1007/978-1-4419-7436-5_10,
© Springer Science+Business Media, LLC 2011

INTRODUCTION

This chapter concerns practical aspects of monitoring spinal motor systems (monitoring of cranial motor nerves is discussed in Chap. 11). It discusses techniques for stimulation of the motor cortex and the spinal cord, and for recording of transcranial motor evoked potentials (Tc-MEP).

The traditional method for intraoperative monitoring of the function of the spinal cord has been to record somatosensory evoked potentials (SSEP), as described in Chap. 6. The sensory pathways that are monitored by recording SSEP occupy the dorsal and lateral portions of the spinal cord, while the motor pathways occupy the ventral portion (see Chap. 9). The ventral portion of the spinal cord has a different blood supply than the dorsal portion of the spinal cord. The motor tracts can, therefore, be injured without the sensory pathways being affected. This means that monitoring of the SSEP does not detect changes in the function of the ventral (motor) part of the spinal cord, and the descending motor tracts can be injured without causing any changes in the SSEP. It is, therefore, important to monitor spinal motor systems (using MEP recording) during operations in which the spinal cord is at risk of being manipulated.

Technical difficulties, mainly related to producing a satisfactory activation of the motor tracts of the spinal cord in an anesthetized patient, have delayed the general use of monitoring of spinal motor systems. Recent developments of techniques for transcranial electrical stimulation (TES) and TMS of the motor cortex and the design of suitable anesthetic techniques have made it easier to activate spinal motor systems in anesthetized individuals. These techniques have provided the basis for general and practical use of intraoperative monitoring of spinal motor systems. Monitoring of SSEP is, however, still used, and it is necessary for reducing the risks of injury to the dorsal part of the spinal cord in operations where the spinal cord is being manipulated. This

means that both motor and sensory monitoring must be done in operations where the spinal cord is at risk of being injured.

Before monitoring of the motor pathways became technically possible and only SSEP were monitored, it was reported that the risk of injury to the motor portion of the spinal cord was low if SSEP monitoring was combined with selective wake-up tests (1). These techniques came into sporadic use in the 1970s, mostly at university hospitals and large clinical centers. Widespread use of this method did not occur until the 1990s. The reason for the success of SSEP monitoring in reducing the risk of motor deficits may be that these early investigators were sensitive to small reversible changes in the SSEP that often occur when the motor pathways are injured. Such functional changes in the sensory part of the spinal cord when the motor parts are injured may be explained by the fact that changes in function of one part of the spinal cord can spread throughout the spinal cord as a "spinal shock." The SSEP responses, however, normalize after a short period giving the false impression of improvement.

Now, it is common to monitor both SSEP and motor systems in operations where the spinal cord is at risk of being injured. For monitoring the motor system, the focus has been on the corticospinal system (lateral system), while monitoring of the medial system (see Chap. 9) is performed only sporadically. While there is no doubt that introduction of intraoperative monitoring in operations where there is risk of injury to the spinal cord has reduced the occurrence of such complications as paraplegia, it is difficult to determine exactly the percentage decrease of this risk. The reason is mainly that the incidence of permanent deficits associated with operations on the spine and spinal cord that occurred before the introduction of any form of monitoring was used is not known. Be that as it may, SSEP-only monitoring has been estimated to decrease complications by 50–60% (2). Another obstacle in obtaining valid assessment of the benefit from monitoring is that it is not possible to use the commonly used methods for assessment of gain from medical treatment, namely, randomized controlled trials. This method was deemed unethical because of the known benefits of these monitoring techniques (see Chap. 19).

In addition to SSEP and Tc-MEP monitoring techniques, Vedran Deletis and Ron Leppanen have described more complex methods for monitoring the spinal cord, such as the use of collision techniques (3–5) (see also (6, 7)) and the use of lower extremity muscle reflexes such as the H-reflex and F-response (8, 9).

Electrical stimulation of the spinal cord has been described for monitoring motor systems. However, it may activate pathways other than the motor pathways, such as sensory systems, and this type of monitoring is, therefore, not a monitor of pure motor systems alone. Conventional methods for monitoring motor systems also exclude unconscious proprioception that is essential for normal control of movements. Loss of the function of this system can have severe consequences regarding normal movements such as walking and keeping posture.

This chapter discusses practical aspects of monitoring the motor system of the spinal cord using electrical or magnetic stimulation (TES and TMS) of the motor cortex. Monitoring of muscle reflexes, which is sensitive to changes in the function of several parts of the spinal cord, will also be discussed in this chapter.

MONITORING THE CORTICOSPINAL SYSTEM

Transcranial magnetic or electrical stimulation of the motor cortex is now the most common method used for activating the primary motor cortices for monitoring the motor portion of the spinal cord (10). It must, however, be kept in mind that the anatomical pathways involved during monitoring of Tc-MEP, when accomplished in the conventional way by recording from muscles of the distal limbs, are the lateral motor systems (11) (see Chap. 9). This type of monitoring leaves the system that

innervates the muscles of the proximal limbs and muscles of the trunk essentially unmonitored (the medial system). Injuries to the parts of the spinal cord that control these muscles can, therefore, occur without any changes in the response of the corticospinal system; as yet, the clinical significance of this fact has not been explored. It is known, however, that injury to the medial system can have devastating consequences.

TRANSCRANIAL STIMULATION OF THE MOTOR PATHWAYS

Monitoring of Tc-MEP is a non-invasive method that makes use of either electrical impulses applied through electrodes placed on the scalp (TES) or by strong magnetic impulses (TMS). Transcranial stimulation of the motor cortex was described many years ago (12–14), and TES was, in fact, first described by Gualterotti and Paterson in 1954 (15). However, the use of these methods in the operating room is complicated by several factors; one of which is the effect of anesthesia (16, 17) and the considerable variation among patients (18). TES has now been perfected into a clinically reliable method for activating and monitoring motor pathways in operations where the spinal cord is at risk of being injured. (5, 10, 19, 20). TES is also employed in other operations where motor system activation is utilized in intraoperative monitoring.

With the advent of various types of anesthesia, there are now several anesthesia regimens available that help make the use of TES in the anesthetized patient possible (17) (see Chap. 16). TES is the preferred method for activating the motor system intraoperatively (5, 10, 21) because the practical use of TMS (22) is hampered by technical obstacles, and it is rarely used now in routine operations.

When stimulating the motor cortex to elicit descending neural activity in the spinal cord, it is important to consider that motor activity can be elicited by stimulation of not only the primary motor area, but also by stimulation of the SMA and the PMA. It is also possible to elicit muscle responses by stimulating the somato-sensory cortex. The anatomical location of these three main cortical motor areas varies somewhat among adult individuals, but it is of great importance to take into account the location of the motor cortex in relation to the coronal suture changes with age during childhood. A study showed that the location increased by 1.5 mm per year between two months and 8.6 years of age (*23*). Anomalies in the descending (corticospinal) pathways have also been reported (*24*) (see page 180).

Transcranial Magnetic Stimulation of the Motor Cortex

TMS of the motor cortex makes use of strong impulses of magnetic fields to induce electrical current in the motor cortex. The impulses of a magnetic field are generated by passing strong electrical impulses of current through a coil (**Fig. 10.1**). Many different designs of such coils have been described, and several of these are now commercially available.

Magnetic stimulation of the nervous system is an attractive method for eliciting neural activity in descending motor tracts of the spinal cord, but unfortunately, TMS has several drawbacks that have limited its use in the operating room for cortical stimulation.

It is difficult to accommodate the large coil in an operating room setting and it can be quite bulky; another disadvantage is related to the difficulties to generate a rapid succession of magnetic impulses, as is required, to overcome the effect of anesthesia (*16, 26*) when recording electromyographic (EMG) potentials.

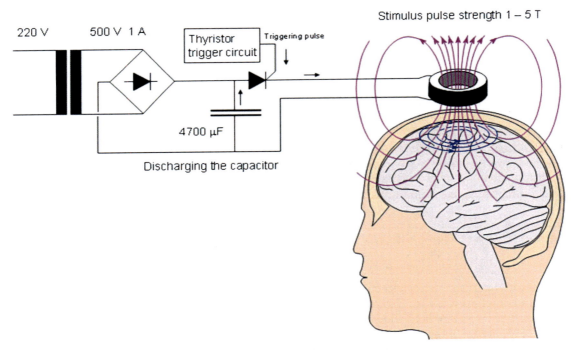

Figure 10.1: Diagram of the underlying principle of TMS: The strong current in the coil produces a magnetic field perpendicularly to the plane of the coil. The magnetic field passes unimpeded through the skull and induces oppositely directed electric current in the brain (Adapted with permission from the web-version of the book: Jaako Malmivuo & Robert Plonsey: *Bioelectromagnetism – Principles and Application of Bioelectric and Biomagnetic Fields*, Oxford University Press, New York, 1995), (Reprinted from: (*25*) with permission from Springer).

When TMS was introduced in the operating room in the late 1980s, the greatest problem was the suppression of the recorded responses by the effect of anesthesia. While it was easy (and pain free) to elicit muscles contractions of arms or legs in the conscious individual, it was not possible or was unreliable to elicit any muscle contractions in the anesthetized individual. Trains of impulses can reduce these problems, but it is difficult to generate a train of magnetic impulses.

Other deterrents in the use of magnetic stimulation in the operating room include the fear that magnetic stimulation might activate vast regions of the brain at the same time and thereby, possibly lead to epileptic seizures or other adverse effects. These worries, however, seem to have been exaggerated, although in rare cases epileptic seizures may indeed have been induced by magnetic stimulation in patients with a history of epilepsy. Additionally, there has been concern that the generated magnetic fields may cause iron and steel instruments to move or affect other electronic devices in the operating room.

Because of these severe drawbacks, TMS has been almost entirely replaced by TES for use in the operating room, but it is used extensively for the clinical laboratory for diagnostic purposes and for treatment.

TMS can be used to induce electrical currents in brain tissue, and it can be used in conscious humans without causing any noticeable discomfort or risks. It is, therefore, used for diagnostic purposes and for treatment of certain disorders such as depression. TMS (14, 27) can activate the motor cortex and elicit volleys of neural activity in the corticospinal tract in a similar way as those elicited by electrical stimulation of the motor cortex (28, 29). Thus, electrical current induced by magnetic stimulation evokes potentials that can be recorded from the spinal cord as D and I waves similar to those seen in the response to electrical stimulation of the motor cortex (**Fig. 9.17**) (28).

The orientation of the magnetic field influences its effectiveness in stimulating different populations of cells in the motor cortex (30).

The site of activation may be at the spike trigger zone of these neurons, or the fibers of the deep layers of the cortex may be activated, depending on the orientation of the magnetic field.

Because stimulation of the motor cortex for eliciting activity in the descending motor tracts depends on the orientation of the magnetic field, it is important to position the coil correctly (31).

The strong magnetic field that is generated can cause large stimulus artifacts that may interfere with the recorded responses. In the laboratory, it is possible to eliminate stimulus artifacts by injecting an appropriate amount of current (of opposite phase) into the recording circuit (27), but such methods are usually too elaborate to be used in the operating room. It has been shown that it is possible to record adequately clean responses, elicited by magnetic stimuli, from face muscles even though the recording site is close to the location of the stimulating coil provided that appropriate precautions are taken (32). Leads from the recording electrodes should be straight and point away from the patient. Artifacts should be prevented from overloading the amplifiers by keeping the amplification very low (see Chap. 18). It is also important to use electronic filters that are set wide and to use computer programs to remove the artifacts before the recorded potentials are subjected to further (digital) filtering using finite impulse response zero-phase filters (see Chap. 18). Those precautions, together with the use of finite impulse response digital filters, reduce the time-smearing of the artifacts so that the artifacts do not overlap in time with the responses.

Transcranial Electrical Stimulation of the Motor Cortex

TES of the motor cortex requires that a large voltage be applied to the stimulating electrodes placed on the scalp. Depending on the type of electrodes used, several hundred volts may be necessary to obtain a response, which is unacceptably painful in the conscious patient. This limits the possibility of obtaining pre- and postoperative recordings using techniques similar to those used intraoperatively, but is not an obstacle intraoperatively because patients are anesthetized.

Practical Use of Electrical Stimulation of the Motor Cortex

Although gold cup EEG electrodes may be used, Corkscrew electrodes are commonly used for TES (*10*), or more recently, subdermal electrodes (*33*) have come into favor. It was mentioned earlier (see page 47) that stimulators used for activating neural tissue (peripheral nerves and cells or fiber tracts in the CNS) may be either constant current or constant voltage generators (*34–36*) (for a theoretical treatment of constant current stimulation see (*37*)). Constant current stimulators for TES have the advantage that the current delivered to the head is independent of the electrode impedance and the impedance of the electrode-tissue interface. This is important for two reasons: first, the probability of injury to tissue depends on current density. With constant current stimulation, the level of current administered is under the control of the operator, and it will not suddenly change during a surgical procedure if the electrode impedance changes; second, the degree of activation of a cable-like axon is proportional to the gradient of the current traveling (*38*) along the axon. Since the current traveling along the axon is proportional to the total current produced by the stimulator, the neurophysiological effects of constant current stimulation will be independent of the electrode impedance and the impedance of the electrode tissue interface. Of course, this does not guarantee that the current delivered to neural structures is independent of changes in the impedance of other structures such as the scalp and brain, which may cause shunting of electrical current. Changes in geometry of the skull or presence of air inside the skull, supplanting some of the cerebrospinal fluid (CSF), can also affect the current flow through the cortical tissue that is to be activated. (For a more detailed discussion of constant current stimulation, see Chap. 18).

Electrode Placement. For stimulation of upper extremities, the electrodes should be placed at C_3-C_4 locations (10–20 system, **Fig. 6.1**), and at C_1–C_2 for lower extremities. It is generally assumed that anodal (positive) current applied to the surface of the cortex is more effective than cathodal (negative) current for activating descending motor tracts (*27*) (For a theoretical analysis of TES of the motor cortex see (*37*)). Cathodal current elicits a more variable response, and the threshold is higher.

Since the anode is the effective stimulating electrode, at least for weaker stimulation, it should be placed on C_1 or C_3 to elicit a response in the right limbs, and C_2 or C_4 for activating muscles on left limbs. Stimulation (**Fig. 10.2**) at these locations elicits clear D and I waves from the corticospinal tract as seen when recorded from the spinal cord (Chap. 9). Electrode placement with the anode at the vertex (C_z), and the cathode at a location that is 6 cm anterior to the anode emphasizes the I waves and produces D waves of a lower amplitude than stimulation with electrodes placed at C_1-C_2 and C_3-C_4 (see Chap. 9, **Fig. 9.23**).

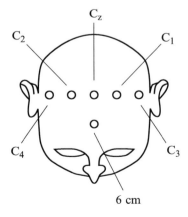

Figure 10.2: Electrode placement for TES of the cerebral motor cortex. (Reprinted from: (*10*) with permission from Elsevier).

Electrical impulses applied to the scalp (TES) activate fibers in the cerebral cortex rather than cell bodies (39). The efficacy of stimulation depends on the orientation of the axons in relation to the generated current vector, which in turn depends on the electrode montage. Electrode placements at C_3-C_4 for upper extremity stimulation or C_z'-F_z for lower extremities produces vertically oriented current vectors that are ideal for stimulation of the descending axons of the motor cortex that eventually form the corticospinal tract. Placing the stimulating electrodes closer together creates more horizontally oriented current vectors, thus, activating cortical fibers that generate I waves in the corticospinal tract. Increasing the stimulus strength deepens the penetration of the electrical current in the brain, stimulating cells at deeper layers of the motor cortex and therefore, activating different parts of the corticospinal tract.

Using short pulse widths of 50–100 µS in rapid succession[1] with inter-pulse intervals as short as 2 ms can elicit D waves (40). Constant voltage stimulation offers the possibility of a fast charge delivery (41). When eliciting MEP through transcranial stimulation, fast and slow charges provide similar intra-individual variability, but fast charge stimulation seems to be more efficient and requires approximately 35% less total charge for the same response as stimulation with slow change. The latency of the response is not different for the two kinds of stimulation (42).

Anesthesia

As with TMS, the success in eliciting responses from TES requires adequate anesthesia as discussed in Chap. 9, page 189, and Chap. 16.

Safety Concerns in Transcranial Electrical Stimulation

The practical use of TES caused considerable concern regarding safety when it was introduced in the operating room. TES uses high-voltage stimulation, as much as 1,500 V at times. This may cause direct tissue damage, cause seizures, and the stimulus current may directly cause contractions of muscles of the head, such as the temporalis muscle, and result in tongue lacerations or even jaw fractures.

Kindling, the eliciting of seizure activity from repeated stimulation of brain tissue, has been shown to occur in animal experiments, but has not been reported in humans in connection with TES. The risk of inducing seizures by TES in patients with epilepsy is not higher than it is in patients who do not have epilepsy (43). McDonald reports only five occurrences of seizures in a study of 15,000 cases monitored using TES, and some of those non-published seizures were not related to TES (44). The low risk of TES may be because this form of stimulation mainly activates descending vertical fibers and perhaps hyperpolarizes horizontally oriented axons in the cerebral cortex. Other forms of cortical stimulation, such as bipolar electrical stimulation, have a higher risk of seizures.

The risks from activating nearby muscles, in particular the temporalis muscles and the masseter muscle are real. These muscles, are some of the strongest muscles of the human body, and they can produce strong bite forces. Jaw clenching may also occur with single-pulse stimulation, which indicates that both corticobulbar activation by pulse-trains and direct stimulation of the motor branches of the trigeminal nerve may be involved. The muscular force from the spread of current in TES increases proportionally

---

[1] Digitimer D185: 1000V maximum voltage output (set by user); 1.5 A maximum current output, Risetime of 0.1A per microsecond, 50 µS pulse duration, 1–9 pulses with user defined interpulse interval, Reversible output polarity switch, User defined trigger facilities permit integration with popular EMG recording equipment. Digitimer Ltd, 37 Hydeway, Welwyn Garden City, Hertfordshire, AL7 3BE, England

with the number of impulses that are delivered within a short interval of stimulation (Journee, personal communication, 2009).

The activation of mastication muscles depends on how the stimulating electrodes are placed. When placed at C_3 and C_4, the masseter contractions were most pronounced when compared to stimulation at C_z'/F_z, C_3/C_z or C_4/C_z montages. When the stimulating electrodes are placed at C_3/C_4, TES may produce stronger biting than with electrodes placed at C_1/C_2 because the electrodes are closer to the facial and trigeminal nerves (21). TES may also induce contractions of muscles that are innervated by the facial nerve.

These problems can largely be avoided by proper placement of bite blocks, but lip lacerations and tongue bites are likely to occur when precautions, such as bite blocks, are not adequately used. Bite injuries due to jaw muscle contractions during TES are the most common, but still infrequent complications (44). Complications mentioned by McDonald's study included 29-tongue or lip lacerations, two scalp burns, five cardiac arrhythmias, and one mandible fracture in 15,000 operations.

DIRECT STIMULATION OF THE MOTOR CORTEX

In operations where the motor cortex is exposed, it is possible to stimulate the cortex directly by placing grid electrodes on the surface of the cortex (**Fig. 10.3**) or by using a

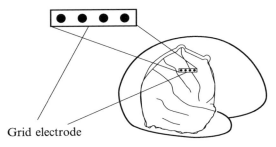

Grid electrode

Figure 10.3: Placement of electrodes over the exposed cerebral motor cortex for electrical stimulation. (Based on (10) with permission from Elsevier).

small, bipolar stimulator. Such direct electrical stimulation can elicit responses in descending motor pathways in a similar way as transcranial stimulation (28).

When stimulation of the motor cortex is described, most (if not all) authors refer to the primary motor cortex (M1). However, as discussed in Chap. 9, the corticospinal tract contains nerve fibers that originate in premotor cortical areas (PMA and SMA) and the somatosensory cortex (S1) (45). Little is known about the representation of these cortical areas in the spinal tracts, except for the ventral corticospinal tract, the axons of which are assumed to originate in PMA and SMA.

RECORDING OF THE RESPONSE TO ELECTRICAL OR MAGNETIC STIMULATION

D waves are so named because they are assumed to be elicited by direct activation of corticospinal fibers, whereas I waves are the result of indirect activation of corticospinal fibers through transsynaptic activation (46). The D waves are negative peaks that are assumed to be generated by activity in the dorsal corticospinal tract (47). Similar waves are observed in response to TMS and in response to direct electrical stimulation of the exposed cortical surface (48).

The I waves are later components in the response from descending motor tracts in the spinal cord that are evoked by stimulation of the primary motor cortex through cortico-cortical connections (see Chap. 9). The I waves consist of a volley of waves that were first identified in animal experiments (49) and in humans (50). These waves are negative peaks that are generated in the dorsal corticospinal tract; usually, four negative peaks (N_2, N_3, N_4, and N_5) can be identified. Contributions to these I waves may also come from the ventral corticospinal tract that is located in the anterior (ventral) funiculus. This latter tract has bilateral contributions from motor cortices (see Chap. 9). The D and I waves recorded in humans are similar to those described in animals (28, 48).

The D and I waves are not affected by muscle relaxants (*16*), but their latencies increase after cooling of the spinal cord with minimal effect on the amplitude of the recorded potentials (*51*). This is in accordance with the fact that these responses are the result of propagated activity in fiber tracts. The I waves are affected by anesthesia (*16*) (see Chap. 9).

Practical Aspects of Recording D and I Waves

The response from the descending motor tracts (corticospinal tract) can be recorded from the spinal cord using epidural electrodes. The subsequent muscle responses can be recorded as EMG potentials from selected muscles.

TES of the motor pathways in humans generates D and I waves in the descending corticospinal tracts (see Chap. 9). These waves can be recorded from electrodes placed in the epidural space of the spinal cord (**Fig. 10.4**) (*52*).

A commonly used epidural electrode for recording D and I waves, type JX-3002, has three platinum-iridium recording cylinders placed 18 mm apart. The electrode has double lumen that allows flushing the recording area with saline (*10*). Such epidural catheter electrodes can be placed percutaneously, which is favored in procedures performed by Japanese surgeons (*53*). Centers in the USA favor placing the recording electrode epidurally after laminectomy, etc. (*10*). It is also possible to use a standard four contact depth electrode.[2]

The presence of the D waves in the response to transcranial stimulation in humans indicates that the applied stimulation indeed activates the motor pathways and that the descending corticospinal tract is intact proximally (centrally) to the site where they are recorded. The latency of the D wave increases when the recording site in the epidural space in the spinal cord is moved caudally, which is in good agreement with the assumption that the D wave is generated by propagated impulses in descending motor tracts as has been shown in animal experiments (*28, 54*).

Since it is normal practice to stimulate only one side of the brain at a time, namely, the side to which the anode of the stimulating electrodes is applied, it is expected that the D wave will be from only one side and that the D waves mainly reflect activity in the dorsal corticospinal tract. It is not known how much of the recorded D wave is from the anterior corticospinal tract

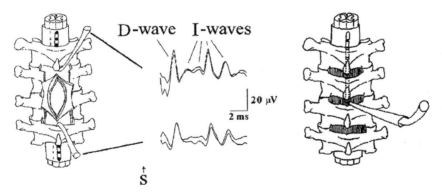

Figure. 10.4: Recording of the response from the spinal cord in an operation for a spinal cord tumor, using two catheter electrodes each with three cylinder electrodes, one placed caudal and one placed rostral (for control purposes) to the surgical field. The *top recording* shows the response that approaches the tumor region, and the *lower recordings* show the response having passed the tumor region. The *right illustration* shows placement of an epidural electrode in an operation where the spinal cord was not exposed. (Adapted from: (*10, 52*) with permission from Elsevier).

---

[2] AD-TECH Medical Instrument Corporation 1901 William Street Racine WI 53404 USA.

and whether other tracts also contribute to the response. In addition to activating the descending corticospinal tract, electrical and magnetic stimulation activates other descending motor tracts that may contribute to the recorded D waves, such as the medial motor tracts.

Interpretation of Recorded Responses

Certain guidelines for risk of paralysis have stated that a decrease of the amplitude of the D wave to 50% of its original amplitude does not imply a noticeable risk of paralysis. It has been assumed that if the amplitude of the D wave declines more than 50%, it indicates a high risk of paralysis (paraplegia for the lower spinal cord and quadriplegia for cervical tumors) (55). Other investigators have regarded a decrease of more than 50% to be a sign that predicts poor outcome, but different criteria should be applied to different surgical procedures (56). If the D waves recorded from the spinal cord decrease to 50% of their original amplitude, it may mean that 50% of the total number of fibers is rendered non-conducting, which may be tolerated, but this assumption seems to assume that there is a reserve of 50%.

No doubt, people do have fiber reserves in fiber tracts (e.g., the corticospinal tract), which means that a certain number of nerve fibers can be lost without any signs of deficits. However, the size of these reserves is different for different individuals, and the reserves generally decrease with age. This means that a tolerable decline in the number of functioning axons in a fiber tract, such as the corticospinal tract, varies among individuals. It does not seem to be realistic to set a certain value of decrease in the amplitude of recorded response as acceptable (corresponding to a certain loss of active nerve fibers; see discussion about how much change can be tolerated, criteria for alarm, in Chap. 17).

If the stimulation activates both sides of the corticospinal tract and only one side is affected by surgical manipulations, total conduction block in that part of the corticospinal tract will only cause a reduction of 50% in the recorded potentials assuming that the other side has normal conduction and that the two sides contribute equally to the recorded responses. This means that 100% of the corticospinal tract on the affected side can completely cease to conduct nerve impulses and the recorded potentials can still be within the acceptable limit of 50% of normal amplitude. Therefore, the generally accepted limit of a 50% decrease in the amplitude of the D wave is ambiguous, and it has been shown that such changes may cause motor deficits (56). It may be true that a 50% loss of conduction of corticospinal fibers is the limit for a successful outcome (without noticeable motor deficits) in many individuals if it occurs evenly on the tracts on both sides. On the other hand, if it is caused by 100% loss of fibers on one side and 0% on the other side, the amplitude of the recorded potentials will decrease only 50%. This simple example sets the 50% rule in doubt, and it calls for lower limits that are related to a person's age and other individual factors such as the person's general health.

Recording of Muscle Evoked Potentials

Recording of muscle responses (EMG responses) from distal limb muscles elicited by cortical stimulation can also be of value in monitoring the corticospinal tract, although some investigators regard monitoring of D waves of superior importance because preservation of D waves has proven to be the strongest predictor of maintained integrity of the corticospinal system (56). While the D waves are little affected by anesthesia, the EMG responses are attenuated or abolished by many anesthetics and are, of course, abolished by neuromuscular blockade or reduced in amplitude by partial neuromuscular blockade (16).

Monitoring spinal cord function on the basis of recordings of muscle activity that is elicited by transcranial stimulation is also an effective method for detecting injury to the spinal cord, provided that appropriate stimulus and recording parameters are used, but this technique does suffer from the disadvantage that muscle relaxants cannot be used. It is, however, more difficult to obtain EMG responses than responses directly taken from the spinal cord because recordings of EMG potentials depend on the excitability of alpha motoneurons, which is decreased by anesthetics (because of reduced facilitatory input from high CNS centers, and other parts of the spinal cord, see Chap. 9). It is also important that the recording is made from appropriate muscles, and attention must be paid to the patients' preoperative conditions regarding paresis or paralysis of specific muscle groups.

Since it has been customary to select the corticospinal system for recordings of EMG potentials, the recordings are often made from muscles on the distal extremities such as the hand (**Fig. 10.5**). Small hand muscles are most appropriate to record from, because many corticospinal fibers converge on their motoneurons. For the lower extremities, the abductor hallucis brevis is the optimal muscle from which EMG potentials may be recorded because its motoneurons are richly innervated by corticospinal fibers (*10*). The tibialis anterior is an alternative muscle to use. Recordings are typically performed with needle electrodes or wire hook electrodes in specific muscles, although the advantages of using needle electrodes rather than surface electrodes for recording Tc-MEP have not been evaluated.

Studies have shown that a single, electrical stimulus applied to the scalp to stimulate the motor cortex can elicit a stronger muscle contraction than a single shock to the respective peripheral nerve. These results, obtained in individuals with no neurologic deficits, were interpreted to show that a single shock to the motor cortex could give rise to a train of impulses in a motor nerve and hence, stronger contraction than a single stimulus to a peripheral nerve.

Interpretation of EMG Potentials. One of the major problems with the use of Tc-MEP is determining warning criteria on the basis of changes in the EMG responses. One problem lies in the fact that there is a large inherent variability in the amplitude of the muscle responses. Another problem lies in the fact that muscle responses are often polyphasic and extended over time, so that it is difficult to quantify them. Most neurophysiologists now use one of two methods to avoid this latter problem.

One approach, the threshold method (*57*), involves measuring the lowest level of stimulation for which muscle evoked potentials (MEP) can be obtained. An increase in threshold by more than, for example, 100 V for TES may be regarded as significant. One considerable problem with this approach is determining how much the stimulus intensity can be increased to obtain a response before it is a sign of significant change in function.

Another approach assumes that a significant change has occurred only if the MEP disappear entirely. This seems to be a too crude criterion. In operations for intramedullary spinal cord tumors, the disappearance of EMG potentials is regarded as a temporary phenomenon that does not affect outcome if the amplitude of the D wave remains above 50% of its baseline.

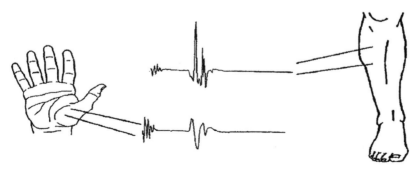

Figure 10.5: Recording of motor evoked potentials from muscles (EMG potentials) elicited by trains of electrical impulses applied to the motor cortex. (Adapted from: (*10, 52*) with permission from Elsevier).

The lack of good solutions to these problems has been an obstacle to the acceptance of the use of EMG recordings together with transcranial stimulation of the spinal motor system.

MONITORING OF THE MEDIAL SYSTEM

Monitoring of D and I waves as well as monitoring of the response from muscles on distal limbs concerns the corticospinal tract (lateral system) only, and thus, acts to protect only control of those muscles that are innervated by the corticospinal tract from paralysis or paresis. The other descending tracts (medial system) that innervate proximal limb muscles and the trunk (see Chap. 9) have so far, not been monitored routinely. As discussed above, it would be important also to monitor the medial system, which can be made by recording EMG potentials from trunk muscles or muscles on proximal limbs.

Loss of distal limb mobility is the most obvious postoperative deficit observed because the examination is commonly made with the patient in bed, and because of that, deficits of the trunk muscles are not as readily observed. However, neurologists who allow a longer postoperative interval before examining patients (when they are ambulatory), find that some patients may have problems walking and keeping posture after spinal cord operations although they have few observed deficits in the use of their distal limbs. The observed deficits of trunk muscles must then be caused by injuries to the medial motor system of descending motor tracts in the spinal cord (see Chap. 9).

The importance of the corticospinal system (lateral spinal motor system) has increased during evolution and is probably of greater importance in humans than in other primates because the corticospinal system provides the ability for fine movements of hands (fingers) and feet. However, the importance of one of the tracts of the medial system, the vestibulospinal tract, is obvious from experience with individuals who have lost their vestibular function due to

conditions such as vestibular neuronitis, or from ototoxic antibiotics. Such individuals experience severe deficits that can be related to motor function, which is arbitrated by the medial system, affecting balance, posture, and the ability to walk and other functions of trunk muscles. Although these symptoms decrease with time, and may totally disappear in young individuals (due to reorganization of the nervous system through activation of neural plasticity), the deficits that are caused by loss of function related to the vestibulospinal tract indicate that at least one part of the medial descending system is essential. While little is known about the functional importance of the other tracts of the medial motor system, the deficits experienced from the loss of function of the vestibulospinal system indicate that there is a need to specifically monitor the medial system in addition to monitoring the corticospinal system.

STIMULATION AND RECORDING FROM THE SPINAL CORD

In the discussion above of monitoring the spinal cord, the descending activity was generated by stimulation of the cerebral motor cortices, and the recordings were made either from the surface of the spinal cord or from muscles. Another technique makes use of electrical stimulation of the spinal cord while recording the responses from specific muscles (EMG) (58) or from peripheral nerves (59).

Several forms of intraoperative electrical stimulation of the spinal cord have been described. One method makes use of electrical stimulation of the spinal cord and recording of the responses from a different location of the spinal cord. This method, promoted by the Japanese neurosurgeon Tamaki (53), makes use of recordings of stimulus-elicited potentials from the spinal cord, independent of the anatomical location of their sources. This means that any fiber tract, descending or ascending, will be represented in such recordings, but to an extent that depends on the exact placement of the stimulating and recording electrodes.

Stimulation of the spinal cord via needles placed percutaneously in decorticated spinous processes or by epidurally placed electrodes can activate the entire spinal cord in a nonspecific way, and both motor and sensory pathways can be activated in that way. Thus, both the dorsal column (sensory) and the corticospinal tracts (motor) have been suggested to contribute to such responses. These responses are thus, non-specific, and their value for intraoperative monitoring of the spinal cord has been questioned (*60*).

Kai and his coworkers (*61*) have shown in animal studies that neurogenic MEP (NMEP) that were elicited by such electrical stimulation of the spinal cord could be recorded from peripheral nerves. The recorded potentials consist of large-amplitude motor components, which have shorter latencies than the longer latency and small-amplitude polyphasic sensory potentials (*61*). These investigators concluded that these potentials yield more information about the condition of the spinal cord when it is subjected to surgical manipulations.

In recent years, questions have arisen as to the accuracy, or the interpretation, of recordings of the response to direct stimulation of the spinal cord. More detailed studies of the recorded potentials elicited by stimulation of the spinal cord using collision techniques have shown that the responses to spinal cord stimulation mainly reflect transmission in the dorsal column, thus mainly testing the sensory pathway and not the motor pathways. A polyphasic component in the response that may be caused by transmission in motor pathways rarely could be seen.

Collision studies that are often used in the physiological laboratory have found use in the operating room for better differentiation among different tracts that are stimulated. One of the first to publish results using collision techniques was Leppanen 1999 (*3*). Deletis (*4*) used collision techniques to map the spinal cord (see Figure. 13.5, Chap. 13).

Collision studies have suggested that the descending volleys of activity that result from percutaneous spinal stimulation are primarily, but not totally, composed of descending antidromic sensory components (*3, 62*). The source of these potentials is the dorsal column pathways that generate components of the SSEP, rather than motor components. These results are supported by clinical studies (*63*).

Monitoring F and H Responses

Yet another method of monitoring the function of the spinal cord makes use of stimulation of a peripheral, mixed nerve and recording EMG responses from muscles innervated by the nerve. Two (or three) different responses can be recorded, one of which (M-wave) is the direct response by orthodromic activation of motor fibers. Stimulating the sensory part of a mixed nerve may also elicit an H-response because stimulation of proprioceptive fibers activates the monosynaptic stretch reflex activating the alpha motoneurons (see Chap. 9) (**Fig. 10.6**). The antidromic volley elicited in the motor fibers that terminate in the alpha motoneuron can also elicit a third kind of response, the F response, which is caused by backfiring of motoneurons (*9, 64*).

It is seen that the response of the H-reflex reaches a peak before the direct response saturates. The reason for the decrease in the H-response is that when the stimulus is increased above a certain value, motor nerve fibers become activated to the point of stimulation, which prevents activation again when the volley from the alpha motoneuron arrives. Monitoring of the H-reflex (**Fig. 10.7**) can provide information about the condition of the spinal horn, and the F-response is a measure of the excitability of the alpha motoneuron.

MONITORING DURING SPECIFIC SURGICAL PROCEDURES

The methods described above for monitoring the motor system are suitable for many different kinds of operations that affect the spinal cord. When monitoring specific kinds of operations, slightly different variations of these methods are often used.

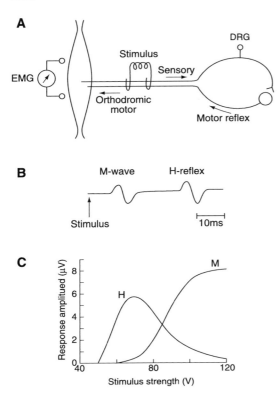

A

EMG

Stimulus

Sensory

DRG

Orthodromic motor

Motor reflex

B

M-wave   H-reflex

Stimulus   10ms

C

Response amplitude (µV)

H

M

40   80   120

Stimulus strength (V)

Figure 10.6: Schematic illustration of recording of the H-reflex response. (**A**) A mixed peripheral nerve containing both motor and proprioceptive fibers from muscle spindles is stimulated electrically, eliciting activity that progresses both distally, eliciting a direct muscle contraction (M-wave), and proximally, activating the monosynaptic stretch reflex that causes another and later muscle response (the H-reflex). (**B**) Recording of the direct muscle (M-wave) and the H-reflex from electrodes placed on the muscle. (**C**) Amplitude of the M-wave and H-reflex as a function of the stimulus intensity. The H-response is separated in time, and the amplitudes of these two responses have different relationships to the stimulus intensity. (Reprinted from (*65*) with the permission of Cambridge University Press).

Scoliosis Operations and Removal of Spinal Cord Tumors

TES is now in common use for monitoring of operations on the spinal cord such as during tumor removal, trauma, and for correcting spinal deformities such as scoliosis. D waves may be recorded from the spinal cord, and EMG responses may be recorded from muscles that are innervated by ventral roots that leave the spinal cord at levels below the location at which the operation is performed. EMG potentials are usually recorded from muscles on distal limbs, such as hands or feet, depending on the location on the spinal cord where the operation is performed.

The question regarding how large a change can be tolerated has been much debated. This question was also discussed in connection with monitoring sensory evoked potentials (see page 14). With regard to the monitoring of motor systems, it has been a rule that preservation of the D wave to at least 50% of its preoperative amplitude is important, but loss of the EMG potentials has been regarded to be less serious and not a reason to abort the operation or change its course.

As mentioned earlier (page 107, 119 and 180), abnormalities in certain disorders, such as scoliosis, are not limited to bone structures, but may affect the anatomy of the motor nervous system, and in some individuals, the descending corticospinal tract and the ascending dorsal column medial lemniscus tracts have been reported to not cross in the medulla (*24*). Other parts of a patient's neuroanatomy may also be abnormal to an extent that it must be taken into account in monitoring. Such abnormalities may affect intraoperative monitoring, but produce no noticeable symptoms and may not appear on imaging studies.

Patients, who have prior spinal cord lesions from surgery, trauma, or from radiation therapy, may also have D waves that are difficult to interpret because of the resulting pathology of the spinal cord. Surgical manipulations, such as correction of deformities of the spine, which occurs in patients with scoliosis, may cause the position of the spinal cord to shift and result in

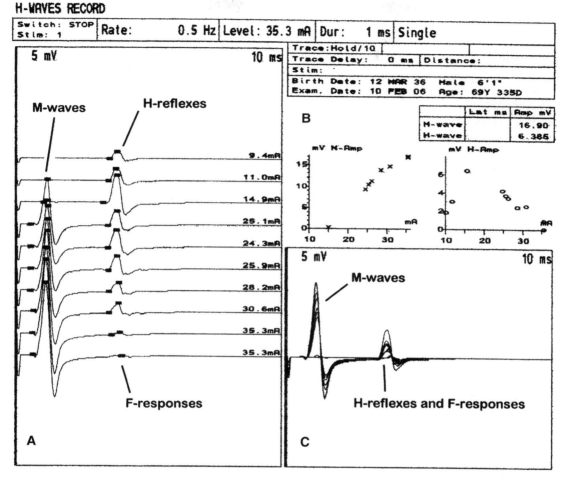

Figure 10.7: Intraoperative recording of the responses of the gastrocnemius H-reflex. (**A** and **B**) At low-intensity stimulation, the H-reflex appears first, and the amplitude peaks when the M-wave appears. Higher-intensity stimulation results in the M-wave amplitude increasing, and the H-reflex is replaced by the F-response. (**C**) The H-reflex is reproducible and of short latency, short duration, and simple configuration (Reprinted from: (*64*) with permission from Springer).

changes in the recorded potentials without any sign of injury to the spinal cord. As mentioned by Deletis and Sala (*56*), such different spatial relationships between the position of the recording electrode and the spinal cord may cause a change in the D wave without a concomitant change in muscle responses or in the SSEP. Such anatomical changes may, therefore, cause ambiguities in interpretation of results of spinal cord monitoring.

Placement of Pedicle Screws for Spinal Fixation

Pedicle screws are used for anchoring spinal instrumentation and are used in many different kinds of operations on the spine. Placement of pedicle screws implies a risk of injuring spinal roots and possibly the spinal cord. It is, therefore, important to be able to determine the location of the tip of a pedicle screw while it is being inserted. Without monitoring, the risk of

neurological deficits from pedicle screw placement procedures is rather high (66). Without
intraoperative neurophysiological monitoring,
incidences of neurologic injuries have been
reported from 1% to 11%, and other factors can
increase the rate of complications to as much as
40%. Imaging (fluoroscopy) is in common use,
but this technique has problems in the form of
false positives and false negatives.

Calancie et al. (67) described how to guide
and evaluate the placement of pedicle screws
using electrophysiological techniques. These
methods involve applying electrical impulses
through the screw and recording triggered electromyographic (tEMG) potentials from appropriate muscle groups. Such neurophysiological
methods are more effective than using imaging
techniques to guide and evaluate pedicle screw
placement.

There are two ways in which the proximity
of a pedicle screw to a spinal root can be determined using neurophysiological techniques.
One method makes use of recording EMG
potentials from a muscle that is innervated by
the motor nerve root that is at risk of being
damaged (68, 69), while electrical stimulation
is applied to the pedicle screw (which is supposed to be electrically conducting) (Fig. 10.8).
Another method is based on monitoring spontaneous motor activity by free-running EMG
recordings.

In pedicle screw placement, an opening is
first made in the pedicle of a vertebra by a surgical instrument (called an awl) for placement

of the screw. Calancie et al. (67) used tEMG
recordings and square, constant current
impulses of 200 μS duration, presented at a rate
of 3.1 pps, and applied to the instrument used
to create the opening. A constant current of
7 mA was applied in this "exploratory," initial
phase. If the bony wall is penetrated, adjacent
cranial nerves could be activated by the applied
current impulses, and could result in tEMG
responses. When the pedicle screw is inserted
into the opening after no breech in the bony
wall had been found, the screw is tested again
for breech by applying the same impulses to
the screw, but at 10 mA. If that test results in
recorded tEMG potentials, it is recommended
that the screw be repositioned (71). Current
practice is to give a warning when a 10 mA
stimulation gives a response, as this value is
still in general use (Richard Toleikis, personal
communication, 2010). Lowering the threshold
would cause fewer false positive responses for
breeching the wall of the opening, but lowering
the threshold would increase the likelihood of
false negative results.

The safe threshold current has been discussed, and it no doubt varies between individuals. Both the patient's age and gender play
roles. Younger patients have higher thresholds
than older patients; for example, older women
with osteoporosis have thresholds in the tens
of mA of current, while younger women have
higher thresholds. (Richard Toleikis, personal
communication, 2010).

Studies indicate that a stimulus threshold
higher than 11 mA results in a higher probability that the pedicle screw has been placed correctly, than when the threshold is lower.
However, there are exceptions to these findings. For example, individuals with osteoporosis are likely to have lower thresholds. In
addition, the threshold of a response to electrical stimulation also depends on which parts of
the spine the screw is inserted, e.g., lower values may be regarded as guideline for pedicle
screws inserted in the thoracic spine.

The threshold value is also influenced by the
stimulation technique. When recording spontaneous (free-running) EMG potentials, it is

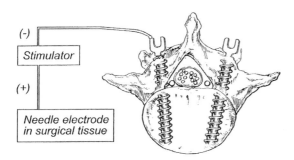

Figure 10.8: Principles of stimulation of a
pedicle screw with electrical impulses (Reprinted
from: (70) with permission from Elsevier).

assumed that the nerve root is sensitive to mechanical stimulation. Electrical stimulation of the pedicle screw is probably better than mechanical manipulation of the screw because the former technique can test the proximity of the pedicle screw to the spinal root by determining the threshold of the electrical stimulation.

It may be helpful to determine the bone threshold before inserting the screw. This can be accomplished by stimulating the lamina close to the pedicle by a hand-held electrode. Triggered EMG responses are observed from muscles that are innervated by motor nerves that originate from the spinal segment where the pedicle screw is to be placed, and which is being stimulated. The threshold may be approximately 25 mA with considerable individual variations. Most investigators have used constant current stimulation for that purpose (8, 70).

The current applied to a pedicle screw can take many paths other than the one through the wall of the opening in which the screw is inserted (**Fig. 10.9**), and worse, the electrical conductivity in these paths is likely to vary during an operation in accordance with how wet the environment is. Different degrees of wetness in the surgical field can affect how much current is shunted away (**Fig. 10.10**) (70). This means that the current that can reach neural tissue varies, and if the shunting is large, the current may not be sufficient to stimulate cranial nerves, and thus, injury by the screw may not be detected.

This is similar to that experienced when stimulating intracranial structures, such as the facial nerve, in operations for vestibular schwannoma that is discussed in Chap. 11. The remedy for the problem is to use a constant voltage stimulator rather than a constant current source (35, 74). Using a constant voltage source will make the electrical current that is delivered to a nerve root independent of the shunting from variable wetness of the surgical field where the stimulation is performed.

While many studies have been concerned with pedicle screw testing and results regarding complications in conventional spine operations, only a few studies have examined minimally invasive procedures. In such procedures, there are difficulties in testing safe screw placements because the screw is placed percutaneously, which does not allow the surgeon to visualize the pedicle in which the screw is placed or visualize the surrounding structures. The surrounding tissue shunts stimulus current, which makes it unclear how much current is passed through the screw, and how much is shunted away to the wall of the opening in the bone. This uncertainty, together with the general praxis of using constant current stimulation, makes placement of pedicle screws in

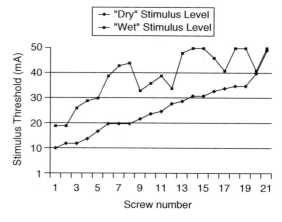

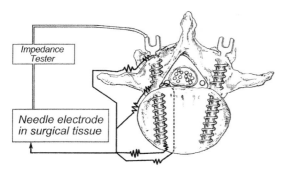

Figure 10.9: Illustration of different current paths that will "steal" stimulus current from the nerve root. (Reprinted from: (70) with permission from Elsevier).

Figure 10.10: Illustration of how the threshold of EMG responses depends on how wet the surgical field is. (Reprinted from: (70) (Modified from (72), Reprinted from: (73) with permission from Elsevier)).

minimally invasive procedures difficult in which shunting of current by surrounding tissue is a greater problem. These factors make the risk of injuring spinal nerves greater than when pedicle screws are placed during conventional, open surgery operations.

STIMULATION OF CERVICAL MOTOR ROOTS

Magnetic stimulation of cervical motor roots is a practical way to elicit neural activity in motor nerves (75). This method is used for diagnostic purposes and is beginning to find practical use in intraoperative monitoring. When interpreting the results of such stimulation, it must be remembered that nerves have regions that are sensitive to magnetic stimulation. One of the most important sensitive regions is the area surrounding a "bend" in a nerve (76, 77). Another such region is the location where a nerve travels between two surroundings with different electrical conductivity such as bone and fluid. This occurs when a nerve enters or emerges from an opening in a bone (foramen). Nerves from the lower spine form the cauda equina, and these nerves bend sharply when they exit the spine. Magnetic stimulation will, therefore, preferentially activate the area of the nerve that is bent (30, 32, 78), and consequently, moving the stimulating coil along the nerve and its root will yield a response with the same latency because it activates the nerve at the same location (where it is bent). Nerves that are not bent or do not have surroundings with different conductivities are difficult to activate using magnetic fields.

EFFECTS OF ANESTHESIA ON MONITORING SPINAL MOTOR SYSTEMS

Anesthesia has a profound effect on motor evoked potentials (MEP) (16, 17, 26, 79). The effect is greatest on muscle responses (EMG), and it is least on early epidural responses

(D waves). There is considerable dose dependent effect on I waves from anesthesia. Anesthesia in general is discussed in Chap. 16.

Effects on Epidural Responses to Stimulation of the Motor Cortex

A study of the effect of isoflurane on the epidural response (D and I waves) of the spinal cord elicited by electrical stimulation of the motor cortex, in a baboon under ketamine anesthesia, shows that the D waves are only marginally affected by isoflurane, but the amplitude of the I waves decreases when the concentration is increased from 0.3% to 2.1% (16) (**Fig. 10.11**). The I waves are abolished at higher concentrations of the anesthetics.

Nitrous oxide also attenuates I waves in the epidural responses in a similar way as isoflurane and has little effect on the D waves (16) (**Fig. 10.12**).

Muscle relaxants, having their major site of action at the neuromuscular junction, attenuate or abolish muscle responses, but have little effect on other electrophysiological recordings such as epidural recordings of D and I waves. Epidural recordings of the response to transcranial cortical or spinal stimulation are often

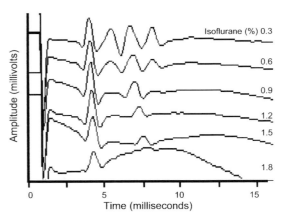

Figure 10.11: The effect of increasing isoflurane concentrations on the epidural response to single impulse transcranial electrical motor cortex stimulation in a Ketamine anesthetized baboon (Reprinted from: (16) with permission from Elsevier).

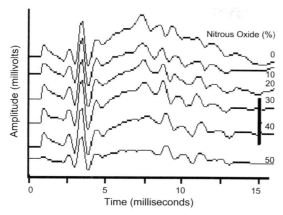

Figure 10.12: The effect of increasing nitrous oxide concentrations on the epidural response to single impulse transcranial electrical motor cortex stimulation in a Ketamine anesthetized baboon. Note that although the D wave is maintained, the I waves are lost in a similar way as from isoflurane. (Reprinted from: (*16*) with permission from Elsevier).

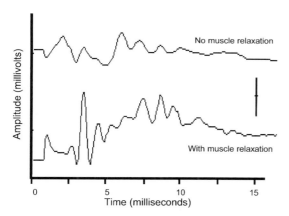

Figure 10.13: Recorded responses from the epidural space to TES of the motor cortex with (*below*) and without (*top*) muscle relaxation. Note the muscle artifact obscures the identification of I waves. (Reprinted from: (*16*) with permission from Elsevier).

contaminated by activity in overlying muscle. Since muscle relaxants abolish such unwanted noise (**Fig. 10.13**), muscle relaxants may in fact improve the quality of recordings of D and I

waves because they dampen the muscle activity that interferes with the recorded responses.

In **Fig. 10.13**, the amplifier utilized had automatic gain control that adjusted the amplification so that the display accurately filled the range of the display. This means that the high content of muscle activity acted as background noise for the recording reducing the automatically controlled amplification, and this is why the D and I waves in the upper graph are not discernable. When the noise is no longer present (lower graph), the D and I waves become clearly visible and appear to have larger amplitudes because the gain of the amplifier has increased due to the absence of the noise (EMG potentials).

Effects on EMG Activity

The choice of anesthesia is probably more important for recordings of cortically elicited MEP (compound muscle action potential, CMAP) than for any other modality of intraoperative monitoring. The level and the kind of anesthesia that is used affect the ability of cortical stimulation to elicit motor responses in different ways, but there may also be individual variations regarding the excitability of the motor system that should not be overlooked. The focus has been on the excitability of the motor cortex, but it seems more likely that the problems are related to the effect of anesthetics on the excitability of spinal cord neurons including the alpha motoneurons. The excitability of spinal cord neurons depends on many factors including facilitatory effect from the internal spinal cord neural circuits, and in particular, from descending facilitatory input to the spinal cord from the reticular formation through the reticulospinal tract (see Chap. 9). The descending activity in the corticospinal tract that produces the I waves also facilitates alpha motoneurons.

Inhalation agents may affect MEP elicited by a single impulse to the motor cortices to an extent that the response cannot be recorded (*16, 80*). The effect of inhalation agents increases with the concentration, but even low concentrations (for example, less than 0.2–0.5% isoflurane) affect the MEP (*16*) (**Fig. 10.14**).

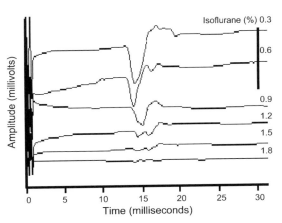

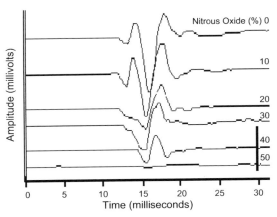

Figure 10.14: The effect of increasing isoflurane concentrations on the compound muscle action potential (CMAP) in response to a single impulse, transcranial electrical motor cortex stimulation in a ketamine anesthetized baboon. (Reprinted from: (*16*) with permission from Elsevier).

Figure 10.15: The effect of increasing nitrous oxide concentrations on the CMAP in response to a single impulse, transcranial electrical motor cortex stimulation in a Ketamine anesthetized baboon. As can be seen, the amplitude is progressively decreased with increasing concentrations similar to isoflurane. (Reprinted from: (*16*) with permission from Elsevier).

Nitrous oxide is a common component of general anesthesia and has been used in combination with opioids in operations where cortically elicited muscle responses are recorded. It has also been used to supplement intravenous based anesthetics such as Propofol or etomidate (*16, 81*). Nitrous oxide depresses transcranial evoked muscle responses, and it produces more profound changes in Tc-MEP than any other inhalation anesthetic agent when compared at equipotent anesthetic concentrations (*81*). The effect of nitrous oxide increases with its concentration (**Fig. 10.15**), mimicking the effects of isoflurane (i.e., loss of compound muscle response (**Fig. 10.15**) and I waves at higher concentrations, (**Fig. 10.11**)).

Studies have suggested that etomidate is an excellent agent for induction of anesthesia and for use during monitoring of transcranial evoked motor potentials (*16*). Etomidate has the least degree of amplitude depression of MEP (*82*). Like other anesthetics, its effect on motor evoked potentials increases with increasing concentration (**Fig. 10.16**), but at low doses it causes an increase of the amplitude of the

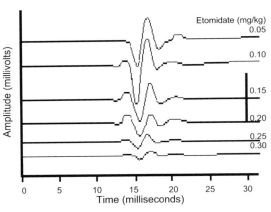

Figure 10.16: The effect of increasing doses of etomidate on the CMAP in response to transcranial electrical motor cortex stimulation in a ketamine anesthetized baboon. Note an initial increase in the amplitude of the CMAP at low doses, but after the initial increase, the amplitude progressively decreases with increasing concentrations of etomidate similar to the effect of isoflurane. (Reprinted from: (*16*) with permission from Elsevier).

motor responses, and this effect is more prominent for transcranial magnetic evoked responses than transcranial electrical evoked responses. Etomidate has little effect on epidural-recorded D waves.

Propofol is a sedative-hypnotic, intravenous agent that is rapidly metabolized. Propofol is in extensive use, and it is often combined with other agents such as opioids in total intravenous anesthesia (TIVA). It has a similar effect on the EEG as barbiturates, and it has a depressant effect on motor response amplitudes. Increasing concentrations of Propofol have a similar effect on Tc-MEP as inhalation agents, namely, a loss of compound motor action potentials and I waves at higher concentrations (*16*) (**Fig. 10.17**).

Clearly, the choice of anesthesia makes a marked difference in the ability to record MEP following transcranial stimulation of the motor tracts. Studies have suggested that the muscle response elicited by TMS can be more sensitive to the inhalation agents than responses elicited by TES (*79*). It appears that the best technique for monitoring of MEP is TIVA. Current TIVA drug combinations usually include opioids with

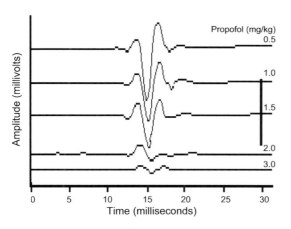

Figure 10.17: Effect of increasing doses of Propofol on the CMAP in response to a single impulse transcranial electrical motor cortex stimulation in a Ketamine anesthetized baboon. (Reprinted from: (*16*) with permission from Elsevier).

Ketamine, etomidate, or closely titrated Propofol infusions (*16*) (see Chap. 16).

MECHANISMS OF SUPPRESSION OF MOTOR RESPONSES BY ANESTHETICS

The fact that the D wave is resistant to anesthetic depression means that the descending activity in the corticospinal tract is unaffected by anesthesia, which in turn means that the excitatory synaptic input to the alpha motoneurons is probably also intact. The propriospinal interneurons that relay most of the descending activity in the corticospinal tracts to the alpha motoneurons (see Chap. 9) are unlikely to be so sensitive to anesthesia that they interrupt transmission of motor activity to the alpha motoneurons (*80*). This has been taken to support the hypothesis that the depression of the MEP from anesthetics is caused by an inability to activate the alpha motoneuron (*83*). This hypothesis is further supported by the fact that the H reflex is also suppressed by halogenated inhalation anesthetics (*84*).

This means that even in an anesthetized patient, information from the motor cortex (such as that elicited by electrical stimulation) arrives at the propriospinal neurons and the alpha motoneurons with little noticeable effect from most forms of anesthesia.

There are at least two reasons for this decreased excitability at the spinal cord level from anesthesia: it can be caused by local effect on synaptic excitability of alpha motoneurons and propriospinal neurons (the only two neurons involved in the activation of muscles from the corticospinal pathways (see Figure. 9.12)) or, it can be caused by reduced facilitatory input to the alpha motoneurons from spinal or sources in the brain. It seems more likely that the effect of anesthetics on muscle responses would be caused by depression of the synapses on the alpha motoneurons, but it may more likely be caused by reduction of the excitability of the alpha motoneurons caused by reduction in neural activity that normally facilitates activation of alpha motoneurons rather than a direct effect on synaptic transmission to the motoneurons.

Facilitatory influence normally arrives at alpha motoneurons from central structures such as the reticular formation through the reticulospinal tract that has facilitatory influence on alpha motoneurons through spinal motoneurons. The activity from the reticular formation that is generated by long chains of neurons, and thus, sensitive to anesthesia, is important for the excitability of alpha motoneurons (65, 85).

Reduced facilitatory input to alpha motoneurons decreases their sensitivity in such a way that a larger EPSP is required to activate these motoneurons. That is most likely the main reason why a single impulse to the cerebral cortex cannot generate an EPSP of sufficient amplitude to reach the higher firing thresholds needed in the anesthetized patient. Decreased influence on alpha motoneurons from local spinal circuits that normally enhance the excitability of the motoneurons may also contribute to the effect of anesthetics. The spinal cord in itself also provides facilitation of alpha motoneurons, much of which is generated by long chains of neurons and, therefore, it is sensitive to the administration of anesthetics such as those used for general anesthesia.

Activating other systems in the spinal cord may also facilitate responses from cortical stimulation in anesthetized individuals. For example, the facilitatory effect of activation of the monosynaptic stretch reflex (H-reflex) can help to overcome the anesthetic effect (86).

I waves that also normally provide facilitatory influence on the alpha motoneurons are likewise suppressed by commonly used anesthetics and that most likely also contributes to the suppression of alpha motoneurons. I waves appear to be necessary for producing myogenic responses in the unanesthetized state (87).

This means that input from the reticular activating system effects the motor system and the sensory system in much the same way (88), and normal excitability of both the sensory and motor systems, thus, depends on both the degree of wakefulness and activity from the brainstem reticular system. This is important for intraoperative monitoring of the motor system because anesthesia that decreases wakefulness by reducing the output of the reticular formation reduces the facilitatory input to motor systems inducing paralysis, which is one of the factors that causes the well-known difficulties in evoking motor responses by cortical stimulation in the anesthetized individual (16, 79).

There is no doubt that eliciting a motor response is complex. Excitatory and inhibitory input to alpha motoneurons arrives from many different parts of the CNS and interacts. Some input is from motor centers, but other input arrives from, for example, the reticular formation and from sensory systems including the somatosensory cortex. This means that monitoring of the spinal motor system using stimulation of the motor cortex may in fact be affected by the function of a mixture of sensory and motor pathways that may change with the type and dosage of the anesthetic agents used.

How to Overcome Lack of Facilitatory Input to Alpha Motoneurons?

The most common way to overcome suppression of motor activity, in addition to selecting anesthetics, is to apply multiple impulses in rapid succession for stimulating the motor cortex. Such stimulation elicits multiple D waves (and possibly I waves), and temporal summation of this activity at the alpha motoneuron causes EPSP of sufficient amplitude to reach the threshold of alpha motoneurons (89), resulting in a peripheral nerve and motor response (**Fig. 10.18**). Such repeated stimulation can cause (temporal) summation of EPSP at the alpha motoneurons to such an extent that the membrane potential can exceed the threshold even with a lack of facilitatory input (90). Technically, it is easy to generate a suitable train of electrical impulses for stimulating the motor cortex (TES), but it is difficult to generate trains of magnetic impulses (TMS) in a rapid succession, which is another reason that

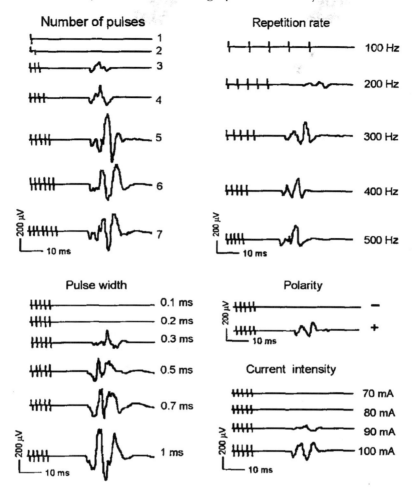

Figure 10.18: Influence of varying stimulation parameters on MEPs recorded from the thenar muscle and elicited by TES with stimulating electrodes placed at C_3+2 cm or C_4+2 cm. The inter-stimulus interval was 2 ms, and constant current of 100 mA was used. (Reprinted from: (*90*) with permission from Elsevier).

TES is now the preferred method for activating the motor system in the operating room.

The effect of temporal integration decreases as the interval between the successive stimuli increases, and the optimal effect is achieved when intervals of 1–2 ms are used, but it can be effective for intervals up to 10 ms (*89, 90*) (see **Fig. 10.18**). The optimal interstimulus interval may vary with the anesthetic effect (*26*). If inhalation agents are used with this multi-pulse technique, a "tuning" of the stimulation interstimulus interval (ISI) may improve the effectiveness of the monitoring.

Often, other phenomena can be observed when attempting to elicit motor responses by stimulation of the motor cortices. Thus, a train of impulses applied to the scalp may not elicit a response, but after repeated stimulation, it may lead to a muscle response (**Fig. 10.19**). This effect is different from simple temporal summation of the EPSP, and it is

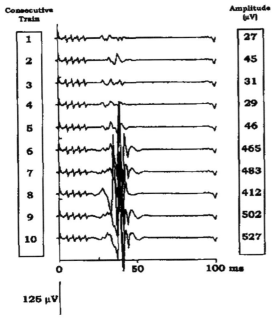

Figure 10.19: Response from the right abductor hallucis brevis muscle in response to repeated presentations of trains consisting of five stimuli, duration 0.1 ms, intensity 288 mA, repeated at a rate of 1 per second, anode over C3 and cathode over C4 (Reprinted from: (*10*) with permission from Elsevier).

likely to involve complex neural circuits in the brain.

Muscle Relaxants

Any form of muscle relaxation brought about by a muscle endplate blocker (such as curare-like agents) or by depolarizing agents (succinylcholine) affect the stimulus-elicited EMG potentials. Partial muscle blockade accomplished by muscle endplate blocking agents have their greatest effect on responses that follow the initial response, and the shorter the time between stimuli, the greater the effect on the following responses. Continuous activity, such as mechanical-elicited or injury-elicited (spontaneous) EMG activity, is attenuated more than single responses. If a short-acting endplate blocking agent is used, it is important

to be aware that the paralyzing action disappears gradually and at a rate that differs from patient to patient and from muscle group to muscle group. The rate at which muscle function is regained depends on the age, weight, etc. of the patient, other diseases that may be present, or other medications that may have been administered. During the time that the muscle relaxing effect is decreasing, stimulation of a motor nerve with a train of electrical shocks will give rise to a relatively normal muscle contraction in response to the initial electrical stimulus, but the response to subsequent impulses will be less than normal.

The effect of muscle relaxants of the endplate blocking type can be shortened ("reversed") by agents, such as neostigmine, that inhibit the breakdown of acetylcholine and, thereby, make better use of the acetylcholine receptor sites that are not blocked by the muscle relaxant that is used. However, a prerequisite for the use of such "reversing" agents is that a fair amount of muscle response (10–20%) has returned before attempting to reverse the effect of the muscle relaxants. It is important to note that reversing the effect of the muscle relaxants does not immediately return the muscle function to normal.

Some investigators (*16*) have advocated the use of partial neuromuscular blockade that reduces the amplitude of the muscle response, a controlled degree of blockade (10–20% of single twitch remaining, or 2 of 4 twitches remaining in a "train of four" response). However, there are several problems associated with partial muscle relaxation. First of all, it is difficult to keep a stable level of relaxation. Secondly, it is questionable if a level of relaxation that is sufficient to provide protection from the patient moving or even more importantly, from coughing, will allow monitoring of some muscles, for example, the facial muscles. It seems to require a greater amount of muscle relaxant drugs to relax the diaphragm than striate muscles such as those of the face. This means that one might need nearly total relaxation of the facial muscles and perhaps spinal muscles in order to provide any meaningful relaxation of the diaphragm. Therefore, others have been reluctant to advocate the use of partial muscle relaxation when muscle responses are to be recorded and have recommended total absence of muscle relaxing agents in the anesthesia regimen when monitoring depend on recordings of EMG potentials.

REFERENCES

1. Brown RH and CL Nash (1979) Current status of spinal cord monitoring. Spine 4:466–78.
2. Nuwer MR, EG Dawson, LG Carlson et al (1995) Somatosensory evoked potential spinal cord monitoring reduces neurologic deficits after scoliosis surgery: Results of a large multicenter study. Electroenceph Clin Neurophys 96:6–11.
3. Leppanen R, R Madigan, C Sears et al (1999) Intraoperative collision studies demonstrate descending spinal cord stimulation evoked potentials and ascending somatosensory evoked potentials are medicated through common pathways. J Clin Neurophysiol 16:170.
4. Deletis V and AB Camargo (2001) Interventional neurophysiological mapping and monitoring during spinal cord procedures. Stereotact Funct Neurosurg 77:25–8.
5. Deletis V and JL Shils (2004) *Neurophysiology in Neurosurgery*. Amsterdam: Academic Press.
6. Sala F, MJ Krzan and V Deletis (2002) Intraoperative neurophysiological monitoring in pediatric neurosurgery: Why, when, how? Childs Nerv Syst. 18:264–87.
7. Sala F, P Lanteri and A Bricolo (2004) Motor evoked potential monitoring for spinal cord and brain stem surgery. Adv Tech Stand Neurosurg 29:133–69.
8. Maguire J, S Wallace, R Madiga et al (1995) Evaluation of intrapedicular screw position using intraoperative evoked electromyography. Spine 20:1068–74.
9. Leppanen R, J Maguire, S Wallace et al (1995) Intraoperative lower extremity reflex muscle activity as an adjunct to conventional somatosensory-evoked potentials and descending neurogenic monitoring in idiopathic scoliosis. Spine 20:1872–7.
10. Deletis V (2002) Intraoperative neurophysiology and methodologies used to monitor the functional integrity of the motor system, in *Neurophysiology in Neurosurgery*, V Deletis and JL Shils, Editors. Academic Press: Amsterdam. 25–51.
11. Kuypers HGJM (1981) Anatomy of the descending pathways, in *Handbook of physiology – the nervous system*, JM Brookhart and VB Mountcastle, Editors. American Physiological Society: Bethesda, MD. 597–666.
12. Merton PA and HB Morton (1980) Electrical stimulation of human motor and visual cortex through the scalp. J Physiol 305:9–10P.
13. Marsden CD, PA Merton and HB Morton (1983) Direct electrical stimulation of corticospinal pathways through the intact scalp in human subjects. Adv Neurol 39:387–91.
14. Barker AT, R Jalinous and IL Freeston (1985) Non-invasive magnetic stimulation of the human motor cortex. Lancet 1:1106–7.
15. Gualtierotti T and AS Patterson (1954) Electrical stimualtion of the unexpeosed cerebral cortex. J Physiol 125:278–91.
16. Sloan T (2002) Anesthesia and motor evoked potential monitoring, in *Neurophysiology in Neurosurgery*, V Deletis and JL Shils, Editors. Elsevier Science: Amsterdam. 451–74.
17. Sloan TB and EJ Heyer (2002) Anesthesia for intraoperative neurophysiologic monitoring of the spinal cord. J Clin Neurophysiol 19:430–43.
18. Daube J and C Harper (1989) Surgical monitoring of cranial and peripheral nerves, in *Neuromonitoring in Surgery*, J Desmedt, Editor. Elsevier Science Publishers: Amesterdam. 115–38.
19. Tabaraud F, JM Boulesteix, D Moulies et al (1993) Monitoring of the motor pathway during spinal surgery. Spine 18:546–50.
20. Burke D, R Hicks, J Stephen et al (1992) Assessment of corticospinal and somatosensory conduction simultaneously during scoliosis surgery. Electroenceph Clin Neurophysiol 85:388–96.
21. MacDonald D (2006) Intraoperative motor evoked potential monitoring: Overview and update. J Clin Monit Comput 20:347–77.
22. Edmonds HL, MPJ Paloheimo, MH Backmann et al (1989) Transcranial magnetic motor evoked potentials (tc MMEP) for functional monitoring of motor pathways during scoliosis surgery. Spine 14:683–6.
23. Rivet D, D O'Brien, T Park et al (2004) Distance of the motor cortex from the coronal suture as a function of age. Pediatr Neurosurg 40:215–9.

24. MacDonald D, L Streletz, Z Al-Zayed et al (2004) Intraoperative neurophysiologic discovery of uncrossed sensory and motor pathways in a patient with horizontal gaze palsy and scoliosis. Clin Neurophysiol. 115:576–82.

25. Møller AR, B Langguth, D De Ridder et al (2010) Textbook of Tinnitus. New York: Springer.

26. Sloan TB and JN Rogers (1996) Inhalational anesthesia alters the optimal interstimulus interval for multipulse transcranial motor evoked potentials in the baboon. J Neurosurg Anesth 8:346.

27. Amassian VE, GJ Quirk and M Stewart (1990) A comparison of corticospinal activation by magnetic coil and electrical stimulation of monkey motor cortex. Electroenceph Clin Neurophys 77:390–401.

28. Kitagawa H and AR Møller (1994) Conduction pathways and generators of magnetic evoked spinal cord potentials: A study in monkeys. Electroenceph Clin Neurophys 93:57–67.

29. Edgeley SA, JA Eyre, R Lemon et al (1990) Excitation of the corticospinal tract by electromagnetic and electrical stimulation of the scalp in the macaque monkey. J Physiol 425:301–20.

30. Amassian VE, L Eberle, PJ Maccabee et al (1992) Modelling magnetic coil excitation of human cerebral cortex with a peripheral nerve immersed in a brain-shaped volume conductor: The significance of fiber bending in excitation. Electroenceph Clin Neurophysiol 85:291–301.

31. Werhahn KJ, JKY Fong, BU Meyer et al (1994) The effect of magnetic coil orientation on the latency of surface EMG and single motor unit responses in the first dorsal interosseous muscle. Electroenceph Clin Neurophysiol 93:138–46.

32. Schmid UD, AR Møller and J Schmid (1992) Transcranial magnetic stimulation of the facial nerve: Intraoperative study on the effect of stimulus parameters on the excitation site in man. Muscle and Nerve 15:829–36.

33. Krammer MJ, S Wolf, DB Schul et al (2009) Significance of intraoperative motor function monitoring using transcranial electrical motor evoked potentials (MEP) in patients with spinal and cranial lesions near the motor pathways. Br J Neurosurg 23:48–55.

34. Yingling C and J Gardi (1992) Intraoperative monitoring of facial and cochlear nerves during acoustic neuroma surgery. Otolaryngol Clin North Am 25:413–48.

35. Møller AR and PJ Jannetta (1984) Preservation of facial function during removal of acoustic neuromas: Use of monopolar constant voltage stimulation and EMG. J Neurosurg 61:757–60.

36. Prass R and H Lueders (1985) Constant-current versus constant-voltage stimulation. J Neurosurg 62:622–3.

37. Stecker MM (2005) Transcranial electric stimulation of motor pathways: A theoretical analysis. Comput Biol Med 35:133–55.

38. Rattay F (1987) Ways to approximate current-distance relations for electrical stimulated fibres. J Theor Biol 125:339–49.

39. Nowak LG and J Bullier (1998) Axons, but not cell bodies, are activated by electrical stimulation in cortical gray matter. I. Evidence from chronaxie measurements. Exp Brain Res 118:477–88.

40. Novak K, AB De Camargo, M Neuwirth et al (2004) The refractory period of fast conducting corticospinal tract axons in man and its implications for intraoperative monitoring of motor evoked potentials. Clin Neurophysiol 115:1931–41.

41. Journée HL (2004) The Biological Interface and Hardware of Electrical Stimulation., in *Neurophysiology in Neurosurgery*, V Deletis and JL Shils, Editors. Academic Press: Amsterdam. 128–31.

42. Hausmann ON, K Min, N Boos et al (2002) Transcranial electrical stimulation: Significance of fast versus slow charge delivery for intraoperative monitoring. Clin Neurophysiol 113:1532–5.

43. Szelényi A, Joksimovic B and V Seifert (2007) Intraoperative risk of seizures associated with transient direct cortical stimulation in patients with symptomatic epilepsy. J Clin Neurophysiol 24:39–43.

44. MacDonald DB (2002) Safety of intraoperative transcranial electrical stimulation motor evoked potential monitoring. J Clin Neurophysiol 19:416–29.

45. Schieber MH, (2007) Comparative anatomy and physiology of the corticospinal system., in *Handb Clin Neurol*. 15–37.

46. Day BL, PD Thompson, JPR Dick et al (1987) Different sites of action of electrical and magnetic stimulation of the human brain. Neurosci Lett 75:101–6.

47. Kernel D and CP Wu (1967) Responses of the pyramidal tract to stimulation of the baboon's motor cortex. J Physiol (Lond) 191:653–72.

48. Katayama Y, T Tsubokawa, S Maejima et al (1988) Corticospinal direct response in humans: Identification of the motor cortex during intracranial surgery under general anesthesia. J Neurol Neurosurg Psych iat 51:50–9.

49. Amassian VE, M Stewart, GJ Quirk et al (1987) Physiologic basis of motor effects of a transient stimulus to cerebral cortex. Neurosurg. 20:74–93.

50. Tsubokawa T (1987) Clinical value of multi-modality spinal cord evoked potentials for prognosis of spinal cord injury, in *Thoracic and Lumbar Spine and Spinal Cord Injuries*, RP Vigouroux and P Harris, Editors. Springer-Verlag: New York. 65–92.

51. Deletis V (1993) Intraoperative monitoring of the functional integrety of the motor pathways, in *Advances in neurology: Electrical and magnetic stimulation of the brain*, O Devinsky, A Beric and M Dogali, Editors. Raven Press: New York. 201–14.

52. Deletis V, Z Rodi and VE Amassian (2001) Neurophysiological mechanisms underlying motor evoked potentials (MEPs) elicited by a train of electrical stimuli: Part 2. Relationship between epidurally and muscle recorded MEPs in man. Clin Neurophysiol 112:445–52.

53. Tamaki T, H Takano and K Takakuwa (1985) Spinal cord monitoring: Basic principles and experimental aspects. Cent Nerv Syst Trauma 2:137–49.

54. Patton HC and VE Amassian (1960) The pyramidal tract: Its excitation and functions, in *Handbook of Physiology and Neurophysiology, Vol 11*. American Physiology Society: Washington, D.C. 837–61.

55. Kothbauer KF (2002) Motor evoked potential monitoring for intramedullary spinal cord tumor surgery, in *Neurophysiology in Neurosurgery*, V Deletis and JL Shils, Editors. Academic Press: Amsterdam. 73–92.

56. Deletis V and F Sala (2008) Intraoperative neurophysiological monitoring of the spinal cord during spinal cord and spine surgery: A review focus on the corticospinal tracts. Clin Neurophysiol 119:248–64.

57. Calancie B, W Harris, JG Broton et al (1998) "Threshold-level" multipulse transcranial electrical stimulation of motor cortex for intraoperative monitoring of spinal motor tracts: Description of method and comparison to somatosensory evoked potential monitoring. J Neurosurg 90:457–70.

58. Machida M, MC Weinstein, T Yamada et al (1985) Spinal cord monitoring: Electrophsysiological measures of sensory and motor function during spinal surgery. Spine 10:407–13.

59. Owen JH, KH Bridwell, R Grubb et al (1991) The clinical application of neurogenic motor evoked potentials to monitor spinal cord function during surgery. Spine 16:S385–90.

60. Koyanagi I, Y Iwasaki, T Isy et al (1993) Spinal cord evoked potential monitoring after spinal cord stimualtion durong surgery of spinal cord tumors. Neurosurgery 33:451–60.

61. Kai Y, JH Owen, LG Lenke et al (1993) Use of sciatic neurogenic motor evoked potentials versus spinal potentials to predict early-onset neurologic deficits when intervention is still possible during overdistraction. Spine 18:1134–9.

62. Toleikis JR, JP Skelly, AO Carlvin et al (2000) Spinally elicited peripheral nerve responses are sensory rather than motor. Clin Neurophysiol 111:736–42.

63. Minahan RE, JP Sepkuly, RP Lesser et al (2001) Anterior spinal cord injury with preserved neurogenic "motor"-evoked potentials. Clin Neurophysiol 112:1442–50.

64. Leppanen R (2006) Intraoperative applications of the H-reflex and Fresponse: A tutorial. J Clin Monit Comput 20:267–304.

65. Møller AR (2006) Neural plasticity and disorders of the nervous system. Cambridge: Cambridge University Press.

66. Thomsen K, FB Christensen, SP Eiskjaer et al (1997) The effect of pedicle screw instrumentation on functional outcome and fusion rates in posterolateral lumbar spinal fusions: A prospective randomized clinical study. Spine 22:2813–22.

67. Calancie B, N Lebwohl, P Madsen et al (1992) Intraoperative evoked EMG monitoring in an animal model. A new technique for evaluating pedicle screw placement. Spine 17:1229–35.

68. Bose B, LR Wierzbowski and AK Sestokas (2002) Neurophysiologic monitoring of spinal nerve root function during instrumented posterior lumbar spine surgery. Spine 27:1444–50.

69. Toleikis JR, JP Skelly, AO Carlvin et al (2000) The usefulness of electrical stimulation for assessing pedicle screw placements. J Spin Disord 13:283–9.

70. Toleikis JR, (2002) Neurophysiological monitoring during pedicle screw placement, in *Neurophysiology in Neurosurgrey*, V Deletis and JL Shils, Editors. Elsevier: Amsterdam. 231–64.

71. Calancie B, P Madsen and N Lebwohl (1994) Stimulus evoked EMG monitoring during trans-pedicular lumbosacral spine instrumentation. Spine 19:2780–86.

72. Kretchmann HJ and W Weinrich (1999) *Neurofunctional systems*. Thieme: New York.

73. Shils JL, M Tagliati and RL Alterman (2002) Neurophysiological monitoring during neurosur-gery for movement disorders, in *Neurophysiology in Neurosurgery*, V Deletis and JL Shils, Editors. Academic Press: Amsterdam. 405–48.

74. Yingling C (1994) Intraoperative monitoring in skull base surgery, in *Neurotology*, RK Jackler and DE Brackmann, Editors. 1994, Mosby: St. Louis. 967–1002.

75. Mills KR, C McLeod, J Sheffy et al (1993) The optimal current direction for excitation of human cervical motor roots with a double coil magnetic stimulator. Electroenceph Clin Neurophysiol 89:138–44.

76. Kimura J, A Mitsudome, T Yamada et al (1984) Stationary peaks from moving source in far-field recordings. Electroenceph Clin Neurophys 58:351–61.

77. Lueders H, RP Lesser, JR Hahn et al (1983) Subcortical somatosensory evoked potentials to median nerve stimulation. Brain 106:341–72.

78. Schmid UD, AR Møller and J Schmid (1992) The excitation site of the trigeminal nerve to transcranial magnetic stimulation varies and lies proximal or distal to the foramen ovale: An intraoperative electrophysiological study in man. Neurosci Lett 141:265–8.

79. Sloan T and D Angell, (1993) Differential effect of isoflurane on motor evoked potentials elic-ited by transcortical electric or magnetic stimu-lation, in *Handbook of Spinal Cord Monitoring*, SS Jones et al, Editors. Kluwer Academic Publishers: Hingham, MA. 362–7.

80. Yamada H, EE Transfeldt, T Tamaki et al (1994) The effects of volatile anesthetics on the relative amplitudes and latencies of spinal and muscle

81. Sloan T, (1996) Evoked potentials, in *A Textbook of Neuroanesthesia with Neurosurgical and Neuroscience Perspectives*, MS Albin, Editor. McGraw-Hill: New York. 221–76.

82. Glassman SD, CB Shields, RD Linden et al (1993) Anesthetic effects on motor evoked potentials in dogs. Spine 18:1083–9.

83. Loughnan B, S Anderson, M Hetreed et al (1989) Effects of halothane on motor evoked potential recorded in the extradural space. Br J Anaesth 63:561–4.

84. Mavroudakis N, A Vandesteene and E Brunko (1994) Spinal and brain-stem SEPs and H reflex during enflurane anesthesia. Electroencephalogr clin Neurophysiol 92:82–5.

85. Hicks R, I Woodforth, M Crawford et al (1992) Some effects of isoflurane on I waves of the motor evoked potential. Br J Anaesth 69:130–6.

86. Taniguchi M, J Schram and C Cedzich, (1991) Recording of myogenic motor evoked potential (mMEP) under general anesthesia, in *Intraoperative Neurophysiological Monitoring*, J Schramm and AR Møller, Editors. Springer Verlag: Berlin. 72–87.

87. Amassian VE, M Stewart, GJ Quirk et al (1987) Physiological basis of motor effects on a tran-sient stimulation to cerebral cortex. Neurosurgery 20:74–93.

88. Møller AR (2003) Sensory Systems: Anatomy and Physiology. Amsterdam: Academic Press.

89. Taylor BA, ME Fennelly, A Taylor et al (1993) Temporal summation – the key to motor evoked potential spinalo cord monitoring in humans. J Neurology 56:104–6.

90. Neuloh G and J Schramm (2002) Intraoperative neurophysiological mapping and monioring for supratentorial procedures, in *Neurophysiology in Neurosurgery*, J Deletis and JL Shils, Editors. Elsevier: Amsterdam. 339–401.

potentials evoked by transcranial magnetic stimulation. Spine 19:1512–7.

11

Practical Aspects of Monitoring Cranial Motor Nerves

INTRODUCTION

Cranial motor nerves are at risk of being injured during many different kinds of neurosurgical operations of the skull base, such as operations to remove different kinds of tumors. (Regarding the anatomy and function of cranial nerves, see Appendix B.) Cranial motor nerves can also be at risk during operations on the vascular system of the brain. The risk of postoperative impairment or loss of function of cranial motor nerves as a result of surgical manipulations can be reduced by appropriate use of intraoperative neurophysiological monitoring. Methods are available for monitoring the motor function of CN III, CN IV, CN V, CN VI, CN IX, CN X, CN XI, and CN XII.

When any one of these nerves are involved in tumors, or when regions of the brain that are close to these nerves are manipulated or dissected, proper identification of the nerves intracranially is a prerequisite for preserving their functions.

It may also be of value to monitor the extracranial (peripheral) branches of some of the cranial nerves such as the facial nerve (CN VII), which may be at risk in operations involving the face that may place the branches of the facial nerve at risk for sustaining injury. The peripheral (extracranial) course of the facial nerve may be at risk of being injured during operations that involve the parotid gland. During operations in the chest and on the thyroid gland, the recurrence nerve (a branch of the vagus nerve, CN X) may sustain injury.

From: *Intraoperative Neurophysiological Monitoring: Third Edition*
By A.R. Møller, DOI 10.1007/978-1-4419-7436-5_11,
© Springer Science+Business Media, LLC 2011

Extracranial branches of CN IX, CN X, and CN XI may be at risk of being injured during operations around the jugular foramen, such as for example, to remove tumors in that region. Carotid endarterectomy may also involve some of these lower cranial nerves. Some lower cranial motor nerves may sustain injuries along their extracranial course during surgical operations in the upper neck.

This chapter describes how state-of-the-art electrophysiological methods can be used for intraoperative monitoring of cranial motor systems in different kinds of surgical operations. Methods to monitor cranial motor nerves are described, and discussions are presented regarding the benefits of such monitoring during neurosurgical operations in which these particular nerves are at risk of being injured. Monitoring of sensory cranial nerves (CN II, CN V, and CN VIII) is covered in Chaps 6–8.

This chapter will begin with a discussion of facial nerve monitoring, because the techniques used are applicable to monitoring other cranial motor nerves.

MONITORING OF THE FACIAL NERVE

The facial nerve may be injured in a variety of operations, but most frequently, it occurs during operations to remove vestibular schwannoma.[1] Loss of facial function is a major handicap. Cosmetically it is disastrous, but from a practical point of view, a total loss of facial nerve function on one side makes it difficult to eat. Additionally, eye problems, such as injury to the cornea, can occur due to reduced or absent tear production and the loss of the ability to close the eyelid properly. Artificial tear solutions must be used to avoid drying of the cornea, which would result in eye pain and the risk of impaired vision due to corneal bruises. Implanting a (gold) spring in the eyelid that facilitates automatic closing of the eyelid by

using gravitational force is helpful, but there is no doubt that loss of facial nerve function dramatically changes the life of anyone, and even a moderate impairment of facial function can be a severe handicap. Therefore, no effort should be spared to preserve the function of the facial nerve during operations in which it is being manipulated.

Intraoperative neurophysiological monitoring of the function of the facial nerve is rewarding in that it can make a major difference in the outcome of an operation in which the facial nerve is involved or is being manipulated. Introduction of intraoperative monitoring in operations for vestibular schwannoma had a major impact on the quality of life of individuals who had vestibular schwannoma removed surgically. Before introduction of intraoperative monitoring of the facial nerve in operations to remove vestibular schwannoma, most surgeons did not even attempt to save the facial nerve when operating on large tumors – they knew they would not succeed, and it was not unusual to lose facial function even during removal of small tumors. In fact, before the introduction of facial nerve monitoring, most people with tumors larger than 2.5 cm in diameter lost facial function or had severe weakness of the mimic muscles after removal of such tumors.

Introduction of facial nerve monitoring changed the situation radically, and it became possible to save facial function even in operations of large vestibular schwannoma.

Vestibular schwannoma, earlier known as acoustic tumors, comprise the great majority of the tumors in the cerebellopontine angle (CPA). The proximity between the facial nerve (CN VII) and the eighth cranial nerve (CN VIII), from which these tumors originate, places the facial nerve at risk when a vestibular schwannoma is being removed. Additionally, the anatomical proximity of the facial nerve to the eighth cranial nerve causes the tumor to "engulf" the facial nerve. Often, a tumor may have caused injury to the facial nerve prior to surgical intervention;

---

[1]Vestibular schwannoma is now the official name for tumors of the eighth nerve that previously were (and still are) called acoustic tumors.

therefore, some individuals with vestibular schwannoma may have slight facial weakness before they are operated upon. Even in patients in whom the facial nerve is not directly involved in the tumor, there is a risk of injuring the facial nerve due to surgical manipulations in connection with removal of the tumor.

Facial Nerve Monitoring in Removal of Vestibular Schwannoma

Intraoperative monitoring of facial nerve function during operations to remove vestibular schwannoma was introduced in some hospitals in the early 1980s, and it has been officially recognized as a valuable adjunct to such operations since 1991 when it was stated in a "Consensus Statement" of the National Institutes of Health Consensus Development Conference (held December 11–13, 1991) that, "There is a consensus that intraoperative real-time neurologic monitoring improves the surgical management of vestibular schwannoma, including the preservation of facial nerve function and possibly improves hearing preservation by the use of intraoperative auditory brainstem response monitoring. New approaches to monitoring acoustic nerve function may provide more rapid feedback to the surgeon, thus enhancing their usefulness." The statement continues: "Intraoperative monitoring of cranial nerves V, VI, IX, X, and XI also has been described, but the full benefits of this monitoring remains to be determined." (1).

The "Conclusion and Recommendation" of this report offers an unambiguous endorsement of intraoperative monitoring as an adjunct to surgical therapy for vestibular schwannoma: "The benefit of routine intraoperative monitoring of the facial nerve has been clearly established. This technique should be included in surgical therapy of vestibular schwannoma. Routine monitoring of other cranial nerves should be considered" (Consensus Statement 1991, page 19). Since the publication of the Consensus Statement, the benefit of intraoperative monitoring of the facial nerve has been confirmed in many subsequent studies, see for example (2, 3).

Even with intraoperative monitoring, there is a risk of the facial nerve being destroyed during tumor removal. The risk is greater when a tumor has grown to such a size that it is engulfing the facial nerve, or the nerve has become embedded in the tumor capsule. The surgical removal of a tumor may result in a total and permanent loss of facial function even in patients in whom the facial nerve is located outside the tumor capsule.

The most common reason for surgical damage to the facial nerve is that the surgeon did not know exactly where the facial nerve was located. Another reason is that tumors often divide the facial nerve so that different parts of the nerve become located in different parts of a tumor. Adequate use of intraoperative monitoring makes it possible to locate all parts of the facial nerve in most operations for vestibular schwannoma, even for large tumors.

Damage to the facial nerve may occur even during removal of relatively small vestibular schwannoma if the surgeon does not locate the facial nerve. When a tumor is larger than 2.5 cm in diameter, there is a substantial possibility that the facial nerve has been displaced and often has been divided by the tumor. Thus, removal of tumors larger than 2.5 cm has a higher risk of impairment or permanent loss of facial function than the removal of smaller tumors.

Improvements in surgical techniques and the introduction of intraoperative monitoring of facial function have improved this situation considerably, and the facial nerve is now rarely severely damaged during removal of tumors of 2.5 cm or smaller when using intraoperative neurophysiological monitoring and facial function is normally preserved even after removal of large tumors.

Electrical stimulation of the facial nerve intracranially using a hand-held stimulating electrode, in conjunction with recording facial muscle contractions, has proven to be an important tool in identifying the nerve during removal of vestibular schwannoma. In the past, mechanical sensors were used to detect the contraction of facial muscles (4, 5), but recording of EMG potentials from facial muscles is now the most common way to record facial muscle activity, and thus, determine the degree of activation of the facial nerve (6–14).

Regardless of how facial muscle contractions are recorded, all these methods involve probing the surgical field for the presence of the facial nerve using a hand-held stimulating electrode. In the beginning of an operation, the task is to find regions of the tumor where there are no parts of the facial nerve present so that large pieces of the tumor can be removed without injuring the facial nerve. Later, when most of a tumor has been removed, the task becomes to find all parts of the facial nerve.

Although intraoperative monitoring of the function of the facial nerve was described as early as 1898 (see Krauze, 1912 (15)), and electrical stimulation in connection with visual detection of contractions of the facial muscles was described more than half a century ago (16, 17), some investigators recognized that there was a need for better ways to detect contractions of facial muscles. To address this need, Delgado et al. (6) developed a method to record electrophysiological responses from facial muscles (EMG); these investigators displayed and photographed EMG potentials on an oscilloscope, which were observed by an assistant. They did not, however, use this method to help locate the facial nerve in the surgical field, but rather, to compare the waveform of the EMG recorded during the operation for the purpose of detecting injuries to the facial nerve. A few years later, Sugita and Kubayashi (4) described a way to make the contractions of facial muscles audible by using small accelerometers placed on the face to record the movements of the facial muscles. The electrical potentials generated by the accelerometers could then be amplified and presented through a loudspeaker. Later, other investigators described different methods to record facial movements in order to detect activation of the facial nerve (5, 18) using sensors that recorded movements of face muscles.

It was not until the mid-1980s that intraoperative monitoring of facial function, as we know it now, came into general use during removal of vestibular schwannoma. Recording facial EMG is the current, prevailing method for recording facial muscle activity in operations to remove vestibular schwannoma, and presenting facial EMG recordings through a loudspeaker is now commonly included when operating near the facial nerve.

Recording Facial EMG. Since the purpose of monitoring facial nerve function during operations to remove vestibular schwannoma is to identify all parts of the facial nerve, EMG potentials may be recorded differentially on a single channel, with one electrode placed in the mentalis/orbicularis oris muscles of the lower face and the other electrode placed in the orbicularis oculi/superior frontalis muscles to represent the upper face (**Fig. 11.1**). Such electrode placement makes it possible to record EMG activity that is elicited by electrical stimulation of the facial nerve intracranially from muscles that represent most of the branches of the facial nerve. Such electrode placement also makes it possible to monitor muscle activity that results from mechanical stimulation of the facial nerve and activity that results from injury to the facial nerve (continuous activity) (19). Needle electrodes, such as platinum needle electrodes, or similar disposable needle electrodes are suitable for such recordings as are wire hook electrodes. The electrodes should be secured by a good quality adhesive tape with micropores (for example, Blenderm surgical tape[TM2]).

Some investigators have advocated recording facial muscle activity from two or more of the muscle groups that are innervated by different branches of the facial nerve independently, on separate recording channels (20). However, such dual recording has little advantage over a single-channel recording obtained differentially

---

[2]3M Center, St. Paul, MN 55144–1000.

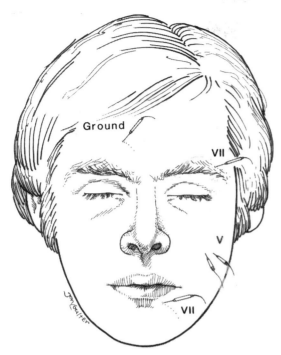

Figure 11.1: Schematic drawing showing the placement of electrodes for recording responses from the facial muscles. The two electrodes marked VII are to be connected to an EMG amplifier. Also shown is the placement of electrodes for selective recording from the masseter muscle for monitoring the motor portion of the trigeminal nerve (CN V).

between electrodes placed as described above, which provides information relevant to the preservation of the function of all branches of the facial nerve. The purpose of facial nerve monitoring is not to find which part of the facial nerve innervates the lower face and which part innervates the upper face; the purpose is to find and preserve any part of the facial nerve.

When the facial muscle responses are recorded differentially between electrodes placed in the upper and lower face (**Fig. 11.1**), the responses from mastication muscles will also

be included in the recording. The mastication muscles are innervated by the motor portion of the trigeminal nerve. A tumor can push the facial nerve rostrally so that its location becomes close to the trigeminal nerve, and when operating on a large vestibular schwannoma, it may not be totally obvious from visual inspection of the surgical field which of the two nerves, the facial or the trigeminal, is being stimulated. Electrical stimulation of the nerve with a hand-held stimulating electrode, while observing the latency of the EMG potentials elicited by stimulating one of the two nerves, reveals whether it is the facial nerve or the trigeminal nerve. The latency of the response obtained when stimulating the trigeminal nerve is much shorter than that obtained from stimulating the facial nerve (**Fig. 11.2**).

Electrical stimulation of the motor portion of CN V intracranially elicits a muscle response in the masseter muscle with a latency of less than 2 ms, while the earliest response from the facial muscles to stimulation of the facial nerve intracranially is approximately 6 ms (7 ms to its first peak, see **Fig. 11.2**). Thus, EMG responses that appear with latencies longer than 5 ms are inevitably caused by contraction of facial muscles; while EMG responses with latencies shorter than 3 ms are caused by contraction of the masseter muscles or the temporalis muscles, and thus, a result of stimulation of the trigeminal motor nerve.

Separate recordings from muscles innervated by the trigeminal nerve can be made by placing electrodes in the masseter muscles as shown in **Fig. 11.1**. This offers the best possibility to discriminate between muscle activity from the trigeminal nerves and that from the facial nerve evoked by electrical or mechanical stimulation, as well as spontaneous activity that may be a sign of injury.

Audible, recorded EMG activity is important because it provides valuable feedback to the surgeon and helps the surgeon to avoid injuring the facial nerve during removal of tumor tissue located in close proximity to the facial nerve.

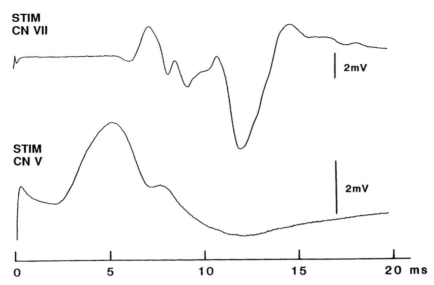

Figure 11.2: *Upper curve:* EMG potentials recorded differentially from electrodes placed in the superior orbicularis oculi/frontalis muscles and in the mentalis/orbicularis oris muscles in response to electrical stimulation of the facial nerve intracranially using a monopolar electrode. The stimuli were rectangular impulses of 150-µS duration presented at 5 pps and the stimulus strength was 1.0 V. *Lower curve:* EMG responses recorded from the same electrodes as shown in the upper curve of this figure, but when the motor portion of the fifth nerve was stimulated intracranially. The stimuli were rectangular impulses of 150-µS duration presented at 5 pps and the stimulus strength was 1.2 V.

However, it is important that the audio amplifier should be equipped with circuitry that suppresses the stimulus artifact (*14*).

There are complex computer-controlled systems on the market that allow an EMG signal to trigger a tone signal. Such systems are supposed to require little or no human interaction, and the surgeon is assumed to get all-important information from the "beeps" emitted when the EMG potentials exceed certain amplitude. However, converting the EMG signal into tone signals offers little, if any, advantage over listening to the recorded EMG signals using a simple system consisting of an amplifier and a (computer) display. On the contrary, the recorded EMG potentials, when made audible, directly provide much valuable information that cannot be conveyed by such tone signals.

It is also questionable if monitoring without an experienced physiologist being present in the operating room offers the full advantage of facial nerve monitoring.

In the beginning of an operation to remove a large vestibular schwannoma, electrical stimulation can be used to find regions of the tumor that do not contain any portion of the facial nerve. This enables the surgeon to remove large portions of the tumor without risk of injuring the facial nerve, and it reduces operating time considerably. As removal of the tumor progresses, the goal is to continually identify the facial nerve so that surgical injury to the nerve can be avoided.

For finding a region of a tumor where there is no nerve present, a monopolar stimulating electrode connected to a stimulator that produces a relatively constant voltage of electrical stimulation is suitable (*14*). When this technique is used in the first part of an operation to remove a medium-to-large tumor, considerable time is saved because large portions of the tumor can be removed with little risk of injuring the facial nerve (*14*). The fact that a tumor often displaces and sometimes divides the facial nerve makes it imperative to test a tumor for the presence of the facial nerve before removal of any part of the tumor is performed. Thus, a tumor mass located in the CPA should never be removed without first probing the portion of the tumor in question with the facial nerve stimulator, and the tumor removal should only precede if it is found to be unresponsive to electrical stimulation.

When the facial nerve is involved in a tumor, nerve tissue often cannot be distinguished visually from the surrounding tumor tissue, and the only way to identify all parts of a nerve is by electrical stimulation. Such electrical probing of the surgical field must be made frequently so that the location of the nerve (and regions that do not contain any parts of the facial nerve) is always known during all phases of the tumor removal.

The facial nerve often extends over a sizeable portion of large tumors, and it may have many separate fascicles and may appear diffuse. It is, therefore, necessary to probe all parts of the tumor with the electrical stimulator to ensure that the entire facial nerve has been correctly identified, and any nerve tissue that gives a facial response must be identified before tumor tissue is removed.

Some investigators have promoted the use of a bipolar stimulating electrode in connection with operations to remove vestibular schwannoma (*21*). A bipolar stimulating electrode has a greater spatial selectivity and is useful for finding the exact location of the facial nerve. A bipolar electrode is also ideal for determining which of two nerves located close to each other is the facial nerve. A bipolar stimulating electrode, however, is not suited for identifying regions of a tumor where no portion of the

facial nerve is present because a bipolar electrode is too spatially selective. It would be ideal to have both monopolar and bipolar stimulating electrodes available during operations to remove vestibular schwannoma, but if simplicity is important, a monopolar electrode is the best choice.

Careful monitoring of facial muscle function should also be performed during removal of the portions of a tumor located inside the internal auditory meatus, and the facial nerve should be identified by electrical stimulation.

Another advantage from displaying the facial EMG response on a computer screen (in addition to making it possible to obtain latency measurements) is the possibility to observe the waveform of the response and determine its amplitude. When using supramaximal stimulation of the facial nerve, the amplitude of the EMG response is an approximate measure of how many nerve fibers have been activated (see Chap. 2). Observing the change (reduction) in the amplitude of the EMG response during an operation, therefore, provides information about the degree of injury to the facial nerve.

It is important to quickly find the location of the facial nerve. Observing the amplitude of the EMG evoked by the hand-held stimulator can help. If the amplitude increases when the electrode is moved, it means that it is moved in the direction where the facial nerve is located; if it decreases, it is moved away from it. This simple procedure can reduce the time it takes to find the location of the facial nerve, but it requires that an experienced physiologist is present in the operating room to direct this procedure.

It has been suggested that the location of the facial nerve can be determined by probing the surgical field with a surgical instrument, but this is not a suitable way to find the facial nerve. Monitoring facial EMG by touching the facial nerve with a surgical instrument cannot identify the anatomical location of an uninjured facial nerve because manipulation of an uninjured nerve causes little, if any, EMG activity. Only injured nerves are sensitive to mechanical stimulation. There is no substitute for electrical stimulation to find the location of a nerve in the operative field.

Identification of the Location of Injury. An injury to the facial nerve in patients who undergo surgical removal of a vestibular schwannoma is usually focal in nature. The location of the injury along the nerve can be identified by comparing the latencies of the EMG responses to electrical stimulation at different locations along the nerve's intracranial course. The latency of the response typically increases in a step-wise fashion when the stimulating electrode is moved from a location that is distal to the injured section of the nerve to a location that is proximal to the injured section. When stimulation is performed proximal to an injured section of a nerve, the waveform of the recorded EMG potentials is often different (broader with multiple peaks) from those recorded when the nerve is stimulated at a location that is distal to the injured section. When made audible, the sounds of EMG responses are often distinctly different in response to stimulation at two such locations. These differences make it possible to identify the anatomical location of injured portions of the facial nerve.

When electrical stimulation is used to find the anatomical location of a conduction block in the facial nerve, it is important to understand that a nerve is an electrical conductor itself in addition to its ability to carry propagated neural activity. Portions of a nerve that do not conduct propagated nerve impulses can conduct electrical impulses passively. When a monopolar stimulating electrode is used, and the stimulus is set at an intensity that is too high, it is possible that electrical stimulation of an injured part of the facial nerve may elicit an EMG response because the stimulus current is conducted passively to the part of the nerve that is intact and actively conducts propagated nerve activity. When no response is obtained by stimulating the facial nerve at a certain location, the stimulus intensity should not be increased too much because this may result in misleading results due to the passive conduction of the stimulus current.

Identifying the Trigeminal Motor Nerve. The trigeminal nerve (portio minor) innervates the mastication muscles, the temporalis and the masseter muscles, which are large strong muscles. When the trigeminal nerve is activated, these muscles will contract, and depending on the placement of the EMG electrodes for monitoring contractions of the facial muscles, contraction of the mastication muscles may result in recordings of activity by these electrodes although the electrodes were not placed in the mastication muscles. This is especially the case when the electrode placement shown in **Fig. 11.1** is used. EMG activity that is evoked by stimulation of the trigeminal nerve can be distinguished from that evoked by stimulation of the facial nerve on the basis of the latency of the responses (**Fig. 11.2**), even when the EMG activity from facial muscles is recorded on a single channel as shown in **Fig. 11.**1. However, the converse is not true; EMG activity that is caused by injury or evoked by mechanical stimulation of the facial nerve cannot be distinguished from activity caused by injury or evoked by mechanical stimulation of the trigeminal motor nerve by merely observing the response.

Recording from the masseter muscle in a separate channel is the best way to identify the response from stimulating the trigeminal motor nerve (see **Fig. 11.1**). Two needle (or wire) electrodes placed close to each other in the masseter muscle and connected to a differential amplifier can serve that purpose (**Fig. 11.1**). Using an additional recording channel to record from the masseter muscle (**Fig. 11.1**) can make it possible to differentiate between the continuous responses of the muscles that are innervated by the facial nerve and those that are innervated by the trigeminal nerve. With this electrode placement, the additional channel will only record from the masseter muscles, and the facial muscles will not contribute noticeably to the response.

Mechanically-Induced Facial Nerve Activity. When the facial nerve is directly involved in a tumor, it is often very fragile and does not have the visual appearance of a nerve. Seen from a retromastoid approach, the facial nerve emerges from the internal auditory meatus and turns down sharply. Its appearance is often more like wet tissue paper than that of a nerve. Removal of a tumor mass in which such a fragile nerve is embedded is an extremely delicate process. Safe removal of such an adherent tumor can be greatly facilitated by the surgeon if he or she continuously monitors the sound of the EMG responses while operating. A slightly injured nerve is sensitive to mechanical manipulation and gives off neural activity that elicits muscle contractions (EMG activity) when the nerve is being manipulated (*22*). The technique of gently scraping the tumor mass off the facial nerve, while listening to the EMG activity from facial muscles, acts as feedback to the surgeon and can help the surgeon avoid serious and permanent injury to the facial nerve. Removal of tumor tissue that is adherent to the facial nerve will, therefore, cause clear, and often strong EMG activity. By listening to the EMG responses made audible, the surgeon can tell when a manipulation might have caused damage to the nerve, and he or she can then stop or alter the manipulation (*9, 14*).

Mechanical stimulation of an injured motor nerve often causes sustained activity in the respective muscle innervated by the nerve that may last a few seconds, and sometimes longer, after it has been manipulated (*9, 13, 23*). Similar mechanical stimulation of a normal (not injured) nerve may not result in any EMG activity, or it may result in an EMG response that lasts only as long as the manipulation lasts. The mechanically-evoked muscle activity from surgical manipulation will cease within a short time after manipulation of a slightly injured facial nerve is discontinued, but if the nerve is severely injured, the induced muscle activity will continue for many seconds, or even minutes, after cessation of manipulation of the nerve. Such prolonged activity should be a

warning to the surgeon that the manipulation has caused injury to the facial nerve that may impair facial function temporarily, or perhaps even permanently. Individuals who have had several episodes of sustained EMG activity during tumor removal often have more-or-less pronounced facial weakness postoperatively.

Heat as a Cause of Injury to the Facial Nerve. Sustained muscle activity may also result from electrocoagulation when heat spreads to the facial nerve. To reduce the risk of that occurring, electrocoagulation should use the lowest level of coagulation current, and the coagulation should be applied for short periods with intervals to allow for cooling of the tissues adjacent to the site of electrocoagulation, always using only bipolar coagulators.

Drilling the bone of the internal auditory meatus can also cause heat that can spread to the facial nerve and become a risk of injury to the facial nerve as indicated by evoking EMG activity in facial muscles. Efficient cooling by irrigation with fluid of a suitable (low) temperature while drilling the bone of the internal auditory meatus can reduce the risk of injury to the facial nerve. Pre-cooling the bone that is to be drilled may also be beneficial in such situations. Continuously monitoring facial EMG is a valuable tool to detect when the facial nerve has been heated to a degree that poses a risk of permanent injury to the nerve.

Irrigation of a slightly injured facial nerve with saline, at a temperature that is below normal body temperature, often gives rise to facial muscle activity that lasts for many seconds. There is no evidence, however, that such EMG activity is a sign of risk to the function of the facial nerve. Irrigation with a fluid whose temperature is *above* normal body temperature imposes a serious risk to all neural tissue with which the fluid comes into contact, and thus, should be avoided at all times.

The same recording electrodes and equipment used to record evoked EMG potentials can be used for continuous monitoring of the EMG activity from mechanical stimulation of the facial nerve, but it necessitates display of "free-running EMG" during periods when electrical stimulation is suspended. This possibility is included in most commercial intraoperative recording equipment.

Indications for Grafting of the Facial Nerve. In situations where the facial nerve is unresponsive to electrical stimulation at the end of tumor removal, the surgeon must make a decision regarding grafting the facial nerve in the same operation or wait and see if the function of the facial muscles recovers postoperatively. There are advantages in grafting the facial nerve in the actual tumor operation, but it must be remembered that absence of response to electrical stimulation of the facial nerve does not provide information regarding recovery of facial function. Neuropraxia and axonotmesis cannot be distinguished from more severe kinds of nerve injuries (neurotmesis) on the basis of an electrophysiological test. This means that electrophysiological tests cannot provide guidance regarding the prognosis for recovery of the facial nerve. Visual inspection must be the guide for decisions about whether to do a grafting procedure in the tumor operation.

Continuous Monitoring of the Function of the Facial Nerve

It would be a great advantage if it were possible to monitor the facial nerve continuously, in a similar way as, for example, monitoring SSEP, motor evoked potentials, and ABR. The blink reflex would be suitable for continuous monitoring of the integrity of the facial nerve. In conscious individuals, it can be elicited by electrical stimulation of the supraorbital nerve, while recording EMG potentials from the orbicularis oculi, but the blink reflex is normally, totally suppressed by conventional anesthesia when elicited in the conventional way by applying single electrical impulses. The reason it cannot be elicited during surgical anesthesia is that the motoneurons in the facial nucleus cannot be activated, probably for the same reason that the

spinal neurons are difficult to activate during anesthesia (see page 209), namely, absence of the normal facilitatory input to the facial motoneurons.

This assumption is supported by the observation that the blink reflexes can be elicited in individuals with hemifacial spasm on the affected side (*24*). In hemifacial spasm (HFS), the facial motor nucleus is hyperexcitable (*25*) (see Chap. 15), and this hyperexcitability counteracts the synaptic suppression from anesthesia so that the reflex can be elicited. After the offending blood vessel is moved off the facial nerve root, it is no longer possible to elicit the blink reflex as a sign of facial nerve integrity because the hyperexcitability of the facial motonucleus requires the presence of the vascular contact with the facial nerve root (*26*).

There are other ways to compensate for synaptic suppression, and one such way is to apply a train of stimulus impulses instead of a single impulse (*27*) (this method, in connection with suitable anesthesia regimen, is now used routinely for activation of the spinal motor neurons in anesthetized individuals, see Chap. 10). The blink reflex is traditionally evoked by single impulses presented at a rate of 2–5 pulses per second to the supraorbital nerve where it emerges from the foramen orbitalis (*28*). Elicited in this way, the blink reflex response consists of two EMG responses known as the R_1 and R_2, with the R_1 having a latency of approximately 10 ms.

It was recently shown that it is possible to elicit the blink reflex in surgically anesthetized patients using a train of four to seven stimulus impulses applied to the supraorbital nerve when suitable modern anesthesia techniques are used (*27*).

The reason why a train succeeds and a single impulse fails to elicit a response is that a train of impulses generates larger EPSP in the facial motonucleus than a single stimulus impulse because of the effect of temporal summation on the EPSP. The blink reflex elicited by trains of impulses applied to the supraorbital nerve, thereby, provides a method for continuous monitoring of the function of the facial nerve in operations where the facial nerve is at risk of being injured.

In a study of 27 operations, the R_1 response could be elicited in 23 operations. The latencies varied between 12.5 ms and 26.3 ms, thus longer than the normal 10–11 ms for the R_1 response in conscious individuals. The anesthesia used in the patients that were studied differed. One group received desflurane, the other TIVA with Propofol.

The effect of using more than one impulse to elicit the blink reflex is shown in **Fig. 11.3**. It was seen that a single impulse did not yield any response, but the R_1 component of the blink reflex responses (**Fig. 11.3A**) could be obtained when a train of stimuli were presented.

In summary, intraoperative monitoring of facial EMG, elicited by electrical stimulation of the intracranial portion of the facial nerve, is critical in reducing the risk of injury to the facial nerve during operations to remove vestibular schwannoma. Using the techniques just

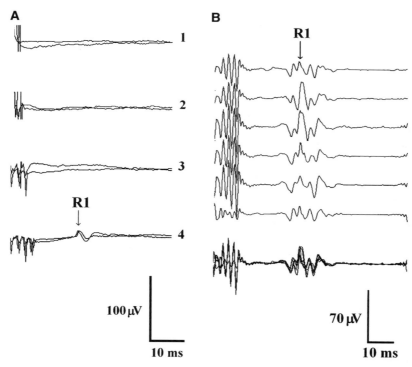

Figure 11.3: The R_1 response of the blink response in a patient operated upon for a trigeminal tumor under desflurane anesthesia. The responses were recorded from the orbicularis oculi muscles. The stimuli were rectangular impulses with a duration of 0.5 ms in trains of 3–5 impulses, separated by 2 ms and applied to the scalp at $C_3(+)$ to $C_4(-)$. (**A**) The effect of increasing the number of impulses in the trains from 1–4. (**B**) Reproducibility of the responses to trains of impulses. The *bottom trace* is a superposition of six responses. The latency of the R_1 response was 26.3 ms. (Reprinted from (*27*) with permission from Elsevier).

described, total tumor removal is often possible with preservation of facial function, even in large vestibular schwannoma. The possibility to achieve continuous monitoring of the facial nerve by using the blink reflex elicited by trains of impulses in connection with suitable anesthetics (27) is a further important development that can improve facial nerve monitoring.

Monitoring the Facial Nerve in Other Operations

It is beneficial to monitor the function of the facial nerve intraoperatively (together with several other cranial nerves (see page 247, 253)) in other operations such as operations in which large tumors of the skull base are resected.

Although vestibular schwannoma are by far the most common type of tumor in the CPA, other tumors may occur in this area, and removal of such tumors may place the facial nerve at risk. However, meningioma in the CPA seldom involve the facial nerve to the same extent as do vestibular schwannoma, but intraoperative monitoring of the facial nerve during operations on meningioma, using a technique similar to that used during removal of vestibular schwannoma, may be beneficial in reducing the risk of injury to the facial nerve from mechanical manipulation or from heat from electrocoagulation.

Epidermoid cysts (or cholesteatoma) and other rare masses may also be located in the CPA, and although they seldom involve the facial nerve directly, the availability of facial nerve stimulation and recording of facial EMG potentials may be useful in their removal, and it may facilitate preservation of the facial nerve in such operations.

Tumors of the facial nerve itself (facial nerve neuroma) occur rarely, and it is generally not possible to save the facial nerve in resection of facial nerve tumors. In such operations, nerve grafting may be made in the same operation. A facial nerve stimulator is helpful in identifying the facial nerve and in finding the

location in order to undertake such nerve grafting.

There are several other operations in which it is valuable to be able to identify the intracranial portion of the facial nerve. Patients with HFS have a blood vessel in close contact with the intracranial portion of their facial nerve near the brainstem (root exit zone, or REZ). It is known that when this blood vessel is moved away from the facial nerve and a soft implant is placed between the vessel and the nerve (microvascular decompression, MVD) such patients are cured of their disease (see Chap. 15). Since monitoring the abnormal muscle response that guides the surgeon in operations for HFS involves recording facial EMG potentials, the same setup can be used for monitoring intraoperative injuries to the facial nerve in patients. Surgical manipulation, and particularly, heating from electrocoagulation, can result in continuous EMG activity. Compression of the facial nerve from, for instance, placing an implant that is too large between the facial nerve and the offending blood vessel can also result in continuous EMG activity.

Another example of an operation where the facial nerve may be at risk is in MVD operations of the eighth or fifth nerve to treat vertigo or trigeminal neuralgia (see Chap. 15). Identification of the facial nerve may be difficult in some of these operations solely on anatomical grounds and visual inspection. Electrical stimulation in connection with recordings of facial EMG potentials offers an easy way to positively identify the facial nerve. This is particularly important when the operation is complicated: for example, when patients have been operated on previously and scar tissue has developed, or when there are other reasons to expect anatomical abnormalities. In such patients, extensive dissection would often be necessary to determine the identity of the different nerves anatomically by visual inspection only, while it is easy to identify the facial nerve by using electrical stimulation.

MONITORING OF OTHER CRANIAL MOTOR NERVES

Skull base tumors are often large by the time they are diagnosed and operated on, and because the anatomy is often greatly distorted, there can be uncertainty about the anatomical location of cranial nerves. During such operations, several cranial motor nerves are monitored. The same technique utilized for identifying the facial nerve, as described above, can also be used for finding the anatomical location of other cranial nerves that may be involved in other skull base tumors. For instance, it was mentioned earlier in this chapter that the responses from the muscles of mastication that are innervated by the motor portion of the trigeminal nerve (CN V) can be observed by recording the muscle response from a pair of recording needle electrodes placed in the masseter muscle (**Fig. 11.1**).

Monitoring of Cranial Nerves III, IV, and VI

Skull base tumors may invade the cavernous sinus and, thereby, directly involve several cranial motor nerves, particularly those innervating the extraocular muscles (CN III, CN IV, and CN VI). Loss of function of the trochlear nerve (CN IV), which innervates the superior oblique muscle, is inconvenient to an individual person, but does not interfere significantly with the use of the eye in question. Loss of function of the abducens nerve (CN VI), which innervates the lateral (or external) rectus muscle, impairs the use of the affected eye noticeably because it prevents from moving the eye laterally from a mid position. Loss of function of the oculomotor nerve (CN III), which innervates the three other extraocular muscles (**Fig. 11.4A**), is a serious complication because it essentially results in functional blindness of the affected eye – it places the eye in a far lateral, downward pointing position from which it cannot be moved. The CN III nerve also innervates the upper eyelid, and paralysis of CN III causes drooping of the eyelid (ptosis). CN III also possesses autonomic fibers that control the size of the pupil and the ciliary muscle that controls accommodation. Loss of these parts of CN III contributes to the impairment of vision of the affected eye.

Tumors of the skull base tend to be large, and they, therefore, often distort the anatomy. For this reason, one of the main purposes of intraoperative neurophysiological monitoring in operations to remove skull base tumors is to aid the surgeon in identifying the anatomical location of the cranial nerves that are involved.

To record EMG potentials from extraocular muscles, needle electrodes or wire hooks may be placed percutaneously in or close to the lateral rectus muscle (CN VI), the inferior rectus muscle (CN III) and the superior oblique muscle (CN IV) (*30*) as shown in **Fig. 11.4B**. It is not necessary that the electrodes penetrate the respective muscles; the electrodes only need to be close to the muscles to produce EMG responses with amplitudes sufficient to be visible on a computer screen without any averaging. Care must be taken not to injure the eye globe. Risks can be minimized by placing the electrodes so that they point away from the globe and secure them in that position using a good-quality plastic adhesive tape (for example, 3M Co.,[3] Blenderm[R]). Reference electrodes are placed on the forehead on the opposite side so that they do not record activity of the facial muscles on the affected side (**Fig. 11.4B**). Wire hook electrodes may be more appropriate for recordings from the extraocular muscles than needle electrodes. Such electrodes can provide monopolar or even bipolar recordings.

Probing the surgical field by a hand-held monopolar stimulating electrode while recording EMG potentials from the extraocular muscles (*30, 31*) is a suitable method for identifying the anatomical location of the cranial nerves that innervate the extraocular muscles. Similar

---

[3]Arrow International, Reading, PA. 1-800-978-9278.

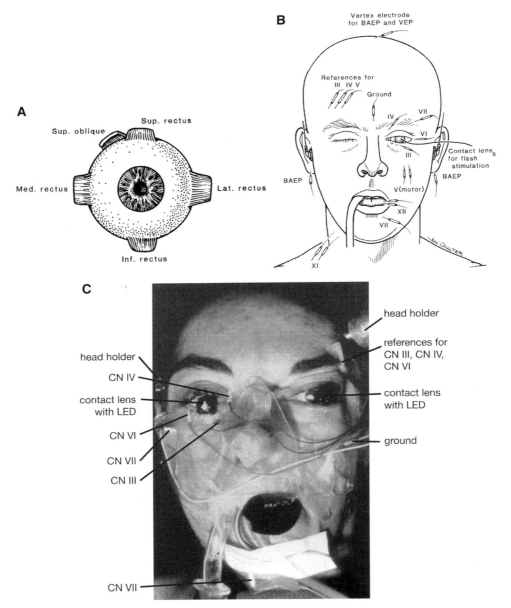

Figure 11.4: (**A**) Anatomy of the orbit showing the extraocular muscles. (**B**) Schematic drawing of placement of electrodes for monitoring cranial nerves. Electrode placements for auditory brainstem responses (ABR) and visual evoked potentials (VEP) were also recorded. Note the earphone and the contact lenses with light-emitting diodes for monitoring visual evoked potentials. (Reprinted from: (*29*) with the permission from McGrawHill). (**C**) Electrode placement in a patient in whom intraoperative recordings were made from the extraocular muscles and the facial muscles. Contact lenses with LEDs are also shown.

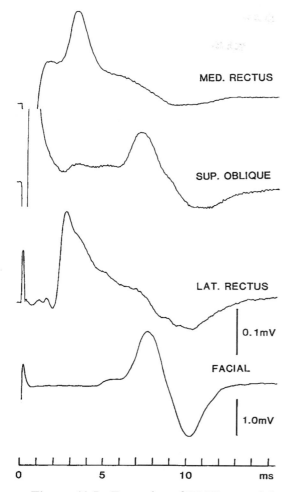

MED. RECTUS

SUP. OBLIQUE

LAT. RECTUS

0.1mV

FACIAL

1.0mV

0   5   10   ms

Figure 11.5: Examples of EMG potentials recorded from the extraocular muscles and from the facial muscles with the recording electrodes placed similar to those in **Fig. 11.4B**. The stimulation was applied to the intracranial portions of the respective nerves using a handheld monopolar stimulating electrode.

stimulation parameters such as those described for stimulation of the facial nerve are suitable, although a slightly higher stimulus strength may be required (1–1.5 V when using impulses of 100 μS duration delivered by a semi-constant voltage stimulator). A bipolar stimulating electrode, used for this purpose, has the

same advantages and disadvantages as described above for monitoring the facial nerve.

The recorded potentials from the extraocular muscles have amplitudes from 0.2 mV to 1 mV (**Fig. 11.5**). In addition to displaying the recorded EMG responses of the respective muscles on a computer screen (**Fig. 11.5**), it is advantageous to make the responses – from one muscle at a time – audible in the same way as described for potentials recorded from the facial muscles (page 238).

Sekiya and coworkers (*32*) have described methods to record EMG potentials from extraocular muscles using noninvasive electrodes. Instead of using needle electrodes or wire electrodes, electrodes (**Fig. 11.6A**) in the form of small wire loops (ring electrodes) placed under the eyelids are used. This method provides an important alternative to using invasive methods to record EMG potentials from the extraocular muscles. The amplitudes of the EMG potentials recorded with these electrodes are somewhat smaller than those that can be recorded from needle electrodes (**Fig. 11.6B**), but the potentials are large enough to be visualized directly on a computer screen without any averaging, and the EMG potentials can be made audible.

MONITORING LOWER CRANIAL MOTOR NERVES

Monitoring of lower cranial nerves (CN IX, CN X, CN XI, and CN XII) (*34–36*) is valuable in connection with operations of many kinds of skull base tumors (*31*). The motor portion of the glossopharyngeal nerve (CN IX) can be monitored intraoperatively (*34–36*), although CN IX only innervates one muscle, the stylopharyngeal muscle. Recording from this muscle, or in its vicinity, can be made by placing a pair of recording electrodes in the soft palate on the same side as the operation. The electrodes should be placed only after the patient is intubated, and all other tubes that are inserted through the mouth are in place. The electrodes

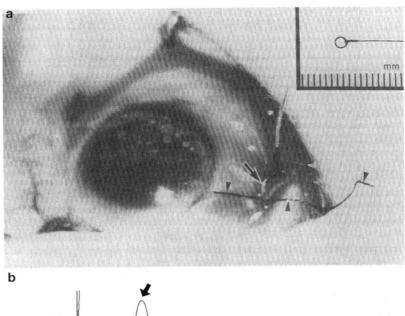

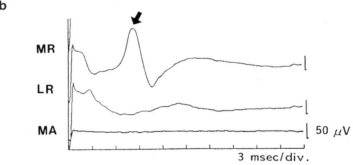

Figure 11.6: (A) Ring electrode for recording EMG potentials from extraocular muscles. (Reprinted from: (*32*)). (**B**) Recordings from two extraocular muscles using the electrode shown in (**A**), and recordings from the masseter muscle. *MR* medial rectus muscles, *LR* lateral rectus muscle, *MA* masseter muscles. (Reprinted from: (*33*) with the permission from Lippincott Williams & Wilkins).

may be secured in place by anchoring the electrode leads to the face by adhesive tape. The anatomical location of the different nerves can be found by using a hand-held electrical stimulating electrode as described for the facial nerve (see page 238). The EMG potentials, recorded in response to simulation of the glossopharyngeal nerve intracranially, typically have latencies of approximately 7 ms (*34*). Because the glossopharyngeal nerve is involved in the control of the vascular system, caution should be exercised when stimulating this nerve

electrically, and cardiovascular signs should be watched closely.

A branch of CN X, the recurrent nerve, is a motor nerve that innervates the laryngeal muscles. Monitoring of the motor portion of the vagus nerve can be performed by recording EMG potentials from larynx musculature, such as the vocalis (*34, 35*). Some investigators have placed EMG electrodes in the laryngeal musculature by visual inspection, but that placement requires the use of a laryngoscope and some technical skill. The electrodes may be placed in

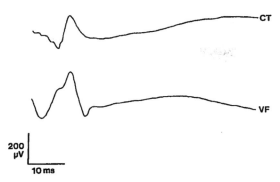

Figure 11.7: Comparison between responses to stimulation of the vagus nerve intracranially in patients undergoing operations where the vagus nerve in the CPA angle was exposed. The recordings were made from electrodes placed in the larynx and in the cricothyroid muscle percutaneously. Simultaneous comparison of the response from the transcricothyroid muscle shown on the upper trace (CT) and endoscopically placed vocal fold electrode response in the lower trace (VF). The amplitude of the responses of the endoscopically placed electrodes is slightly larger than that recorded percutaneously. The stimulus artifact is not shown in these recordings. The onset latency of the response was 4 ms. (Reprinted from: (36) with the permission from Lippincott Williams & Wilkins).

the vocal cords or, even better, in the supraglottic larynx (false vocal cords) (34, 35)

EMG potentials can also be recorded from larynx muscles by electrodes that are placed percutaneous in the cricothyroid muscle (36). The cricothyroid muscle responds to stimulation of both the recurrent laryngeal nerve and the superior laryngeal nerve (which is a branch of CN X) (see **Fig. 11.7**). Verification of correct electrode placement in the conscious patient may be made by having the patient vocalize a high-pitched sound and recording EMG activity, which shows maximal amplitude when the recording electrodes are correctly placed. With experience, it is possible to place such electrodes correctly in anesthetized patients.

Monitoring EMG responses from laryngeal muscles can also be made by recording EMG

potentials from metallic tape wrapped around the tracheal tube, which then acts as EMG electrodes (34).

Because the vagus nerve innervates many systems in the abdomen and is involved with respiratory, cardiac, and intestinal functions, electrical stimulation of CN X should be performed with caution. Great caution should be exercised especially when stimulating the right vagus nerve because the right vagus nerve innervates the heart; electrical stimulation of the right vagus nerve may, therefore, cause a heart block. Heart rate and blood pressure should be monitored.

The spinal accessory nerve (CN XI) can be monitored intraoperatively by recording EMG potentials from the sternocleidomastoid muscle or the trapezius muscle, which are both innervated by CN XI. The EMG responses from these muscles can easily be recorded by placing a pair of electrodes into the respective muscles. When stimulating CN XI electrically, however, there is need for caution because such stimulation may cause a contraction so strong that a rupture of tendons or a dislocation of joints may occur, or the patient might move on the operating table in a way that poses a risk during the time that intracranial procedures are in progress. Only single impulses should be used because trains of impulses can elicit dangerously large muscle contractions because of temporal summation.

The hypoglossal nerve (CN XII) innervates the tongue. If one of the two hypoglossal nerves is severed, atrophy of the tongue will develop on the side of the severed nerve, and if the nerve is damaged or interrupted bilaterally, it causes a serious handicap such as inability to speak or swallow. Monitoring of CN XII can be performed by recording EMG potentials from the tongue (**Fig. 11.8**). Monitoring the hypoglossal nerve should be included when operating in the area of the clivus and foramen magnum; such monitoring can often help save this small nerve from being injured. Recording EMG potentials from the tongue while probing the surgical field with a handheld electrical stimulating electrode makes it possible to locate CN XII. Monitoring

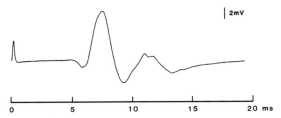

Figure 11.8: Example of EMG recordings from two needle electrodes that were placed on the side of the tongue in response to electrical stimulation of CN XII intracranially. These recordings were obtained during an operation to remove a large chordoma in which the hypoglossal nerve was embedded. The stimuli were rectangular impulses of 150-μS duration presented at 5 pps and the stimulus strength was 1.2 V.

of the response to such stimulation can also verify the integrity of this nerve (*30, 35*).

TMS OF CRANIAL NERVES

TMS has been used for stimulation of the trigeminal and facial nerves during MVD operations for research purposes, but rarely for monitoring purposes. Studies of how impulses of a magnetic field applied by a coil placed outside the head can induce electrical currents in the brain that can stimulate the facial nerve (*37–40*) and the trigeminal nerve (*41*) have provided some insight in the mechanisms of stimulating intracranial nerves by magnetic stimulation.

Monitoring the Extracranial Portion of the Facial Nerve

The facial nerve may be at risk of being injured when it is dissected and manipulated along its peripheral course in the face as well as where it travels in its bony canal (the Fallopian canal) before reaching the stylomastoid foramen. The same technique for identifying the facial nerve as described earlier in this chapter can be used to reduce the risk of injury

to the peripheral branches of the facial nerve. For example, removal of tumors of the parotid gland may result in injury to the facial nerve, but with proper identification of the various branches of the facial nerve that may be involved in the tumor, it is often possible to avoid injury to any branch of the facial nerve (*42*). When the area around a parotid tumor is dissected, a facial nerve stimulator should be used to identify the different branches of the facial nerve.

It is important to note that the latency of the EMG responses to stimulation of the peripheral portion of the facial nerve is much shorter than it is in response to stimulation of the facial nerve intracranially. Thus, a facial nerve stimulator that makes use of an artifact suppression circuit to inactivate the audio amplifier during the period when the artifact occurs may also suppress some of the actual EMG response, if the setting of the duration of the suppression is used for intracranial stimulation of the facial nerve. Displaying of EMG potentials on a computer screen is usually not affected by artifact suppression, and the entire response will show on the screen, even if the duration of artifact suppression is set too long to make it audible.

It is important to identify the facial nerve in other kinds of operations that involve the face. Operations such as those to correct temporomandibular joint disorders may result in injury to a branch of the facial nerve from the incision because the facial nerve sometimes has an abnormal course. The risk posed by the meanderings of the facial nerve can be diminished by mapping the course of the branches of the facial nerve in the region where the incision is to be made. In repairing trauma to the face, it is important to be able to identify all branches of the facial nerve in order to minimize the risks of injuring any part of the facial nerve.

After an accident, or after certain operations, neuroma may form on the facial nerve; an operation may be required simply to remove such neuroma. The location of a neuroma that lies in the path of nerve conduction ("neuroma in continuity") can be determined intraoperatively by recording EMG potentials while stimulating a branch of the nerve electrically at different locations along its path. This is discussed in more detail in Chap. 12 in connection with intraoperative measurements of neural conduction in peripheral nerves.

MONITORING FUNCTIONAL ASPECTS OF THE BRAINSTEM

ABR as an Indicator of Brainstem Manipulations

Nuclei of the brain (gray matter) are more sensitive to ischemia and surgical manipulations than fiber tracts (white matter). Several components of the ABR have their generators in nuclei in the brainstem, and the recorded ABR, therefore, depends on the integrity of several nuclei in addition to fiber tracts in the brainstem. Surgical manipulations and ischemia of the brainstem can, therefore, cause changes in the ABR. This fact makes it possible to detect when the brainstem is surgically manipulated or when there are risks of ischemia of this part of the central nervous system. The changes in ABR that result from brainstem manipulation are more complex than those seen when the auditory nerve has been injured, and these changes are, therefore, more difficult to interpret.

The components of the ABR affected depend on which parts of the brainstem are manipulated. On the basis of knowledge about the neural generators of ABR, it is often possible to relate a certain change in the ABR waveform to specific anatomical structures. Changes (increases) in the interpeak latency (IPL) of peaks I and III of the ABR indicate that lower brainstem structures at the level of the auditory nerve or cochlear nuclei, on the side that is being stimulated, are being affected.

A change in the IPL of peaks I–III is less likely to occur when the ear opposite to the operated side is being stimulated. There is, however, a possibility that manipulation of the brainstem may cause a stretching of CN VIII on the opposite side, or the manipulation may affect the region of the pontomedullary junction of the brainstem and cause changes in the IPL of peaks I–III in the ABR elicited by stimulating the ear opposite to the tumor.

A change (increase) in the IPL of peaks III and V indicates an effect on the lateral lemniscus on the side opposite to the one that is being stimulated and perhaps an effect on the nuclei of the superior olivary complex (SOC) on either side.

When it is not clear which side of the brainstem may be compressed or manipulated in an operation, it is justified to record ABR elicited by stimulating both ears (one at a time, as it serves no purpose to stimulate both ears simultaneously).

Large Vestibular Schwannoma and Skull Base Tumors

Operations on large vestibular schwannoma and tumors of the skull base may involve manipulations of the brainstem that can result in severe complications (page 95). The ABR elicited from the opposite ear often change as a result of brainstem manipulations and brainstem compression, and these ABR changes occur earlier than, for example, cardiovascular changes (43).

Traditionally, changes in cardiovascular function (heart rate and blood pressure) have been used to detect the effect of brainstem manipulations. However, the changes that can be detected in heart rate and blood pressure occur with a certain delay and often only after excessive manipulations. A study that compared changes in ABR with cardiovascular changes showed that ABR in many instances changed before cardiovascular changes could be detected (43). When used to monitor brainstem function in patients who are operated upon to remove large vestibular schwannoma, ABR should be elicited by stimulating the ear opposite to the side of the tumor and recorded in the conventional way. Because patients with large vestibular schwannoma usually do not have any usable hearing on the affected

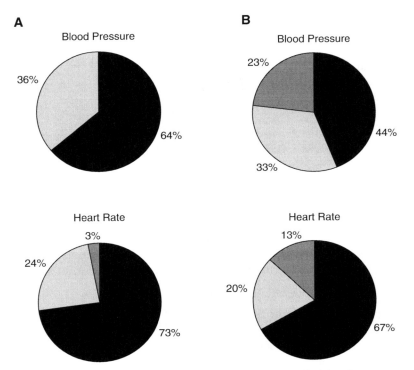

Figure 11.9: Comparison between ABR changes and changes in blood pressure and heart rate during the operation of a large vestibular schwannoma. (**A**) Percentage of manipulation conditions in which the latency of peak V of the ABR increased above the 95% confidence interval before, after, or at the same time as blood pressure and heart rate changes exceeded the 95% confidence interval. (**B**) Percentage of manipulation conditions in which the amplitude of peak V of the ABR decreased above the 95% confidence interval before, after, or at the same time as blood pressure and heart rate changes exceeded the 95% confidence interval. (Reprinted from: (*43*) with the permission from Maney Publishing).

side, it is not helpful to record auditory evoked potentials elicited from the ear on the operative side.

Comparison Between ABR Changes and Cardiac Changes

In a study of patients undergoing removal of large vestibular schwannoma, ABR elicited from the contralateral ear was monitored (*43*). When the observed changes in ABR were compared to changes in blood pressure, it became evident that changes occurred generally in both ABR and blood pressure, but that the changes occurred earlier in the ABR (**Fig. 11.10**). This supports the assumption that intraoperative monitoring of

ABR is beneficial in operations in which the brainstem may be manipulated (*43, 44*).

The results shown in **Fig. 11.9** were obtained by recording data about the changes in different components of the ABR and cardiovascular data that were recorded by the anesthesia team. An example of such recordings for a patient undergoing an operation to remove a large vestibular schwannoma is shown in **Fig. 11.10**.

Comparison of changes in blood pressure and heart rate with changes in the amplitude and latency of peak V of the ABR during operation of large vestibular schwannoma (*43*) have shown that the latency of peak V changed

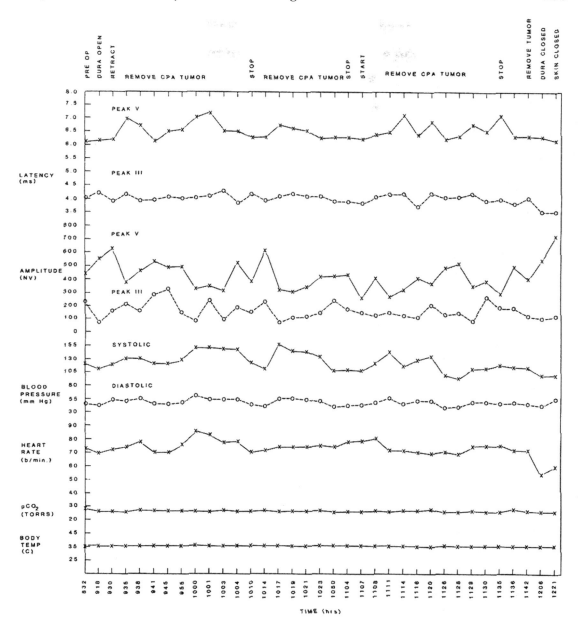

Figure 11.10: Change in the latency and amplitude of peaks III and V in the ABR in response to contralateral stimulation together with changes in cardiac parameter during an operation to remove a vestibular schwannoma. (Reprinted from: (*43*) with the permission from Maney Publishing).

before changes in heart rate in 73% of the cases and at the same time in 24% of the cases. In only 3% of the cases did the heart rate change before the latency of peak V changed (*Fig. 11.9A*). Changes in the latency of peak V occurred before changes in blood pressure in 64% of the operations and at the same time in 36% of the operations. Changes in the amplitude of peak V were slightly less effective compared with changes in heart rate and blood pressure. The amplitude of peak V changed before blood pressure in 44 % of the operations, at the same time in 33% of the operations and in 23 % of the operations, changes in the amplitude of peak V occurred after the blood pressure had changed. When compared with heart rate, changes in the amplitude of peak V occurred before changes in heart rate in 67% of the operations, at the same in 20% of the operations and after heart rate change, in 13% of the operations.

These results showed clearly that intraoperative monitoring of the ABR elicited from the contralateral ear is an important indicator of brainstem manipulation and that it is a valuable supplement to the traditionally used indicators, namely, changes in heart rate and blood pressure.

OTHER ADVANTAGES OF RECORDING AUDITORY EVOKED POTENTIALS INTRAOPERATIVELY

There are advantages of using direct recordings of CAP from the auditory nerve that exceed reducing the risk of hearing loss in the individual patient in whom monitoring is being made. Studies of the changes in the CAP from CN VIII and the cochlear nucleus have provided information that has aided in the development of better surgical methods, thus not only benefitting the individual patient in whom monitoring was performed, but also benefitting the surgical profession.

Recording CAP from CN VIII or from the cochlear nucleus has made it possible to relate the effects to specific surgical events, such as electrocoagulation. This cannot be done using ABR because the time it would take to produce an interpretable recording would make it difficult to determine exactly what step in an operation caused a change in function of the auditory nerve.

In operations in the CPA when the retromastoid approach is used, manipulations of the eighth nerve may occur, for instance, when the cerebellum is retracted. It has been indicated in earlier studies that medial-to-lateral retraction (45, 46) places the eighth nerve at greater risk than does retraction in a caudal-to-rostral direction. This hypothesis has been confirmed by studies of CAP recordings from the auditory nerve (47).

Experience in intraoperative monitoring has also shown that the arachnoid membrane that covers CN VIII may be stretched by retracting the cerebellum, and thereby, stretch the eighth nerve. It was found that changes in auditory evoked potentials that occur during MVD operations can be reduced by opening the arachnoid membrane widely as soon as possible after it has been exposed (Jho and Møller, unpublished observation 1990) – even in operations in which only CN V must be exposed in order to carry out the operation. The reason that it is beneficial to make a large opening in the arachnoid membrane is probably because tensions along the edge of the opening lessen as a result of the large opening or that the arachnoid membrane that is connected to CN VIII can stretch the nerve when, for example, the cerebellum is retracted.

Recording of CAP from the auditory nerve has shown that there are considerable differences in individual susceptibility to mechanical manipulation of the auditory nerve.

These are examples of how intraoperative neurophysiological monitoring can promote the development of surgical methods that are more effective and have less risk.

REFERENCES

1. Anonymous (1991) Acoustic neuroma, NIH consensus development program. Online 1991 Dec 11–13 9:1–24.
2. Jacob A, LLJ Robinson, JS Bortman et al (2007) Nerve of origin, tumor size, hearing preservation, and facial nerve outcomes in 359 vestibular schwannoma resections at a tertiary care academic center. Laryngoscope 117:2087–92.
3. Wilson L, E Lin and A Lalwani (2003) Cost-effectiveness of intraoperative facial nerve monitoring in middle ear or mastoid surgery. Laryngoscope 113:1736–45.

4. Sugita K and S Kobayashi (1982) Technical and instrumental improvements in the surgical treatment of acoustic neurinomas. J Neurosurg 57:747–52.

5. Silverstein H, E Smouha and R Jones (1988) Routine identification of the facial nerve using electrical stimualtion during otological and neurotological surgery. Laryngoscope 98:726–30.

6. Delgado T, W Buchheit, H Rosenholtz et al (1979) Intraoperative monitoring of facial muscle evoked responses obtained by intracranial stimulation of the facial nerve: A more accurate technique for facial nerve dissection. Neurosurgery 4:418–21.

7. Kartush J and K Bouchard, (1992) Intraoperative facial monitoring. Otology, neurotology, and skull base surgery, in *Neuromonitoring in Otology and Head and Neck Surgery*, J Kartush and K Bouchard, Editors. Raven Press: New York. 99–120.

8. Leonetti J, D Brackmann and R Prass (1989) Improved preservation of facial nerve function in the infratemporal approach to the skull base. Otolaryngol Head Neck Surg 101:74–8.

9. Prass RL and H Lueders (1986) Acoustic (loudspeaker) facial electromyographic monitoring. Part I. Neurosurgery 19:392–400.

10. Harner S, J Daube, C Beatty et al (1988) Intraoperative monitoring of the facial nerve. Laryngoscope 98:209–12.

11. Linden R, C Tator, C Benedict et al (1988) Electro-physiological monitoring during acoutic neuroma and other posterior fossa surgery. Le Journal des Sciences Neurologiques 15:73–81.

12. Benecke J, H Calder and G Chadwick (1987) Facial nerve monitoring during acoustic neuroma removal. Laryngoscope 97:697–700.

13. Yingling C and J Gardi (1992) Intraoperative monitoring of facial and cochlear nerves during acoustic neuroma surgery. Otolaryngol Clin North Am 25:413–48.

14. Møller AR and PJ Jannetta (1984) Preservation of facial function during removal of acoustic neuromas: Use of monopolar constant voltage stimulation and EMG. J Neurosurg 61:757–60.

15. Krauze F (1912) Surgery of the Brain and Spinal Cord, First English edition. New York: Rebman Company. 738–43.

16. Olivecrone H (1941) Die Trigeminusneuralgie und iher Behandlung. Nervenartz 14:49–57.

17. Rand RW and TL Kurze (1965) Facial nerve preservation by posterior fossa transmeatal microdissection in total removal of acoustic tumours. J Neurol Neurosurg Psychiat 28:311–6.

18. Shibuya M, N Matsuga, Y Suzuki et al (1993) A newly designed nerve monitor for microneurosurgery: Bipolar constant current nerve stimulator and movement detector with pressure sensor. Acta Neurochir 125:173–6.

19. Prell J, J Rachinger, C Scheller et al (2010) A real-time monitoring system for the facial nerve. Neurosurgery 66:1064–73.

20. Yingling C (1994) Intraoperative monitoring in skull base surgery, in *Neurotology*, RK Jackler and DE Brackmann, Editors. Mosby: St. Louis. 967–1002.

21. Babin RM, HR Jai and BF McCabe (1982) Bipolar localization of the facial nerve in the internal auditory canal, in *Disorders of the Facial Nerve: Anatomy, Diagnosis, and Management*, MD Graham and WF House, Editors. Raven Press: New York. 3–5.

22. Howe JE, JD Loeser and JH Calvin (1977) Mechanosensitivity of dorsal root ganglia and chronically injured axons: A physiologic basis for radically pain of nerve root compression. Pain 3:25–41.

23. Daube J and C Harper (1989) Surgical monitoring of cranial and peripheral nerves, in *Neuromonitoring in Surgery*, J Desmedt, Editor. Elsevier Science Publishers: Amesterdam. 115–38.

24. Møller AR and PJ Jannetta (1986) Blink reflex in patients with hemifacial spasm: Observations during microvascular decompression operations. J Neurol Sci 72:171–82.

25. Møller AR and PJ Jannetta (1986) Physiological abnormalities in hemifacial spasm studied during microvascular decompression operations. Exp Neurol 93:584–600.

26. Møller AR (1991) Interaction between the blink reflex and the abnormal muscle response in patients with hemifacial spasm: Results of intraoperative recordings. J Neurol Sci 101:114–23.

27. Deletis V, J Urriza, S Ulkatan et al (2009) The feasibility of recording blink reflexes under general anesthesia. Muscle Nerve 39:642–6.

28. Kugelberg E (1952) Facial reflexes. Brain 75:385–96.

29. Møller AR (1990) Intraoperative monitoring of evoked potentials: An update, in *Neurosurgery Update I. Diagnosis, Operative Technique, and Neuro-oncology*, RH Wilkins and SS Rengachary, Editors. McGraw-Hill Inc: New York. 169–76.

30. Møller AR (1987) Electrophysiological monitoring of cranial nerves in operations in the skull base, in *Tumors of the Cranial Base: Diagnosis and Treatment*, LN Sekhar and VL Schramm Jr, Editors. Futura Publishing Co: Mt. Kisco, New York. 123–32.

31. Sekhar LN and AR Møller (1986) Operative management of tumors involving the cavernous sinus. J Neurosurg 64: 879–89.

32. Sekiya T, T Hatayama, T Iwabuchi et al (1992) A ring electrode to record extraocular muscle activities during skull base surgery. Acta Neurochir 117:66–9.

33. Sekiya T, T Hatayama, T Iwabushi et al (1993) Intraoperative recordings of evoked extraocular muscle activities to monitor ocular motor function. Neurosurgery 32:227–35.

34. Lanser M, R Jackler and C Yingling (1992) Regional monitoring of the lower (ninth through twelfth) cranial nerves, in: Intraoperative Monitoring in Otology and Head and Neck Surgery, J Kartush and K Bouchard, Editors. Raven Press: New York. 131–50.

35. Yingling CD and YA Ashram (2005) Intraoperative monitoring of cranial nerves in skull base surgery, in *Neurotology, 2nd Edition*, RK Jackler and D Brackmann, Editors. Elsevier-Mosby: Philadelphia. 958–93.

36. Stechison M (1995) Vagus nerve monitoring – A comparison of percutaneous versus vocal fold electrode recording. Otol Neurotol 16:703–6.

37. Schmid UD, AR Møller and J Schmid (1992) Transcranial magnetic stimulation of the facial nerve: Intraoperative study on the effect of stimulus parameters on the excitation site in man. Muscle and Nerve 15: 829–36.

38. Maccabee PJ, VE Amassian, RQ Cracco et al (1988) Intracranial stimulation of the facial nerve in human with the magnetic coil. Electroenceph Clin Neurophysiol 70:350–4.

39. Rösler KM, CW Hess and UD Schmid (1989) Investigation of facial motor pathways by electrical and magnetic stimulation: Sites and mechanisms of excitation. J Neurol Neurosurg Psychiatry 52:1149–56.

40. Schmid U, A Møller and J Schmid (1995) Transcranial magnetic stimulation of the trigeminal nerve: intraoperative study on stimulation characteristics in man. Muscle Nerve 18:487–94.

41. Schmid UD, AR Møller and J Schmid (1992) The excitation site of the trigeminal nerve to transcranial magnetic stimulation varies and lies proximal or distal to the foramen ovale: An intraoperative electrophysiological study in man. Neurosci Lett 141:265–8.

42. Schwartz D and S Rosenberg (1992) Facial nerve monitoring during parotidectomy, in *Intraoperative Monitoring in Otology and Head and Neck Surgery*, J Kartush and K Bouchard, Editors. Raven Press: New York. 121–30.

43. Angelo R and AR Møller (1996) Contralateral evoked brainstem auditory potentials as an indicator of intraoperative brainstem manipulation in cerebellopontine angle tumors. Neurol Res 18:528–40.

44. Fischer C (1989) Brainstem auditory evoked potential (BAEP) monitoring in posterior fossa surgery, in *Neuromonitoring in Surgery*, J Desmedt Editor. Elsevier Science Publishers: Amsterdam. 191–218.

45. Gardner WJ (1962) Concerning the mechanism of trigeminal neuralgia and hemifacial spasm. J Neurosurg 19:947–58.

46. Jannetta P (1981) Hemifacial spasm, in *The Cranial Nerves*, M Samii and P Jannetta, Editors. Springer-Verlag: Heidelberg, West Germany. 484–93.

47. Møller AR and PJ Jannetta (1983) Monitoring auditory functions during cranial nerve microvascular decompression operations by direct recording from the eighth nerve. J Neurosurg 59:493–9.

PART IV

PERIPHERAL NERVES

Chapter 12
  Anatomy and Physiology of Peripheral Nerves
Chapter 13
  Practical Aspects of Monitoring Peripheral Nerves

  This section will discuss monitoring the function of peripheral nerves through intraoperative techniques. Perhaps of greater importance will be the discussion regarding diagnostic aids in operations to repair injured peripheral nerves and their intraoperative application through the use of electrophysiological methods. This assignment of importance stems from the fact that the severity of lesions of peripheral nerves cannot be assessed by visual inspection and that intraoperative physiological diagnosis is essential for deciding the strategy of an operation. While such tasks can be performed with basic neurophysiological equipment, the interpretation of the results of recordings from peripheral nerves requires detailed knowledge about the anatomy and the normal function of peripheral nerves. Understanding the effect of various forms of insults on the function of peripheral nerves is also important for providing intraoperative electrophysiological support during surgical repair of injured nerves.

  Chapter 12 describes the anatomy of peripheral nerves and some of the most common pathologies. Chapter 13 discusses the use of intraoperative monitoring of peripheral nerves (the use of neurophysiology for diagnosis of lesions of peripheral nerves is discussed in Chap. 15).

12

Anatomy and Physiology of Peripheral Nerves

INTRODUCTION

This chapter describes the normal anatomy and function of somatic peripheral nerves and different forms of injuries that can occur from trauma and other forms of insults. Since intraoperative monitoring of nerves of the autonomic nerves has not found practical use, this topic is not covered in detail. Chapter 13 provides a description of the practical aspects of intraoperative monitoring and diagnosis of pathologies of peripheral nerves.

ANATOMY

Peripheral nerves of the body are spinal nerves that originate or terminate in the spinal cord; some cranial nerves that originate or terminate in the brainstem also give rise to peripheral nerves (cranial nerves are discussed

in Chap. 11). Most peripheral nerves contain somatic motor fibers, sensory nerve fibers, proprioceptive fibers, pain fibers, and some spinal nerves contain visceral and autonomic nerve fibers. In general, sensory fibers of peripheral nerves enter the spinal cord as dorsal roots, and motor fibers exit the spinal cord as ventral roots.

Classification of Peripheral Nerves

Sensory and motor nerves are mostly composed of myelinated nerve fibers. Most mixed nerves also contain nerve fibers that carry pain signals and fibers that belong to the autonomic nervous system. While sensory and motor nerves and some pain fibers are myelinated fibers, some pain fibers and autonomic fibers are unmyelinated.

Myelinated fibers can be divided into three main groups according to the diameter of their axons, usually labeled Aα, Aβ, and Aδ fibers. Unmyelinated fibers are C-fibers. The conduction velocity of nerve fibers is proportional to the diameter of their axons (**Table 12.1**). Motor nerve fibers belong to the Aα groups, and most

From: *Intraoperative Neurophysiological Monitoring: Third Edition,*
By A.R. Møller, DOI 10.1007/978-1-4419-7436-5_12,
© Springer Science+Business Media, LLC 2011

Table 12.1
Conduction velocity in nerve fibers of different types

Fiber type	Function	Average axon diameter (mm)	Average conduction velocity (m/s)
Aα	Motor nerves, primary Muscle-spindle afferents	15	100 (70–120)
Aβ	Mechanoreceptor afferents	8	50 (30–70)
Aδ	Temperature and pain afferents	<3	15 (12–30)
C	Pain afferents Sympathetic postganglionic fibers	~1	1 (0.5–2)

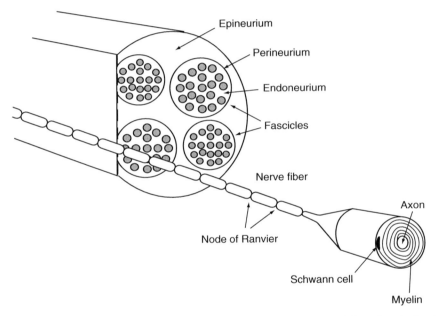

Figure 12.1: Anatomy of a typical peripheral portion of a nerve. After Sunderland 1981 (*1*); (Reprinted (*2*) with the permission of Cambridge University Press).

sensory nerves belong to the Aβ fiber types, while pain fibers belong to the Aδ and C groups.

When peripheral nerves enter or exit the spinal cord or the brainstem, the myelin changes from peripheral myelin to central myelin. Central myelin is generated by oligodendrocytes, while Schwann cells generate the myelin of the peripheral portion of nerves. The transition

zone between the peripheral and the central part of nerves occurs near their entry to the central nervous system (CNS) and is known as the Obersteiner–Redlich zone.

Axons of the peripheral portion of nerves are covered by endoneurium to form nerve fibers, and nerve fibers are organized in bundles (fascicles) that are covered by a sheath of perineurium (**Fig. 12.1**). The peripheral portion

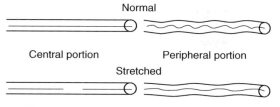

Figure 12.2: Effect of traction and injury on the central and the peripheral portion of a nerve. After Sunderland 1981 (*1*); (Reprinted from (*2*) with permission from Cambridge University Press).

of nerves may consist of a single funiculus, or it can be composed of several funiculi (bundles) that are covered by perineurium. Epineurium covers nerve trunks (*1*).

Funiculi in the peripheral portion of nerves have an undulated form (**Fig. 12.2**). This allows the nerves to be stretched without inducing stress on the individual nerve fibers, but traction that exceeds the stretched length of a nerve causes some of the typical injuries, which often occurs as a result of trauma (*1*).

In the central portion of a nerve, the endoneurium, which consists of collagen fibrils, has finer fibrils than in the peripheral portion, and the perineurium and epineurium are absent. The central part of nerves, therefore, lacks some of the protection that peripheral portions have. Since the central portion of nerves lacks a funicular support structure and undulations are absent (**Fig. 12.2**), the central portion of nerves is more fragile, more sensitive to traction and vulnerable to mechanical stress than their peripheral counterparts. This is especially important for spinal nerve roots (and for cranial nerve roots).

The transition zone between the peripheral and central portion of nerves (the Obersteiner–Redlich zone) has been studied especially in cranial nerves, where it has been shown to be sensitive to irritation from, for example, blood vessels (see Chaps. 7 and 15). Visual inspection does not reveal the location of the transition zone, but histological methods clearly show a

difference between the central and the peripheral part of a nerve. This region of nerves is the common anatomical location of Schwannoma, such as vestibular Schwannoma of the auditory vestibular nerve (see page 79, 124, 133, 149, 236). Spinal nerves can also develop Schwannoma, especially in connection with a genetic defect, neurofibromatosis type 2 (NF2).

Sensory Nerves

The fibers of sensory spinal nerves are bipolar nerve fibers that have their cell bodies in the dorsal root ganglia (DRG). Sensory nerves enter the dorsal horn of the spinal cord as dorsal root fibers (see Chap. 5).

Motor Nerves

The motor nerve fibers that leave the spinal cord as ventral spinal roots mostly belong to the Aα group of nerve fibers. The cell bodies (alpha motoneurons) of axons that innervate skeletal muscles are located in lamina IX of the ventral horn of the spinal cord (Chap. 9) (*3*). The nerve fibers that innervate the intrafusal muscle (Aα fibers) travel together with other motor fibers, and their cell bodies are located in lamina IX of the ventral horn of the spinal cord (*3*).

PATHOLOGIES OF NERVES

Trauma can cause specific injuries to nerves, and nerves can be injured because of the ingestion of substance such as alcohol, and by diseases such as diabetes mellitus. Some of these factors can destroy the myelin (demyelination). Inflammation can also cause changes in the morphology and the function of peripheral nerves and age-related changes also affect peripheral and cranial nerves.

Traumatic injuries may affect a limited portion of a (single) nerve (focal injuries), while disorders (and age) more likely affect one or more entire nerves (mononeuropathy or polyneuropathy).

Focal Injuries

Some investigators have classified the focal morphological changes that typically occur in nerves from traumatic injuries into three main types: neurapraxia, axonotmesis, and neurotmesis. Others have divided such injuries in five groups (4) (**Fig. 12.3**).

Neurapraxia is the mildest form of focal lesions of a nerve (Sunderland grade 1 (4)) (**Fig. 12.3**). It involves partial or complete conduction failure without any detectable structural changes. A nerve can recover totally from neurapraxia without any intervention; full function of the nerve returns within a certain time ranging from several hours to a few days.

Stretching or compression of a nerve containing axons of different diameter affects large diameter axons more than smaller ones (while the effect of local anesthetics on nerves is the opposite). Traction or heating can injure nerves

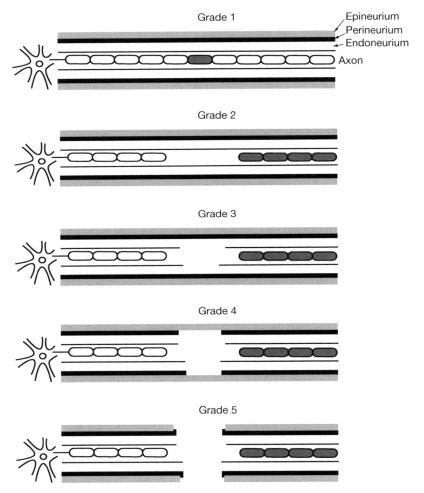

Figure 12.3: Illustration of a nerve with a conduction block without morphological changes (neurapraxia, Sunderland grade 1), and different types of nerve injuries (Sunderland grades 2, 3, 4, and 5) (4) Reprinted from (2) (Reprinted with the permission of Cambridge University Press).

to various degrees, and the injury can be either temporary or permanent.

Interruption of the axons of a nerve without damage to its supporting structures is known as axonotmesis (Sunderland grade 2). Axonotmesis may be caused by insults such as crushing or pinching of a nerve, or it may occur after stretching a nerve. If such lesion occurs distally to the location of the cell body, the parts of the axons that are distal to the lesion will begin to degenerate immediately after the lesion has occurred (Wallerian degeneration[1]) (5). The degeneration of the distal portion is usually complete within 48–72 h after the injury, at which time the nerve no longer conducts nerve impulses. But it is important to keep in mind that the distal portion of the nerve can conduct nerve impulses for some time (24–72 h) after an injury. For bipolar axons, the interruption of axons proximal to the cell body causes similar degeneration of the part of the axons that are proximal to the injury.

If trauma to a nerve also involves the support structure of the nerve, it is known as neurotmesis (Sunderland grades 3, 4 and 5 (4)) (Fig. 12.3) The lightest form of neurotmesis (Grade 3) involves a mixture of axon damage and some damage to the support structure (loss of Schwann cell basal lamina endoneural integrity). This form of injury may resolve by partial regeneration of axons that can occur without intervention, and some function may be regained. Grade 4 describes more serious injuries where scar formation occurs over the entire cross-section of a nerve. In this kind of injury, the continuity of the nerve is maintained, but spontaneous regeneration is blocked by scar tissue. When a total transection of a nerve occurs, it is labeled a Grade 5 injury. This form of injury requires surgical intervention (grafting) to regain function.

Central segment of peripheral nerves are more vulnerable to injuries than the peripheral segment of the nerves because of the lack of support structures, but trauma to the central segment nerves produces similar kinds of injuries as that of the peripheral segment nerves. Because the central nerves lack an undulating form, they are more vulnerable to stretching (Fig. 12.2).

Regeneration of Injured Nerves

When peripheral nerves are injured to the degree that the axons have been interrupted, yet the support structure remains intact (axonotmesis), the axons regenerate. New axons sprout from nerves and begin to grow away from their cell body and toward their normal target using the preserved support structure as a conduit. The regeneration proceeds at a speed of ~1 mm/day, but scar tissue that forms after injuries may act as an obstacle to regeneration. In addition, neurinoma, which can cause various symptoms such as pain, may also result from these sprouting axons.

If the interruption of a bipolar (sensory) axon occurs at a location that is proximal to the cell body, the axon will grow centrally and will make contact with the cells in the spinal cord (or brainstem) to which they were originally connected. Lesions that are located distal to the cell body of axons of sensory nerves cause the axons to grow toward their sensory receptors. New sensory receptors must be created when sensory nerve fibers, such as those innervating cutaneous receptors, reach their normal targets.

Axons of motor nerves that are interrupted grow toward the muscles that the nerves normally innervated, but not all the new motor axons eventually reach their targets and form new motor endplates. Recovery of function after the interruption of axons of a motor nerve requires the formation of new motor endplates. Sprouting of motor nerves consists of multiple fine fibers, many of which would fail to create functional motor endplates. To obtain muscle function, some of these fine filaments must,

---

[1] Wallerian degeneration: Degenerative changes in a segment of a nerve fiber (axon and myelin) that occur when continuity between the nerve fiber and its cell body is interrupted.

therefore, be eliminated which normally occurs over time without any intervention (6). This normally occurs when the outgrowing axon reaches the muscle that it innervated before it was interrupted.

Axons also regenerate (sprout) after more severe injuries to a nerve (neurotmesis), but the success of the sprouts' venture to reach their target depends on the condition of the support structure of the injured nerve. Sufficient regrowth and recovery of function may occur if some of the support structure is intact. Grade 4 and 5 lesions, however, require grafting, either end-to-end or with another nerve, that serves to provide the support structures that can act as conduits for the regenerating axons. Such regenerated nerves have fewer functional nerve fibers than they had before the injury, and many of the new axons activate their targets incorrectly. Misdirected and incomplete regeneration of sensory nerves may cause abnormal sensory input or partial to complete deprivation of input to the CNS (7).

SIGNS OF INJURIES TO NERVES

Intraoperative signs of injuries to peripheral nerves are changes in the response to electrical stimulation, spontaneous or mechanically evoked activity from the motor portion of peripheral nerves, and of course, if the injury is a severe, conduction block.

Slight injury to a peripheral nerve causes decreased conduction velocity that manifests electrophysiologically as increased latencies of compound action potentials (CAP) recorded from one location of a nerve while the nerve is stimulated electrically at another location. Slight injury may also cause a broadening of CAP if the conduction velocity is decreased unevenly among the nerve fibers that make up the nerve in question. More severe injuries

cause greater changes in the waveform of CAP, and a total conduction block results in a single positive deflection when recorded by a monopolar recording electrode (see Chap. 3).

Mechanosensitivity of Injured Nerves

Normal peripheral nerves are rather insensitive to moderate mechanical stimulation, but slightly injured nerves can be very sensitive to mechanical stimulation. Surgical manipulations and touching injured nerves with surgical instruments can result in contraction of muscles that are innervated by the nerve in question (see page 276). Similar mechanical stimulation of an uninjured nerve elicits little or no muscle contractions, which indicates that the sensitivity to mechanical stimulation of a nerve is related to injury.

Clinically, mechanical sensitivity of peripheral nerves is often present in the carpel tunnel syndrome. Tapping on the skin over the median nerve produces a tingling sensation (paresthesia) in the parts of the hand where the skin is innervated by the injured nerve (the Tinel sign[2]). Mechanosensitivity of DRG is also common and involved in some forms of pain (8, 9).

REFERENCES

1. Sunderland S (1981) Cranial nerve injury. Structural and pathophysiological considerations and a classification of nerve injury, in *The Cranial Nerves*, M Samii and PJ Jannetta, Editors. Springer: Heidelberg, Germany. 16–26.
2. Møller AR (2006) *Neural Plasticity and Disorders of the Nervous System.* Cambridge University Press: Cambridge.
3. Brodal P (1998) *The Central Nervous System.* Oxford Press: New York.
4. Sunderland S (1951) A classification of peripheral nerve injuries producing loss of function. Brain 74:491–516.

---

[2] Tinel sign: a tingling sensation from percussion of the skin over a peripheral nerve such as the nerves at the wrist.

5. Chaudhry V and DR Cornblath (1992) Wallerian degeneration in human nerves; Serial electrophysiological studies. Muscle Nerve 15:687–93.
6. Happel L and D Kline (2002) Intraoperative neurophysiology of the peripheral nervous system, in *Neurophysiology in Neurosurgery*, V Deletis and JL Shils, Editors. Academic Press: Amsterdam. 169–95.
7. Lundborg G (2000) Brain plasticity and hand surgery: an overview. J. Hand. Surg. [Br.] 25:242–52.
8. Howe JE, JD Loeser and JH Calvin (1977) Mechanosensitivity of dorsal root ganglia and chronically injured axons: a physiologic basis for radically pain of nerve root compression. Pain 3:25–41.
9. Rasminsky M (1980) Ephaptic transmission between single nerve fibers in the spinal nerve roots of dystrophic mice. J. Physiol. (Lond.) 305:151–69.

13

Practical Aspects of Monitoring Peripheral Nerves

Introduction
Intraoperative Measurement of Nerve Conduction
Recordings of CAP from Peripheral Nerves
Other Methods for Assessing Injuries to Peripheral Nerves
Identification of the Anatomical Location of Nerve Injuries
Assessing Nerve Injuries

INTRODUCTION

Monitoring of neural conduction is important for detecting surgically induced injuries to nerves, and it is a prerequisite for reducing the risks of postoperative deficits. Several different techniques can be used for such monitoring. One method utilizes the stimulation of a nerve and recording compound action potentials (CAP) from another location on the nerve. Other methods use the recording of SSEP, the F-response[1] or the H-response.[2] These methods can be used for detecting partial or complete failure of neural conduction and for the measurements of changes in neural conduction velocity. Such measures are important for detecting injuries caused by surgical manipulations. Similar electrophysiological methods can be used for finding the anatomical location of injuries to nerves. Intraoperative measurement of the conduction of peripheral nerves

plays an important role in guiding the surgeon in repair of injured nerves (see Chap. 15).

INTRAOPERATIVE MEASUREMENT OF NERVE CONDUCTION

The principles of intraoperative measurement of nerve conduction are to stimulate a nerve electrically and record the response from the same nerve at a distance from where it is being stimulated. In the clinic, nerve conduction studies often use recordings of the responses from muscles (electromyography, EMG) in response to electrical stimulation of a mixed nerve (1), but that method only tests motor nerves. If that is performed intraoperatively, it requires the patient to be anesthetized without the use of muscle relaxants. Quantitative information about abnormalities in the function of nerves, including abnormal neural conduction

---

[1] The F-response is caused by backfiring of motoneurons. It is elicited by stimulating mixed nerves electrically and recording from muscles that are innervated by the nerve that is stimulated (1).

[2] The H-reflex is the response of the stretch reflex (4). It is elicited by electrical stimulation of a mixed nerve and the response is recorded from a muscle that is innervated by the nerve.

From: *Intraoperative Neurophysiological Monitoring: Third Edition*,
By A.R. Møller, DOI 10.1007/978-1-4419-7436-5_13,
© Springer Science+Business Media, LLC 2011

velocity, can be better obtained by recording nerve action potentials (CAP). This method can be used to determine the neural conduction velocity in all (large) fibers in a mixed nerve, and it can provide quantitative assessment of the function of peripheral nerves. Such assessments include both motor and sensory fibers, but only large fibers (Aα and Aβ fibers) can be studied in that way. The conduction velocity of slower conducting fibers (Aδ and C fibers in mixed nerves) can be determined by collision techniques and are used in clinical diagnostics, and such methods have also been introduced recently in the operating room (2, 3), but so far, not in general use intraoperatively because of their complexity (see Chap. 10). CAP recording does not require that muscle relaxants be avoided.

Recordings of CAP from Peripheral Nerves

The most characteristic effect on the response from a nerve from insults, such as those that may occur during surgical operation, is increased response latency, indicating that the nerve's conduction velocity is reduced. A decrease in the amplitude of the negative peak (and increased amplitude of the initial positive component) of the recorded CAP in response to supramaximal stimulation is an indication that fewer nerve fibers are currently being activated. Broadening of the negative peak of CAP and the decrease of its amplitude are signs of temporal dispersion of the unit action potentials in the different individual nerve fibers that contribute to CAP. This occurs when the conduction velocity of the different axons of a nerve is affected (decreased) to different degrees.

Since various diseases (such as diabetes mellitus) and age-related changes may cause decreased nerve conduction velocity, the conduction velocity of the nerve suspected to be injured should be compared with the conduction velocity obtained before the operation, or it should be compared with that of another nerve in the region or on the other side of the body of the individual before it can be judged

that surgical injury is the cause of an observed reduced conduction velocity. Obtaining a baseline determination of the conduction velocity of the nerve that is to be monitored is naturally superior to these mentioned methods, but not always possible.

Other Methods for Assessing Injuries to Peripheral Nerves

Methods, such as recording of the F-response or the H-response, can be used for detecting injuries to peripheral nerves. The F-response can be used to monitor the conduction velocity selectively in the motor axons of the proximal part of mixed nerves, while the H-response measures the conduction velocity of both sensory (proprioceptive) and motor fibers. Both of these measures depend on the activation of alpha motoneurons and are affected by anesthesia and muscle relaxants and, therefore, have limited use for intraoperative monitoring. Monitoring of SSEP can be used for detecting changes in conduction velocity of a sensory nerve.

Identification of the Anatomical Location of Nerve Injuries

Measurements of neural conduction velocity in peripheral nerves (sensory, motor, or mixed nerves) can be used to identify the location of a pathology and to determine its nature. Such intraoperative diagnosis can guide the surgeon in operations to repair peripheral nerves, and it is possible to identify the anatomical location of an injured segment of a nerve because of its decreased conduction velocity. (This is discussed in more detail in Chap. 15.)

Assessing Nerve Injuries

When using electrophysiological methods for assessing the location of injury to peripheral nerves, it is important to recognize that the distal portion of a transected peripheral nerve continues to conduct nerve impulses for a period of time up to 72 h after the injury. This means that it is possible to elicit contractions of muscles from electrical stimulation of a motor nerve at locations that are distal to the lesion.

Localizing the Place of Injury. Neurophysiological methods make it possible to localize the exact place where a nerve is injured. This is accomplished by stimulating the nerve in question electrically and recording from different locations along the nerve. Similar basic electrophysiological techniques make it possible to determine if an injured nerve is beginning to regenerate. These methods are superior to other often-used methods involving the recordings of EMG potentials. Decisions about how a particular nerve would best respond to resection and repair compared to more conservative treatment, such as neurolysis, can be made right at the operating table using such basic electrophysiological methods (described in Chap. 15).

Determination of Neural Conduction Velocity. The CAP recorded from a long nerve with a monopolar electrode are triphasic potentials (see Chap. 3), and the latency of the response is usually determined as the time between the onset of the stimulus and the earliest negative peak of the response. The neural conduction velocity of the nerve between these two locations is obtained by dividing the distance between the stimulating and recording electrodes by the value of the latency of the response. The conduction velocity of peripheral nerves is usually given in meters per second (m/s), which corresponds to dividing the distance in millimeters by the latency in milliseconds.

Since neural conduction occurs with almost the same velocity in both directions along a peripheral nerve (the difference being less than 10%), it does not affect the results markedly whether the nerve is stimulated proximal or distal to the location where the recording is being performed.

Measurements of conduction velocity in a peripheral nerve, such as that described above, can be performed without exposing the nerve by properly placing needle electrodes percutaneously for recording and stimulation. This requires a high degree of certainty in identifying the nerve that is to be tested. However, in many cases, for instance, in connection with injuries in the brachial plexus, it is not possible to ensure that the proper nerve is being tested. In such cases, it is necessary to expose the nerve surgically so that the injured nerve can be properly identified, and there is no doubt which nerve is being tested.

REFERENCES

1. Aminoff MJ (1998) Electromyography in clinical practice. New York: Churchill Livingstone.
2. Leppanen R, R Madigan, C Sears et al (1999) Intraoperative collision studies demonstrate descending spinal cord stimulation evoked potentials and ascending somatosensory evoked potentials are medicated through common pathways. J Clin Neurophysiol 16:170.
3. Deletis V and AB Camargo (2001) Interventional neurophysiological mapping and monitoring during spinal cord procedures. Stereotact Funct Neurosurg 77:25–8.
4. Møller AR (2006) Neural plasticity and disorders of the nervous system. Cambridge: Cambridge University Press.

PART V

INTRAOPERATIVE RECORDINGS THAT CAN GUIDE
THE SURGEON IN THE OPERATION

Chapter 14
Identification of Specific Neural Tissue
Chapter 15
Intraoperative Guidance and Diagnosis

The previous sections have emphasized the use of electrophysiological methods in reducing the risk of permanent postoperative neurological deficits as a result of surgical manipulation of neural tissue. In this section, we will discuss a different use of electrophysiology in the operating room, namely, for identification of specific neural structures, beginning with localization of nerves and extending to electrophysiological mapping of the spinal cord and the floor of the fourth ventricle.

The use of intraoperative neurophysiological recordings is not limited to detecting neural injury before becoming permanent; it is gaining greater importance in guiding many kinds of surgical procedures in the area of "functional neurosurgery." Intraoperative *monitoring* is transforming into intraoperative *neurophysiology* because of the possibilities of using neurophysiological techniques to guide the surgeon. New practices, such as guidance in deep brain stimulation (DBS), use of collision techniques etc., are now being introduced in the operating room. It is, therefore, important that the persons who do intraoperative monitoring have sufficient background knowledge of neuroanatomy and neurophysiology, especially with regard to motor systems, to be able to provide such service.

Chapter 15 will discuss practical aspects of how intraoperative neurophysiology can be applied to treatment of various disorders. Disorders such as Parkinson's disease (PD), essential tremor, dystonia, and Gilles de la Tourette's Syndrome are now successfully treated by making lesions or by placing stimulating electrodes for DBS in specific functional parts of the basal ganglia and thalamus. Other diseases such as severe, chronic pain are also treated by DBS. Lesions or stimulating electrodes are positioned using stereotactic techniques, but guidance from recordings of the electrodes and test stimulations are necessary for optimal placement. This implies that the neurophysiologist who is interpreting these intraoperative neurophysiological recordings understands anatomy and physiology of the basal ganglia and how these structures interact with other parts of the motor system (described in Chap. 9). The range of disorders where such guidance can help achieve the therapeutic goal of an operation is rapidly increasing. There is evidence that indicates that such disorders as tinnitus, depression, addiction, and obesity can be treated by DBS.

Chapter 15 also covers mapping of the spinal cord, brainstem, and nerve roots and also discusses how intraoperative neurophysiology can be used for diagnosing lesions of peripheral nerves.

The use of electrophysiology for the purpose of guiding the surgeon in an operation requires other kinds of knowledge and skills than those needed for intraoperative monitoring that is performed for reducing the risk of postoperative neurological deficits. The following chapters provide the physiological and practical basis for that knowledge and those skills.

14

Identification of Specific Neural Tissue

INTRODUCTION

The most direct way that intraoperative neurophysiologic recording may guide the surgeon in an operation is that it can assist in identifying specific structures such as nerves. This is of great importance when trying to identify cranial nerves in cases where the anatomy is distorted by a tumor or other pathologic processes. Previous operations may have changed the anatomy, making it difficult to identify specific nerves solely on the basis of

visual observation in a surgical field. Tumors and malformations of various kinds may have distorted the anatomy so that it becomes difficult to identify specific neural tissue. Similar problems may occur in connection with peripheral nerves.

Intraoperative neurophysiologic recording can help identify structures of the central nervous system (CNS) such as the central fissure that separates the sensory and motor cortical areas. This is of particular importance when a tumor is to be removed or when brain tissue is to be resected in order to treat intractable epileptic seizures. Parts of the cerebral cortex are mapped in operations for epilepsy to avoid removing structures that provide particular

From: *Intraoperative Neurophysiological Monitoring: Third Edition*
By A.R. Møller, DOI 10.1007/978-1-4419-7436-5_14,
© Springer Science+Business Media, LLC 2011

functions that cannot be replaced by the function of other structures. Neurophysiologic methods are also used for mapping the floor of the fourth ventricle and of the spinal cord. Similar methods are used to guide the surgeon in specific operations (see Chap. 15).

LOCALIZATION OF MOTOR NERVES

In this book, we have earlier shown an example of how intraoperative monitoring can reduce the risk of injury to nerves that innervate the extraocular muscles (CN III, CN IV, and CN VI) and the facial nerve (CN VII) (see Chap. 11). In order to do this, the nerves must be localized. Since the anatomy is often distorted because of tumors for which a patient is being operated upon, it is necessary to identify the nerves in each individual patient.

Localization of Cranial Motor Nerves

Cranial motor nerves may become displaced by tumors, such as skull base tumors, that often distort the anatomy to such an extent that it is difficult to identify the nerves visually on the basis of anatomical knowledge alone. Cranial nerves are often directly involved in tumors, thereby adding to the difficulty of identification (1–6). Identifying the facial nerve is particularly important for preservation of facial function in operations for vestibular schwannoma. It is sometimes equally important to be able to identify regions of a tumor where no nerve is apparent so that these regions of the tumor can be removed without injuring the particular nerve (Chap. 11).

Practical Aspects of Identification of Motor Nerves. Since there is usually more than one nerve that needs to be identified, it is beneficial to have the EMG potentials of different muscles displayed in several separate recording channels. Modern equipment allows for displaying many records simultaneously. This allows for many nerves at different anatomical sites to be tested within a short time, and the test can be repeated as often as necessary without causing significant delay of the operation.

It is important to make sure that the stimulator and the EMG amplifiers, as well as the recording electrodes, are functioning adequately. The appearance of a stimulus artifact in the recording of EMG potentials that can be observed, when the hand-held stimulating electrode is first brought into contact with the tissue to be tested, is an important indicator that the entire system is working correctly, but it is not sufficient proof. A small stimulus artifact may be seen even when there is no contact between the stimulator and the patient. The stimulus artifact should increase in amplitude when the stimulating electrode is brought into contact with the tissue in the surgical field if the electrode is delivering an electrical current to the tissue that is being probed. It is advisable, as soon as it is possible during the operation, to test the entire system by stimulating a motor nerve that innervates the muscle from which the EMG potentials are being recorded.

The return electrode for the stimulator may easily become dislodged if it is a hypodermic needle placed directly in the wound. In such a case, there will be no, or only a small, stimulus artifact in the recording. It is, therefore, important during the operation to always check the stimulus artifact whenever electrical stimulation is being performed. To do this, the entire response should be displayed together with the EMG potentials. When an audio monitor is used to make the EMG potentials audible, the initial few milliseconds of the responses are "cut out" to avoid audible interference from the stimulus artifact (see Chap. 18), but this should only be done in the signal that is directed to the audio amplifier and not to the signal that is shown on the computer display.

While it is true that in many cases touching a motor nerve with a surgical instrument results in a stimulation of the nerve and an EMG potential that can be recorded, this does not always happen. In fact, it is only injured nerves that are sensitive to mechanical stimulation. Therefore, one should never rely on such mechanical stimulation for the purpose of locating a cranial motor nerve. Only electrical stimulation should be used for this purpose, and it is important to use the electrical stimulating electrode often when trying to locate a nerve in a surgical field.

Surgical dissecting instruments that can be connected to a nerve stimulator are available (7). Such instruments are helpful for properly identifying a motor nerve by touching it with a surgical instrument without having to take a different instrument (stimulating electrode) for probing the surgical field for the presence of a motor nerve.

Choice of Stimulation. For probing a surgical field to test for the presence of motor nerves, a relatively low-impedance stimulator[1] (3, 8) is the most suitable kind of stimulator. The stimulus impulses that are applied to a nerve should have a negative polarity. Rectangular impulses with duration of 100 microseconds (μs) and a strength of 0.1–0.4 volts (V) will normally elicit EMG responses from muscles that are innervated by a facial nerve when a monopolar stimulating electrode is placed directly in contact with the nerve in question, or in its immediate vicinity. The cranial nerves that innervate the extraocular muscles are slightly less sensitive to electrical stimulation than the facial nerve (see Chap. 11). Should the nerve in question be covered by tissue of any kind, such as the arachnoid membrane, a stimulus strength of 0.8–1.5 V may need to be applied to elicit a response.

Whenever electrical stimulation is used to identify a motor nerve, it must be kept in mind that all surrounding tissue and fluid are good electrical conductors that may conduct the stimulating current to a motor nerve. However, the attenuation and shunting of the stimulus current by the tissue make such remote locations less sensitive to electrical stimulation than a nerve that is located closer to the stimulating electrode. It is, therefore, important to use the lowest possible stimulus strength for localizing a motor nerve. It should be noted that nerves are good electrical conductors themselves. A nerve will (passively) conduct stimulus current

even when it does not conduct nerve impulses (because of injury).

Technique that Can Facilitate Finding a Nerve that Is Embedded in Tissue. The technique for probing tissue with a hand-held stimulating electrode in order to find the location of a motor nerve involves moving the stimulating electrode across the tissue being investigated. If this movement causes the amplitude of the recorded EMG response to increase, then the nerve is located in the direction the electrode was moved. If moving the electrode results in a smaller response, the electrode was moved away from the nerve. Although the use of this method requires close collaboration between the person monitoring the response and the surgeon as well as frequent adjustments of the stimulus strength to keep the response below its maximal amplitude, it can shorten the time taken to locate a nerve in the surgical field considerably.

Bipolar Versus Monopolar Stimulating Electrodes. The use of a bipolar stimulating electrode will result in greater spatial selectivity than using a monopolar electrode (5, 7), but a bipolar stimulating electrode is more difficult to use, and its ability to stimulate a nerve depends on its orientation. In short, a bipolar stimulating electrode is preferable if the purpose is to determine the exact location of a nerve or for determining the identity of each one of two closely located nerves that are clearly visible. A monopolar stimulating electrode is better than a bipolar electrode for searching the location of a nerve in the surgical field.

Injured Nerves. Often it is tempting to increase the stimulus strength when no response is obtained from a stimulating nerve because it is believed that the sensitivity of the nerve has decreased. However, a high stimulus strength may cause stimulation of the normal functioning portion of the nerve by (galvanic) conduction of

---

[1] Even if the stimulator can deliver a (true) constant voltage, the resistance of the stimulating electrode will result in a certain source resistance that is delivered to the tissue. A true constant voltage stimulator means a source without any internal resistance (see Chap. 18).

the stimulus current and thus, give a false impression that the part of the nerve that is stimulated is conducting nerve impulses. This problem is caused by the fact that an injured nerve conducts electrical current even though it does not conduct nerve impulses. The problem is most pronounced when a nerve is free from surrounding tissue or fluid that would otherwise shunt the electrical stimulus current. It is, therefore, important to select a proper stimulus strength – just above normal threshold – when testing a nerve for its ability to conduct nerve impulses.

Mapping the Course of Peripheral Motor Nerves

There are several instances where it is valuable to map the course of peripheral nerves so that a decision can be made as to where exactly an incision can be made. Skin incisions of the face are typical examples of situations where injury may occur to a branch of the facial nerve. The course of the facial nerve varies from individual to individual, and mapping of the different branches of the facial nerve is, therefore, important for determining the exact anatomical location of specific branches of the facial nerve. This can be accomplished by probing the area where it is believed a branch of the nerve is located. Fine needle electrodes placed percutaneously can be used to determine the location of the facial nerve. The return electrode for the stimulator should be placed on the other side of the face. Such mapping can be done by visual observation of contraction of muscles, but more accurate mapping can be made by recording the evoked EMG activity from the respective muscles. The stimulus strength should be small enough to locate a branch of the nerve accurately, but the stimulus strength should be sufficient to avoid missing the nerve. Usually 1.5–2 V is sufficient when using subdermal needle electrodes and when using a semi-constant voltage stimulator. If a constant-current stimulator is used, stimulus strength of 0.2–0.5 mA is suitable. Such mapping is best done in an anesthetized patient, but it is important that the patient is not paralyzed.

Electrical stimulation in connection with recording EMG potentials is valuable for identifying other motor nerves intraoperatively. In operations where a peripheral nerve may be exposed, the surgical field can be probed by a hand-held stimulating electrode, similar to that described for identifying cranial nerves (see Chap. 11). This method for identifying motor nerves is specifically useful in connection with operations that involve the brachial plexus where the courses of the various nerves are complex and there are individual variations. Trauma or previous operations may have altered the anatomy, thereby making it essential to verify the anatomical locations of nerves before operating in areas where nerves may be present.

Safety Concerns

When electrical stimulation is used to identify motor nerves (or for monitoring the integrity of motor nerves), caution should be exercised when the particular nerve innervates large skeletal muscles. Since electrical stimulation may activate all, or nearly all, motor nerve fibers maximally and simultaneously, the contraction may be strong enough to injure the muscle or cause joint dislocations. To avoid this, it is necessary to begin to stimulate motor nerves (for instance, CN XI) with a weaker stimulus and then to increase the stimulus strength slowly while keeping the stimulating electrode in the same position. This procedure must then be repeated for each new anatomical location that is to be tested.

MAPPING OF SENSORY NERVES

Sensory nerves can be localized by applying a sensory stimulus that is specific for the nerve to be identified (e.g., click sounds for the auditory nerve or light flashes for the optic nerve) or an unspecific stimulus (such as electrical stimulation, which has been used for the trigeminal nerve), and then recording CAP from the respective nerve. Recordings can be made with either a monopolar or a bipolar recording electrode. The use of a bipolar recording electrode makes it possible to determine the location of a nerve more accurately than using a monopolar electrode because it has a larger degree of spatial selectivity, and it selectively records potentials that are the result of propagated neural activity. However, it is often difficult to use a bipolar electrode when a nerve is located within a small space intracranially.

When recordings of CAP are made to identify a nerve, the amplitudes and the latencies of the potentials should be noticed. When a recording electrode is placed close to a nerve, the amplitude of the CAP can be expected to be in the range of 10–200 microvolts (μV). Moving the electrode a few millimeters (mm) away from the nerve should reduce the amplitude of the potentials considerably because of the nature of the electrical field generated by the nerve. If the recorded potentials are caused by propagated neural activity in a nerve, the latency of the potentials is expected to change when the recording electrode is moved along the nerve. A bipolar recording electrode will mainly record propagated neural activity when placed on a nerve, which is another reason to use bipolar recording electrodes rather than monopolar electrodes whenever possible (see Chap. 3).

If the amplitude of the recorded CAP is too small to visualize directly and, therefore, subjected to signal averaging to enhance the recorded evoked potentials, it is important to keep in mind that if many responses are averaged, what may be seen may be a far-field response rather than the response from a specific nerve. If the potentials are far-field potentials that are generated by a distant source, then the latency will not change by moving the recording electrode; only the amplitude of the recorded potentials will change. The recording electrode placed on a nerve may pick up electrical potentials that are generated by other structures and passively conducted to the recording site by the nerve from which the recordings are being made.

If electrical stimulation is used, the reference electrode for monopolar recording should be placed as close to the active (recording) electrode as possible in order to reduce the stimulus artifact, but such electrode placement will increase the risk that the reference electrode may pick up evoked potentials from structures that generate evoked potentials in response to the stimulus that is being used. It is not possible to determine from observing the recorded potentials whether they are picked up by the (presumed) active electrode or by the (presumed) reference electrode. (Amplifiers that are used to amplify potentials from nerves and muscles are differential amplifiers that amplify the difference in the electrical potentials that are picked up by the electrodes that are connected to the amplifier's two inputs (see Chap. 18).) The reference electrode must, therefore, be placed at a location where the stimulus cannot be expected to generate evoked potentials of any significant amplitude, compared with those that are recorded by the active electrode (see Chap. 3).

Identifying the Different Branches of the Trigeminal Nerve

Methods for identifying the three different branches of the sensory portion (portio major) of CN V in the posterior fossa using electrophysiologic techniques have been described (9). When a branch of CN V is stimulated electrically by two needle electrodes placed close to the point where the branches emerge from their respective foramina of the head, CAP can be recorded from the intracranial portion of CN V. For practical reasons, it is better to record from the distal branches of the trigeminal nerve while the intracranial portion is stimulated electrically using a bipolar stimulating electrode (9) (**Fig. 14.1**). This method can be used to determine where the different branches of the nerve are located in the intracranial portion of the trigeminal nerve. This is important when parts of the nerve are to be sectioned such as is done for treating trigeminal neuralgias.

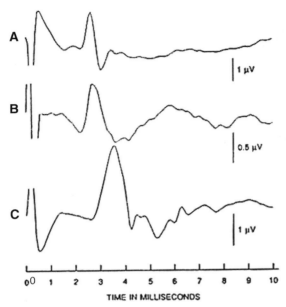

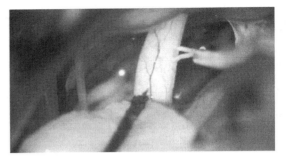

Figure 14.2: Bipolar electrode placed on the exposed eighth cranial nerve.

Figure 14.1: Recording of CAP from the trigeminal foramina (supraorbital, infraorbital, and metal) while stimulating the rostral–medial, medial–lateral, and caudal–lateral portions of the trigeminal nerve intracranially with a monopolar stimulating electrode. The stimulus strength was supramaximal (0.5–1.0 V). The recordings were made from needle electrodes placed in each of the three foramina and connected to each one of three amplifiers. The reference electrodes were placed close to each of the foramina (Reprinted from (9) with the permission from Lippincott Williams & Wilkins).

Identifying the Auditory and the Vestibular Portions of CN VIII

When the central portion of the vestibular nerve is to be severed to treat disorders of the vestibular system, such as the vertigo in Ménière's disease, it is important to determine the anatomical location of the border between the auditory and the vestibular portions of CN VIII. These two portions of CN VIII are located close together near the brainstem. Although the auditory and the vestibular portions of CN VIII usually have slightly different degrees of grayness, it is not always possible to determine the exact location of the demarcation between

these two portions of CN VIII on the basis of visual observations alone. Recording CAP from the auditory nerve in response to click stimulation provides a way to determine the border between these two portions of CN VIII. A monopolar recording electrode does not have sufficient spatial selectivity for such differentiation, and it is necessary to use a bipolar recording technique (10, 11). Placement of a bipolar recording electrode is more demanding than that of a monopolar recording electrode because of the small dimensions of CN VIII and because the intracranial portion of CN VIII is the central part of the nerve that has central myelin and lacks the support structures of its peripheral portion. This makes the central portion of a cranial (and spinal) nerve as fragile as brain tissue. (12) (**Fig. 14.2**). The necessity to have electrodes with narrow tips is also a problem, because such narrow tips can easily cause injury to the auditory–vestibular nerve.

It has been shown that the use of clicks of a relatively low stimulus strength (25 dB sensation level; SL) facilitates discrimination between the vestibular and auditory nerves (10) (**Fig. 14.3**). (These authors defined the used sound levels as 25 dB above the threshold for auditory brainstem responses (ABR), thus probably slightly more than 25 dB above the patient's hearing threshold, SL.) This stimulus level is 30–40 dB lower than that normally used for obtaining ABR in the operating room (usually approximately 65 dB HL at a click repetition

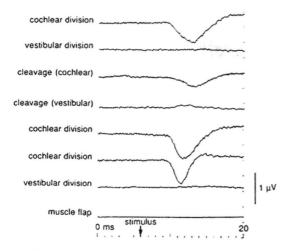

cochlear division

vestibular division

cleavage (cochlear)

cleavage (vestibular)

cochlear division

cochlear division

vestibular division

muscle flap

0 ms   stimulus   20

1 µV

Figure 14.3: Bipolar recordings from the intracranial portion of CN VIII. The stimuli were clicks with an intensity that was 25 dB above the threshold for ABR (Reprinted from (*10*) with permission from Elsevier).

rate of 20 clicks per second, corresponding to about 105 dB PeSPL, see Chap. 7).

Identifying Spinal Dorsal Rootlets that Carry Specific Sensory Input

Spinal cord injuries are often associated with spasticity. This can be treated by medications (such as baclofen) that must be taken daily and have some side effects, or it can be treated surgically by severing a few fascicles of dorsal roots. If such an operation is successful, there is a permanent absence of spasticity (*13, 14*).

When performing such dorsal root neurectomy (rhizotomy) to treat spasticity, it is important to spare parts of the dorsal roots that mediate important functions. Usually, it is the roots from L1 to S2 that are candidates for such selective rhizotomy (*14, 15*), and it is important to spare the parts of the dorsal roots that have important functions. Each dorsal root consists of several rootlets. Electrical stimulation of a nerve at a peripheral location in connection with recording CAP from exposed spinal dorsal roots can be used to test whether a particular rootlet carries important sensory input and should thus, not be sectioned (*15, 16*). For identification of

rootlets that are involved in micturition and sexual function, the dorsal penile or clitoral nerves are stimulated electrically and recording of the elicited CAP is made from each rootlet before it is sectioned (**Fig. 14.4**) (*15*).

The recordings of CAP from the parts of the peripheral nerves in question are best captured by a hand-held bipolar electrode consisting of two wire hooks with a distance of about 5 mm between them. Each rootlet is then lifted up on this hook, so that it is free from fluid and is out of contact with other rootlets, while the respective nerve is stimulated electrically at a peripheral location (*17*) (**Fig. 14.4**).

Because it is a matter of a negative identification of the rootlets (rootlets that do not have a response are supposed to be candidates for being severed), it is important to be sure that the stimulation is adequate to elicit a response and that the recording equipment has adequate sensitivity for the recording. Before any rootlets are severed, some rootlets with a response must be identified in order to ensure that the stimulation is adequate and that the recording equipment works satisfactorily.

MAPPING OF THE SPINAL CORD

Recently, collision techniques have been introduced in the operating room, which make it possible to map the anatomical location of the corticospinal tract (CT) intraoperatively within a surgically exposed spinal cord and provide a semi-quantitative estimate of the number of intact fibers and the number of desynchronized or blocked fibers of the CT (*18, 19*). Collision techniques have been used for many years in animal studies, but it is only recently that this technique has been introduced in intraoperative neurophysiologic monitoring (*18, 20*). The use of the collision technique expands the benefits of monitoring D waves, and it provides information about how D waves are generated (Chaps. 9 and 10). The use of this technique is especially important for proper treatment of patients with intramedullary spinal cord tumors where the anatomy of the spinal

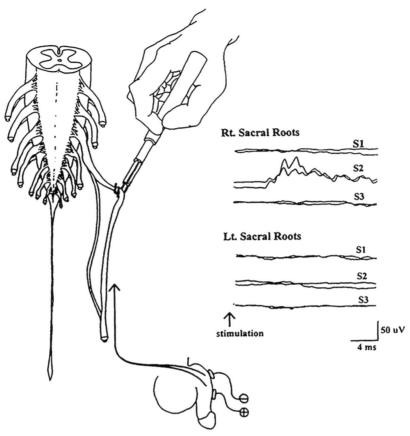

Figure 14.4: Illustration of how dorsal sacral rootlets of the cauda equine can be identified so that specific pudendal afferents can be saved during dorsal root rhizotomies (Reprinted from (*17*) with permission from Lippincott Williams & Wilkins).

cord may be distorted, and the anatomical location of the CT is difficult to determine using visual inspection alone. It may also be beneficial to use collision techniques in scoliosis operations where anatomical abnormalities of the motor and sensory spinal tracts have been observed.

This D wave collision technique involves simultaneous transcranial electrical stimulation (TES) of the motor cortex with stimulation of the CT in the surgically exposed spinal cord (**Fig. 14.5**). Stimulating the exposed spinal cord is done with a small hand-held probe delivering

a 2 mA-intensity stimulus, then simultaneously, TES is used to elicit a descending D wave from the motor cortex (see Chap. 10). This descending D wave collides with the ascending neural activity elicited by stimulation of the spinal cord and which propagates antidromically along the CT (**Fig. 14.5**). The amplitude of the D wave recorded caudal to the collision site decreases because some of the descending activity in the CT that was elicited by transcranial cortical stimulation becomes extinguished by colliding with the ascending activity elicited by stimulation of the CT of the spinal cord. This will only occur when the spinal cord stimulating probe is in close proximity to the CT, and the location of

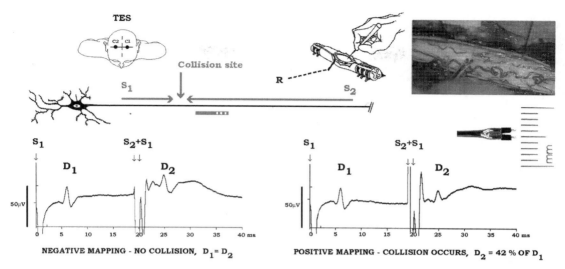

Figure 14.5: Mapping of the corticospinal tract (CT) by D wave collision technique. S1 = transcranial electrical stimulation (TES). S2 = spinal cord electrical stimulation (SpES). D1 = control D wave (TES only). D2 = D wave after combined stimulation of the brain and spinal cord. R = D wave recording electrode in the spinal epidural space. *Left*: negative mapping results (D1 = D2). *Right*: positive mapping results (D wave amplitude significantly diminished after collision). *Right upper corner*: position of hand-held stimulating electrode over exposed spinal cord (Reprinted from (*18, 19*) with permission from Elsevier).

the stimulating electrode that produces such a decrease in the D wave is, therefore, the location of the CT. This technique guides surgeons and allows them to stay clear of the CT.

MAPPING OF THE FLOOR OF THE FOURTH VENTRICLE

Operations inside the brainstem are delicate because of the many important structures that are located within a very small volume of brain tissue. Neurophysiologic methods for electrical stimulation and recording of evoked potentials and EMG potentials are used for mapping the floor of the fourth ventricle to find safe entries to internal structures of the brainstem. Several superficial structures can be identified on the floor of the fourth ventricle using intraoperative neurophysiology (*21–25*) (**Fig. 14.6**). Motor structures can be identified by electrically stimulating the

surface of the floor of the fourth ventricle and recording the EMG responses from muscles that are innervated by the respective motor systems. Using this method, the seventh cranial nerve (CN VII) can be identified where it comes close to the surface of the floor of the fourth ventricle. The hypoglossal nerve (CN XII) can also be identified (**Fig. 14.6**). Both bipolar and monopolar hand-held stimulating electrodes have been used for this purpose. EMG recordings have been made from the orbicularis oculi and orbicularis oris muscles for the facial nerve, and for the hypoglossal nerve, recordings were made from the genioglossal muscle (**Fig. 14.6**). Recording from the lateral side of the tongue would be a better location for recording EMG potentials. Such recordings can distinguish between the left and right hypoglossal nerves, and thus, make it possible to determine which one of the two nerves is being stimulated.

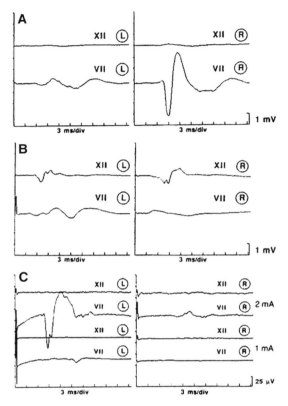

Figure 14.6: Recordings of EMG potentials from muscles innervated by CN VII and CN XII by bipolar electrical stimulation of different locations on the floor of the fourth ventricle. (**A**) Bipolar stimulation of the right facial colliculus and recordings from the genioglossal (CN XII) and orbicularis muscles (CN VII) on both sides. The stimulus current was 0.5 mA. (**B**) Bipolar stimulation at the left trigone of the hypoglossal (CN XII) nerve. (**C**) Bipolar stimulation of the left facial colliculus in the same patient who had a left peripheral facial paresis. The stimulus strength required to evoke a response was 2 mA because of the facial paresis (Reprinted from (21) with permission from Journal of Neurosurgery).

Other investigators have used slightly different methods for localizing structures that are located at, or immediately under, the surface of the floor of the fourth ventricle. Thus, Morota (1995) described similar methods for localizing the facial and the hypoglossal nerves on the

floor of the fourth ventricle. CN IX and CN X can be identified using similar methods (**Fig. 14.7**) (24).

In addition, these investigators used TES for monitoring corticobulbar MEP.

Electrical stimulation of the floor of the fourth ventricle should be done with great caution, and the lowest possible stimulus strength should be used. The stimulus repetition rate should not exceed 10 pps, although 5 pps is generally a better choice, and short duration impulses should be used (50–100 μs duration).

REQUIREMENT OF ELECTRICAL STIMULATION

Selecting the proper kind of electrical stimulation is important for localization of specific structures, and it is important to use the appropriate stimulus strength for localizing neural tissue such as a motor nerve. If the stimulus is too weak, there may be no response, even when the stimulating electrode is close to the nerve or even when it is in contact with the nerve in question. This would result in failure to identify a nerve, which could be disastrous as the surgeon would then be led to believe that there is no nerve present in the region that had been probed, and subsequently manipulate the tissue that contains a nerve or potentially resect a nerve unknowingly. On the contrary, a stimulus that is too strong may spread stimulus current to nerves that are located at a distance from the site of stimulation; this could lead the surgeon to believe that there is a nerve tissue located in areas where there is in fact none.

LOCALIZATION OF THE SOMATOSENSORY AND MOTOR CORTEX (CENTRAL SULCUS)

Localization of the motor and sensory areas of the cerebral cortex can be determined by electrically stimulating the surface of the cortex in a way similar to that done by Penfield and Rasmussen (1950) (26) in their pioneering work on mapping of the cerebral cortex, where

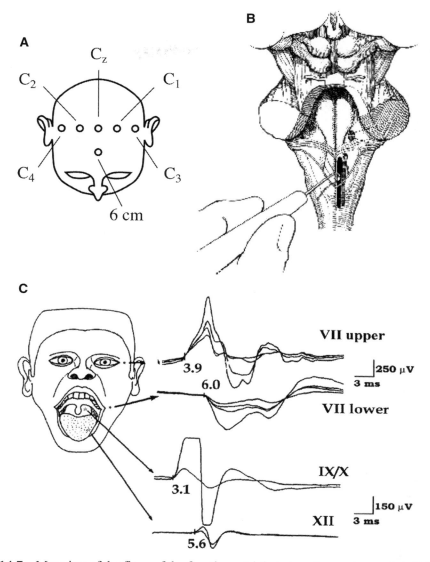

Figure 14.7: Mapping of the floor of the fourth ventricle to localize motor nuclei. (**A**) Placement of stimulating electrodes on the scalp. (**B**) Mapping of the floor of the fourth ventricle using a hand-held stimulating electrode. (**C**) Consecutive recordings of corticobulbar MEPs and recordings from muscles innervating cranial nerves VII, IX/X, and XII (Reprinted from (*24*) with the permission from Lippincott Williams & Wilkins).

they determined the representation of different muscles of the body on the primary motor cortex (M1). The central sulcus (Rolandic fissure) (*27, 28*) separates the primary motor and sensory areas of the cerebral cortex. The location is subject to considerable individual variations, and it can be identified by electrical stimulation of the median while recording the responses from electrodes placed on the surface of the exposed cortex.

This way of localizing the central sulcus is based on the observation that the polarity of the recorded potentials from the sensory and the motor gyri is reversed (**Fig. 14.8**). While

CORTICAL MAPPING

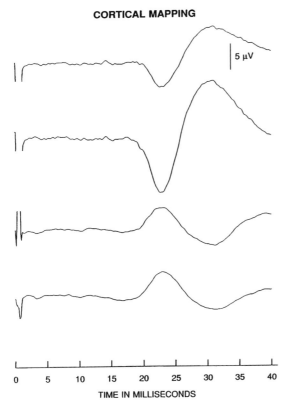

Figure 14.8: Recordings from the exposed surface of the cerebral cortex using four electrodes placed in a straight line with a distance of 1 cm between each of the electrodes, in response to electrical stimulation of the contralateral median nerve at the wrist at a rate of 10 pps. The reference electrode was placed in the wound. The electrode strip was placed in an anterior–posterior direction, with the *upper tracing* originating from the most anterior electrode. The phase reversal of the recordings that occurred between the two middle electrodes indicates that the central sulcus was located between these two electrodes. Thus, the upper two recordings were from the motor area (precentral gyrus), and the lower recordings were from the sensory area of the cerebral cortex. Each recording was the average of 150–250 responses. Negativity is shown as an upward deflection.

stimulating the median nerve in the same way as done to record SSEP from scalp electrodes (see Chap. 6), the exposed surface of the cerebral cortex is mapped by placing on the exposed surface strips of plastic material on which four or more electrodes are mounted, each of which is connected to the input of a separate amplifier. Usually such recording electrodes are placed in a straight line with a distance of 1 cm between each electrode placed perpendicular to what is expected to be the central sulcus.

Stimulation of the median nerve should be done on the side contralateral to the side on which the recordings are being made. The negative peak (**Fig. 14.8**) is assumed to correspond to the N_{20} peak in SSEP, as is seen in scalp recordings contralateral to the side that is stimulated.

Determination of the location of the central sulcus, as described above, is usually made before beginning tumor removal or other relevant operations. If the electrodes are left in place after the central sulcus has been identified, the recordings of the responses from one or more of these electrodes can then be used to monitor the integrity of the somatosensory cortex during tumor removal.

Since the finer details in recordings, such as those shown in **Fig. 14.8**, are not of any interest, filter settings of 30–250 or 30–500 Hz are suitable. The median nerve can be stimulated at a rate of 10 pps, as was described in Chap. 6. The potentials recorded directly from the surface of the somatosensory cortex are of large amplitude, usually well over 5 µV (**Fig. 14.8**), and an interpretable response may be obtained by direct observation of the potentials or after averaging only a few responses, thus requiring less than 10 s of recording time.

Electrical stimulators are of two types: one type delivers a (nearly) constant current independent of the electrical impedance of the electrode and the tissue. The other type of stimulator delivers a constant voltage independent of the electrical impedance in the tissue stimulated (*3, 8*). Which one of these two kinds is most suitable depends on the circumstances. If the shunting of stimulus current varies considerably, the best form of stimulus is constant voltage. If the electrode impedance varies, constant-current stimulation is preferred. The difference between these two types of stimulation is discussed in more detail in Chap. 11.

ANESTHESIA REQUIREMENTS

Since mapping of the floor of the fourth ventricle depends on recording EMG potentials, paralyzing agents cannot be used as a part of the anesthesia regimen (see Chap. 16), but mapping of the spinal cord as described above is little affected by anesthesia and paralyzing agents. The directly recorded potentials from the exposed cortex are affected by anesthesia in a way similar to that of the SSEP that are recorded from electrodes placed on the scalp (in Chap. 6). The amplitude, latency, and waveform of the potentials that are recorded from the exposed cerebral cortex are affected by the level and type of anesthesia, and the way the recorded potentials appear depends on the levels and the kind of anesthesia that is used.

MAPPING CORTICAL AREAS FOR EPILEPSY OPERATIONS

Operations for intractable epilepsy often involve removing regions of the cerebral cortex, and it is imperative to remove as little as possible. The fact that there is considerable individual variation in the anatomical localization of specific cortical areas (29) makes it important to map the cerebral cortex before such operations are undertaken in order to find the exact focus of the epileptic seizure. For that purpose, different forms of recordings (electrocorticography) are used to localize epileptic foci, and for that, arrays of electrodes imbedded in plastic sheets are placed on the cerebral cortex. Recordings are made from many electrodes simultaneously, thus requiring many channels of recordings to be collected.

The placement of the electrode arrays is done in the operating room with the patient under anesthesia. The subsequent recording is usually done over periods of days from the implantation of these semi-permanent electrodes and while the patient is resting in a hospital room.

Mapping of the Insular Cortex

Epileptic foci may also develop deep in the brain, and finding such epileptically active regions deep in the brain has not been possible until recently. It is a different and more difficult task to map structures deep in the brain than mapping the surface of the brain. For example, mapping of the insula cortex has been described recently using b depth electrodes placed using stereotaxic techniques to find which areas of the cortex are the cause of the epileptic seizure (30).

The insular lobe is located under the frontal, parietal, and temporal opercula (see **Fig. 14.9**) (31). This investigator placed electrodes for electrical stimulations in the insular lobe using stereotactic techniques (**Fig. 14.10**). A total of 123 electrode contacts were distributed throughout the insula. When each of 64 of these was activated, clinically detectable responses without subsequent after-discharges were obtained, and 59 of these responses could be confirmed at least once.

These studies were able to pinpoint the anatomical location of epileptic foci and proved important for the surgical treatment of intractable epilepsy. Once found, these areas may be removed surgically. Such implanted depth electrodes are kept in place for a few days while the recordings are done (30).

In addition to making it possible to treat severe epilepsy effectively, the use of this technique provided the opportunity to record from many locations in this structure that are located deep in the brain and also provided results that were of general importance for understanding of the function of the insula (30).

Four major groups of responses were observed: somatosensory responses (19), sensation of warmth/pain (6), viscerosensory

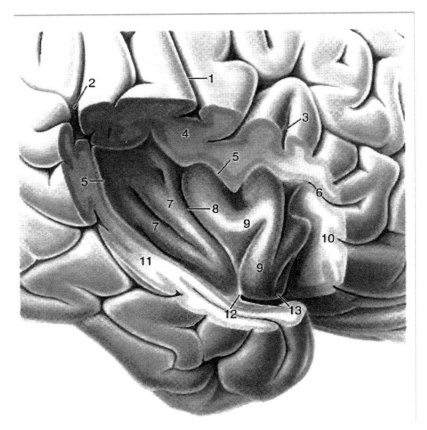

Figure 14.9: Neuroanatomy of the insula. 1, central sulcus; 2, lateral sulcus, posterior branch; 3, lateral sulcus, ascending branch; 4, frontoparietal operculum; 5, lateral sulcus of the insula; 6, lateral sulcus, anterior branch; 7, long gyrus of insula; 8, central sulcus of insula; 9, short gyri of the insula; 10, frontal operculum; 11, temporal operculum; 12, limen insulae; 13, anterior pole of the insula (Reprinted from (*31*) with the permission from Springer).

responses (13), and taste (9). There were also responses that could not be definitely assigned to only one of these qualities, and some (5) responses were reported as taste together with visceral sensations. Stimulation through four of the electrodes gave a combination of the feeling of warmth and general somatosensation.

Mapping for Tumor Removal. Another purpose of mapping of the brain is found in operations where tumors have developed in parts of the brain. In such operations, the purpose of mapping is to localize cortical areas of fundamental importance. Identifying such

important areas that must be spared is done by mapping cortical areas during the operation to remove the tumor, but before tumor removal is begun (see (*32, 33*)). Such mapping is accomplished after large areas of the surface of the cerebral cortex have been exposed, but with the patient being conscious. The stimulation used for mapping is assumed to block function by constantly depolarizing neurons so that they cannot be activated in their normal way.

Penfield pioneered such mapping in the 1930s using a hand-held bipolar stimulating electrode with 60 Hz AC current and appropriately transformed down to a suitable voltage and

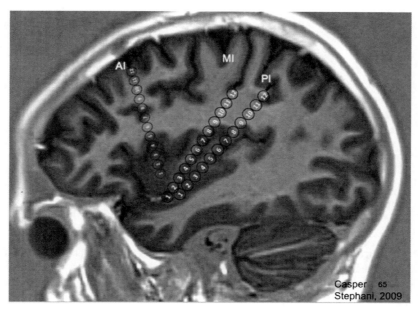

Figure 14.10: Example of depth electrodes in the insular lobe inserted in a dorso-ventral direction in a superimposition of presurgical Brain MRI with postsurgical C-CT (Software iplan-stereotaxy 2.6®, Brainlab) used to determine the location of the electrodes. *AI* anterior insula; *MI* middle insula; *PI* posterior insula. *Numbers* indicate functionally different cortical areas due to results of stimulation. 1, general somatosensation; 2, thermosensation/nociception; 3, gustation; 4, viscerosensation; 5, perception of speech. Stimulus parameters used for mapping the insula were: 1.5–14 mA, pulse width: 0.5 ms, for 3–5 s; 50 Hz (Reprinted from (*30*) with the permission from Dr. Deletis).

isolated from the power line. Similar techniques are still used, but often the stimuli are generated by electronic equipment like other electrical stimuli used for activating neural tissue. When stimulating the motor cortex directly, the use of short pulse trains typically employed in transcranial stimulation is preferred to the long duration 60 Hz stimulation used in the traditional Penfield technique because of the lower risk of seizures. The Penfield technique, however, is still used when cognitive testing is performed (*34*).

Mapping of Language Memory Areas

When operations are aimed at resection of areas of the left temporal lobe and parietal cortex, it is important to avoid specific areas that are critical to language, speaking, and memory (the eloquent cortex[2]). Ojemann did extensive cortical mapping studies in patients undergoing operations for epilepsy using Penfield stimulation methods in conscious patients (*35*).

The anatomical location of these areas, known as parts of the eloquent cortex or brain, varies between individuals (*32, 33, 35*), and their location must, therefore, be determined in each individual patient before an operation is begun in order to preserve their important functions.

The basic principle for such identification is to stimulate a certain area while the patient is performing specific tasks such as speaking or recalling memorized matters, and see if the

---

[2] Eloquent cortex (or brain): those parts of the brain that control speech, motor functions, and senses, the localization of which is important in treating brain tumors. Reprinted from Stedman's Electronic Medical Dictionary Version 7.

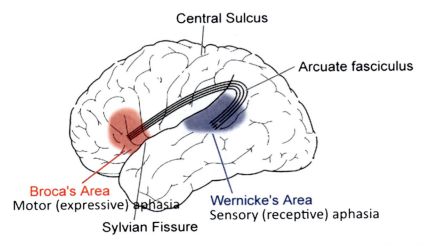

Figure 14.11: Surface of the lateral side of the brain showing the location of the Wernicke and the Broca areas of speech.

stimulation prevents the patient from performing the specific task.

Anatomically, the two areas that are important for hearing, speech, and language are Broca's area and Wernicke's area (**Fig. 14.11**). It is worth noting that the function of these regions is not the same on the two sides; the left side is devoted to speech production, and the right side is more oriented to other functions such as music perception. This means that functions are lost because lesions on the left side cannot be taken over by the right side.

These areas have been referred to as forbidden areas (*37*). When resections are done close to language areas, expressive (Broca) or receptive (Wernicke) language function is often severely compromised. In fact, this deficit has been reported to occur as often as in 60% of operations (*38*); verbal memory deficit occurs at a rate of 50% (*39*). Such deficits are serious and reduce quality of life and limit possibilities of employment.

The medial temporal lobe is associated with long-term memory and should also be preserved.

Many studies have shown that destruction of this region of the temporal lobe bilaterally causes complete loss of episodic memory[3] (see for example, McGaugh (*40*)).

The Penfield technique has been refined over the years (*41*) and is still the most used method for identifying language areas before operations in which cortical areas are to be resected. While it should be possible to do such mapping using functional imaging studies, this has not been relied upon, perhaps because of the lack of sufficient spatial resolution.

In other studies, transcranial magnetic stimulation, TES, and direct cortical stimulation of the motor speech related cortical areas are more modern techniques used to map the speech areas of the cerebral cortex (*42, 43*). In these studies, recordings were made from vocal muscles (primarily in intubated patients under general anesthesia and recording from the cricothyroid muscles) of the patients under general anesthesia (**Fig. 14.12**).

When a positive response was obtained, the stimulation was repeated at least once. Only

---

[3] Episodic memory: the memory of events, times, places, associated emotions and other conception-based knowledge in relation to an experience.

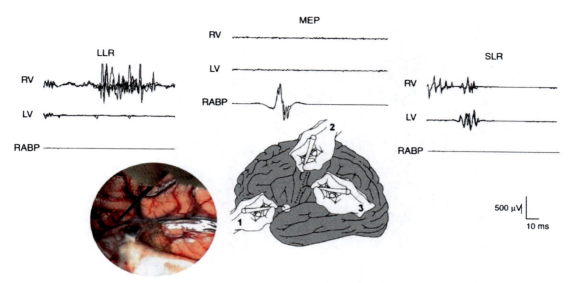

Figure 14.12: Direct cortical stimulation. Schematics of the brain surface with three original responses obtained from vocalis muscle after direct cortical stimulation of the motor speech areas (*LLR* long latency response), primary motor cortex (*SLR* short latency response), and abductor pollicis brevis (APB) muscles after electrical stimulation of the primary motor cortex for small hand muscles. 1, stimulation of the Broca area; 2, stimulation of primary motor cortex; 3, stimulation of primary motor cortex for laryngeal muscles (Reprinted from (*43*) with the permission from Dr. Deletis).

confirmed responses or responses that did correspond to the quality of stimulation of adjacent electrodes were included in the current analysis. Responses with after-discharges were excluded from analysis.

A promising, but very different method to identify which brain areas are activated, is recording of gamma encephalographic activity. Gamma activity is a high-frequency component of the electroencephalogram (frequencies in a band around 40 Hz) that was ignored for many years because of the limitations in old EEG machines that used mechanical penmotors for recording. These machines were just not fast enough to reproduce the gamma activity, which is related to the rhythmic firing of fast-spiking pyramidal cells. Studied in primates and humans, gamma activity has been associated with the coordination of visual and auditory input and sensorimotor activation (*44, 45*).

Gamma activity has been recorded from the exposed cortex as well as from electrodes placed on the scalp. When recorded from the scalp, there is a risk of contamination from EMG activity (*46*).

It has recently been shown that gamma activity is related to language processes as shown in recordings recorded from electrodes placed on the dura (*47*).

Recording of gamma activity is becoming important for studies of connectivity in the brain. For example, electrocorticographic studies during language and memory tasks have recently revealed that the language system is widely distributed in the brain (*48*) by looking at increases in gamma activity during the execution of different tasks. Memory activation is also distributed widely in the brain in areas that are located inferior to the language areas, such as the anterior medial and lateral areas (**Fig. 14.13**).

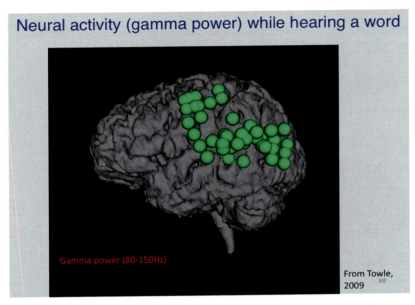

Figure 14.13: Increased gamma activity observed while listening to a spoken word (Reprinted from (*49*) with the permission from Dr. Deletis).

REFERENCES

1. Sekhar LN and AR Møller (1986) Operative management of tumors involving the cavernous sinus. J. Neurosurg. 64:879–89.

2. Møller AR (1987) Electrophysiological monitoring of cranial nerves in operations in the skull base, in *Tumors of the Cranial Base: Diagnosis and Treatment*, LN Sekhar and VL Schramm Jr, Editors. Futura Publishing Co: Mt. Kisco, New York. 123–32.

3. Yingling C (1994) Intraoperative monitoring in skull base surgery, in *Neurotology*, RK Jackler and DE Brackmann, Editors. Mosby: St. Louis. 967–1002.

4. Yingling C and J Gardi (1992) Intraoperative monitoring of facial and cochlear nerves during acoustic neuroma surgery. Otolaryngol. Clin. N. Am. 25:413–48.

5. Lanser M, R Jackler and C Yingling (1992) Regional monitoring of the lower (ninth through twelfth) cranial nerves, in *Intraoperative Monitoring in Otology and Head and Neck Surgery*, J Kartush and K Bouchard, Editors. Raven Press: New York. 131–50.

6. Daube J (1991) Intraoperative monitoring of cranial motor nerves, in *Intraoperative*

Neurophysiologic Monitoring in Neurosurgery, J Schramm and AR Møller, Editors. Springer-Verlag: Heidelberg, Germany. 246–67.

7. Kartush J and K Bouchard (1992) Intraoperative facial monitoring. Otology, neurotology, and skull base surgery, in *Neuromonitoring in Otology and Head and Neck Surgery*, J Kartush and K Bouchard, Editors. Raven Press: New York. 99–120.

8. Møller AR and PJ Jannetta (1984) Preservation of facial function during removal of acoustic neuromas: Use of monopolar constant voltage stimulation and EMG. J. Neurosurg. 61:757–60.

9. Stechison MT, AR Møller and TJ Lovely (1996) Intraoperative mapping of the trigeminal nerve root: Technique and application in the surgical management of facial pain. Neurosurgery 38:76–82.

10. Rosenberg SI, WH Martin, H Pratt et al (1993) Bipolar cochlear nerve recording technique: A preliminary report. Am. J. Otol. 14:362–8.

11. Colletti V and FG Fiorino (1993) Electrophysiologic identification of the cochlear nerve fibers during cerebellopontine angle surgery. Acta Otolaryngol. (Stockh.) 113:746–54.

12. Møller AR, V Colletti and FG Fiorino (1994) Neural conduction velocity of the human auditory nerve: Bipolar recordings from the exposed intracranial portion of the eighth nerve during vestibular nerve section. Electroencephalogr. Clin. Neurophysiol. 92:316–20.

13. Sindou M, G Turano, R Pantieri et al (1994) Intraoperative monitoring of spinal cord SEPs, during microsurgicall DREZotomy (MDT) for pain, spasticity and hyperactive bladder. Stereotact. Funct. Neurosurg. 62:164–70.

14. Sindou M and P Mertens (2002) Selective spinal cord procedures for spasticity and pain, in *Neurophysiology in Neurosurgery*, V Deletis and JL Shils, Editors. Academic Press: Amsterdam. 93–117.

15. Deletis V (2002) Intraoperative neurophysiology and methodologies used to monitor the functional integrity of the motor system, in *Neurophysiology in Neurosurgery*, V Deletis and JL Shils, Editors. Academic Press: Amsterdam. 25–51.

16. Fasano VA, G Broggi and S Zeme (1988) Intraoperative electrical stimulation for functional posterior rhizotomy. Scand. J. Rehab. Med. 17:149–54.

17. Deletis V, DD Vodusek, R Abbott et al (1992) Intraoperative monitoring of the dorsal sacral roots: Minimizing the risk of iatrogenic micturition disorders. Neurosurgery 30:72–5.

18. Deletis V and AB Camargo (2001) Interventional neurophysiological mapping and monitoring during spinal cord procedures. Stereotact. Funct. Neurosurg. 77:25–8.

19. Deletis V and JL Shils (2004) *Neurophysiology in Neurosurgery*. Amsterdam: Academic Press.

20. Leppanen R, R Madigan, C Sears et al (1999) Intraoperative collision studies demonstrate descending spinal cord stimulation evoked potentials and ascending somatosensory evoked potentials are medicated through common pathways. J. Clin. Neurophysiol. 16:170.

21. Strauss C, J Romstock, C Nimsky et al (1993) Intraoperative identification of motor areas or the rhomboid fossa using direct stimulation. J. Neurosurg. 79:393–9.

22. Strauss C (1998) The anatomical aspects of a surgical approach through the floor of the fourth ventricle. Acta Neurochir. (Wien) 140:1099.

23. Sala F and P Lanteri (2003) Brain surgery in motor areas: The invaluable assistance of intraoperative neurophysiological monitoring. J. Neurol. Sci. 47:79–88.

24. Morota N et al (1995) Brainstem mapping: Neurophysiological localization of motor nuclei on the floor of the fourth ventricle. Neurosurgery 37:922–30.

25. Kyoshima K et al (1993) A study of safe entry zones via the floor of the fourth ventricle for brain-stem lesions. J. Neurosurg. 78:987–93.

26. Penfield W and T Rasmussen (1950) The Cerebral Cortex of Man: A Clinical Study of Localization of Function. New York: Macmillan.

27. Lueders H, DS Dinner, RP Lesser et al (1986) Evoked potentials in cortical localization. J. Clin. Neurophysiol. 3:75–84.

28. Goldring S and EM Gregorie (1984) Surgical management of epilepsy using epidural recordings to localize the seizure focus. Review of 100 cases. J. Neurosurg. 60:457–66.

29. Ojemann G, J Ojemann, E Lettich et al (2008) Cortical language localization in left, dominant hemisphere. J. Neurosurg. 108:411–21.

30. Stephani C, G Fernandez Baca-Vaca, M Koubeissi et al (2009) Stimulation of the insula, in *Second Congress, International Society of Intraoperative Neurophysiology*. ISIN: Dubrovnik.

31. Nieuwenhuys R, J Voogd and C van Huijzen (2008) The Human Central Nervous System. New York: Springer.

32. Ojemann GA (2003) The neurobiology of language and verbal memory: Observations from awake neurosurgery. Int. J. Psychophysiol. 48:141–6.

33. Rivet D, D O'Brien, T Park et al (2004) Distance of the motor cortex from the coronal suture as a function of age. Pediatr. Neurosurg. 40:215–9.

34. Ojemann GA (1988) Effect of cortical and subcortical stimulation on human language and verbal memory. Res. Publ. Assoc. Res. Nerv. Ment. Dis. 66:101–15.

35. Ojemann G, J Ojemann, E Lettich et al (1989) Cortical language localization in left, dominant hemisphere. An electrical stimulation mapping investigation in 117 patients. J. Neurosurg. 71:316–26.

36. Penfield W and L Roberts (1959) Speech and Brain-Mechanisms. Princeton: Princeton University Press.

37. Haglund M, M Berger, M Shamseldin et al (1994) Cortical localization of temporal lobe language sites in patients with gliomas. Neurosurgery 34:567–76.

38. Gleissner U, C Helmstaedter, J Schramm, R Sassen et al (2002) Memory outcome after selective amygdalohippocampectomy: A study in 140 patients with temporal lobe epilepsy. Epilepsia 43:87–95.

39. McGaugh J (2000) Memory – a century of consolidation. Science 287:248–51.

40. Lesser R, B Gordon and S Uematsu (1994) Electrical stimulation and language. J. Clin. Neurophysiol. 11:191–204.

41. Deletis V, S Ulkatan, B Cioni et al (2008) Responses elicited in the vocalis muscles after electrical stimulation of motor speech areas. Riv. Med. 14:159–65.

42. Deletis V, I Fernandez-Conejero, S Ulkatan et al (2009) Methodology for intraoperatively eliciting motor evoked potentials in the vocal muscles by electrical stimulation of the corticobulbar tract. Clin. Neurophysiol. 120:336–41.

43. Deletis V (2009) A new contribution to the neurophysiologic exploration of the Broca area, in *Proceedings of the Second Congress, International Society of Intraoperative Neurophysiology*, V Deletis, Editor. ISIN: Dubrovnik. 42–3.

44. Fries P, D Nikolic and W Singer (2007) The gamma cycle. Trends Neurosci. 30:309–16.

45. Creutzfeldt O, G Ojemann and E Lettich (1989) Neuronal activity in the human lateral temporal lobe. I. Response to speech. Exp. Brain Res. 77:451–75.

46. Whitham E, K Pope, S Fitzgibbon et al (2007) Scalp electrical recording during paralysis: Quantitative evidence that EEG frequencies above 20 Hz are contaminated by EMG. Clin. Neurophysiol. 118:1877–88.

47. Crone N, L Hao, J Hart, Jr et al (2001) Electrocorticographic gamma activity during word production in spoken and sign language. Neurology 57:2045–53.

48. Towle VL, HA Yoon, MC Castelle et al (2008) ECoG gamma activity: Differentiating expressive and receptive speech areas. Brain 131:2013–27.

49. Towle VL (2009) Mapping language and memory areas with ECoG, in *Second International Society of Intraoperative Neurophsysiology (ISIN)*, V Deletis, Editor. ISIN: Dubrovnik.

15

Intraoperative Diagnosis and Guidance in an Operation

Introduction

Diagnosis of Injured Peripheral Nerves

Neuroma in Continuity

Localizing the Place of Injury

Identification of the Compressing Vessel in Operations for HFS

The Abnormal Muscle Response

Technique Used to Monitor the Abnormal Muscle Response

Physiologic Guidance for the Placement of Stimulating Electrodes
    and for Making Lesions in the Brain

Implantation of Electrodes in the Basal Ganglia and Thalamus

Basal Ganglia Targets

Monitoring Implantation of Auditory Prostheses

Physiologic Guidance for Placement of ABI

Guidance for Placement of Stimulating Electrodes in Other Parts of the CNS

Anesthesia Requirements

INTRODUCTION

Intraoperative neurophysiologic recordings are beneficial for reducing the risk of postoperative deficits, and similar techniques can be used for the diagnosis of peripheral nerve disorders and for guiding the surgeon in certain operations. Intraoperative measurements of neural conduction and neural conduction velocity can help to determine the nature of a specific pathology and assist in identifying the anatomical location of the pathology in such nerves. Such recordings can guide the surgeon to the proper anatomical location for surgical intervention, and indeed, they may also help the surgeon choose the appropriate surgical intervention.

From: *Intraoperative Neurophysiological Monitoring: Third Edition*
By A.R. Møller, DOI 10.1007/978-1-4419-7436-5_15,
© Springer Science+Business Media, LLC 2011

Hemifacial spasm (HFS) is one of the few disorders where the success of surgical treatment can be monitored through intraoperative neurophysiologic recordings, and this technique is helpful in achieving successful treatment. Intraoperative neurophysiologic recordings are also valuable for intraoperative diagnosis of lesions in peripheral nerves and for guiding placement of lesions deep in the brain and placement of stimulation electrodes for deep brain stimulation (DBS).

DIAGNOSIS OF INJURED PERIPHERAL NERVES

Before the introduction of electrophysiologic methods for assessing neural conduction in injured peripheral nerves, surgeons were confronted with difficult decisions regarding repair of severe nerve injuries on the basis of visual observations and intuition. The introduction of electrophysiologic methods have now made it possible to do functional testing of peripheral nerves in the operating room, and decisions about how to repair such nerves can be based on hard physiologic information.

Neuroma in Continuity

Neuroma in continuity possesses a particular problem regarding choice of optimal treatment. Neuroma in continuity can occur because of injury to peripheral nerves. The condition is caused by incorrect regrowth (sprouting) of regenerating nerve fibers. Accumulation of tangled regenerating nerve fibers (sprouts) builds neuroma that may compress nerve fibers that are unaffected by the lesion or are regenerating normally. Even in small neurinoma, the nerve fibers that pass through it may be interrupted. Conversely, many nerve fibers that pass through a large neurinoma may be conducting effectively, and thus, do not need any surgical intervention. Surgical treatment of neuroma in continuity is especially demanding, and neurophysiologic diagnosis performed intraoperatively is of great importance for the success of repair of such lesions. The severity of lesions of peripheral nerves cannot be assessed by visual inspection, and the aid of intraoperative physiologic diagnosis is essential. If injury to a peripheral nerve has resulted in a neuroma in continuity, it is not possible to

determine preoperatively whether the nerve that is distal to the neuroma has begun to regenerate.

Such information is important for making decisions about whether to perform a nerve graft or to do nothing at all and wait for the nerve to regrow by itself and reach its target (muscles for motor nerves). Such diagnosis can only be obtained by exposing the nerve surgically at the location of the neuroma and making neurophysiologic recordings of neural conduction (1–4).

After a peripheral nerve has been dissected, a neuroma appears as a thickening of the nerve, but it is not possible to determine by visual inspection alone whether there is any neural conduction across the neuroma. However, this can be determined easily by electrically stimulating the nerve on one side of the neuroma and recording the CAP from a location on the nerve on the other side of the neuroma (**Fig. 15.1**). If CAP can be recorded, it is a sign that the nerve conducts nerve impulses through the neuroma, which indicates that the nerve is in the process of regenerating and is growing toward its target. In this case nothing needs to be done. If no CAP can be recorded, there is no neural conduction across the neuroma, and a nerve graft must then be performed to re-establish the function of the nerve.

It may be argued that surgical exploration is unnecessary in such cases, because it would eventually become obvious if the nerve were properly regenerating if a sufficient length of

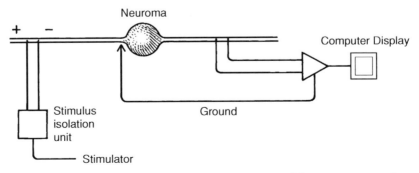

Figure 15.1: Electrical stimulation of a peripheral nerve with a neuroma and recording from the opposite side of the neuroma.

time was allowed to pass. However, if the nerve does not regenerate, it may be too late to perform a nerve graft by the time this fact becomes obvious because the nerve may no longer have the ability to regenerate and, in the case of motor nerves, create new muscle endplates.

Localizing the Place of Injury

Neurophysiologic methods make it possible to localize the exact place where a nerve is injured. This is done by electrically stimulating the nerve in question and recording from a location at a short distance from where the nerve is stimulated. Use of similar basic electrophysiologic techniques makes it possible to determine if an injured nerve is beginning to regenerate. These methods are superior to other often-used methods involving recordings of EMG potentials. Decisions about how a particular nerve would best respond to resection and repair compared to more conservative treatment such as neurolysis can be made right at the operating table using basic electrophysiologic methods.

Practical Aspects of Intraoperative Diagnosing. For such intraoperative diagnosis, both the stimulating and the recording electrodes (**Fig. 15.2A**) should be placed on the same nerve at a small distance from each other. Both stimulating and recording electrodes should be metal hooks (**Fig. 15.2A**). The distance between the stimulating electrodes must be long enough to include a sufficient number of nodes of Ranvier (*4*) (**Fig. 15.2B**).

When a satisfactory response is obtained from a normal nerve, the stimulating–recording electrode assembly can be moved to a section of the nerve whose function is to be diagnosed while keeping the settings for stimulation and recording the same as that used for the normal

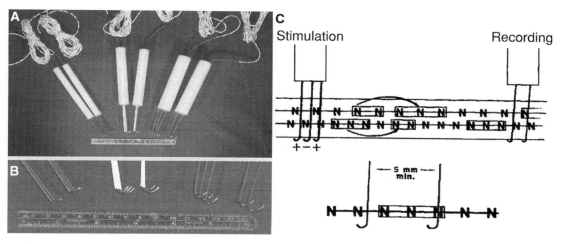

Figure 15.2: (**A**) Electrodes for stimulating and recording compound nerve action potentials (CNAP) can be made in many sizes according to one's needs. Illustrated here, from *left to right*, are miniature, mid-size, and large electrodes. The stimulating electrode contains three contacts, while the recording electrode contains two. The inset enlargement of the electrode tips illustrates the curved hooks on which the exposed nerve can be suspended. The tip separation of the recording electrodes can be adjusted according to the kind of the nerve from which recordings are made. (Reprinted from Ref. (*3*) with permission from Elsevier). (**B**) The distance between the stimulating electrodes must include several nodes of Ranvier of the nerve that is being tested. (**C**) Use of a tripolar stimulating electrode for stimulation in testing a peripheral nerve. (Reprinted from (*4*) with permission from Lippincott Williams & Wilkins).

nerve. If a response is observed, it proves the presence of viable axons. The decision about the treatment of the nerve is made on the basis of these observations. A flowchart for such procedures is shown in **Fig. 15.3**.

For the purpose of finding regions of a peripheral nerve that have abnormal conduction properties, the stimulating and recording electrodes should be moved along the length of the nerve from distal to proximal. When no response is seen from a section of the injured nerve, it is a sign of a conduction block, and this kind of recording procedure makes it possible to discern which part of a nerve has viable axons. This is a totally non-destructive type of testing that can be repeated until the results are satisfactory, and it does not involve risks of damage to regenerating axons.

Nerves may appear by visual inspection to be injured, but electrophysiologic testing could prove otherwise, showing clear signs of axonal continuity. Similarly, lesions that appear to be mild from visual inspection can be functionally severe. This means that physical appearance of a nerve with regard to lesions may be misleading.

Neuromuscular blocking agents can be used during such recordings, and they may even produce an advantage because they prevent muscle activation from the electrical stimulation of intact motor nerves.

Slightly injured nerves have lower conduction velocities than normal nerves, and regenerating nerves have lower conduction velocities than normal nerves because the regenerated nerve fibers have smaller diameters than normal nerve fibers. The effect of a smaller

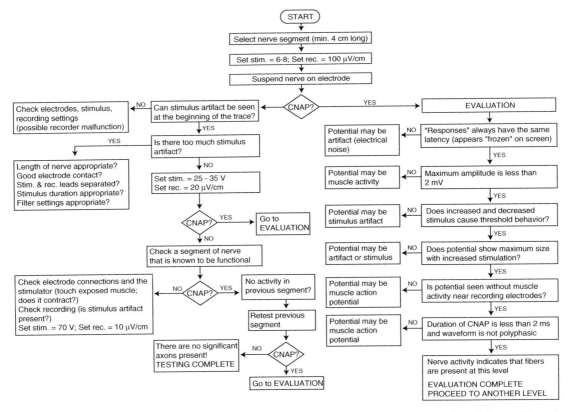

Figure 15.3: Flowchart showing options in peripheral nerve repairs (Reprinted from (*3*) with permission from Elsevier).

diameter of a nerve fiber can be seen when the intensity (current) required to get the maximal response from stimuli of different durations is compared. (It is assumed that rectangular impulses are used as stimuli.) The threshold for electrical stimulation of nerve fibers decreases when the duration of the electrical impulses is increased. A curve of threshold versus duration of the impulses used to stimulate a nerve is shifted toward the right for regenerated fibers (**Fig. 15.4**) because of their smaller diameters. It is seen that the current (intensity) required to achieve maximal response from a nerve is larger for short-duration impulses, and that nerves with regenerated fibers require more current at a certain duration to reach maximal response than normal nerve fibers. (The maximal amplitude of the response (CAP) is obtained when all nerve fibers in the nerve in question are activated.) The difference is exaggerated for regenerated fibers. Therefore, studies of the strength–duration relationship of nerves provide information about the quality of regenerated axons.

Neuropathy of various degrees is common. Elderly individuals normally have fewer active nerve fibers than young people, and the conduction velocity is generally lower. Also, there are usually larger variations in the conduction velocity in the nerve fibers of a peripheral nerve in elderly individuals than that in younger individuals, which causes the CAP to be broader and of lower amplitude in elderly persons than that in young individuals. Pathologies such as diabetes further increase these age-related changes in nerve conduction.

Stimulus and Recording Parameters. It is practical first to apply the stimulation to a nerve, which is known to be normal, and record its response. This sequence will ensure that the equipment is working appropriately and that the patient has normal functions of nerves that are not injured. A stimulus rate of 1–3/s is suitable, and stimulus strengths between 3 and 5 V corresponding 0.5–2 mA can usually activate all large fibers in a mixed nerve. Filters for such recording should be set at ~10 Hz high

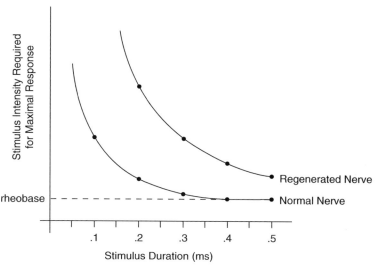

Figure 15.4: Curves showing the relationship between the duration of impulses used to stimulate a nerve electrically and the stimulus intensity required to achieve maximal response (strength–duration curves) for normal and regenerated nerve fibers (Reprinted from (*3*) with permission from Elsevier).

pass and 3 kHz low pass, and a suitable gain of the amplifier should be selected.

The effect of stimulus artifacts on the recorded responses can be diminished by keeping the amplification low so that the stimulus artifact does not overload the amplifier, which will cause the stimulus artifact to be spread out in time (see Chap. 18). The use of good quality stimulus isolation units is important for minimizing the stimulus artifacts. The stimulus artifacts can also be reduced by increasing the distance between stimulating and recording electrodes (to at least 2 cm), and separating the stimulating and recording leads. Placing a ground electrode between the recording and stimulating electrodes (**Fig. 15.1**) may also help to reduce the stimulus artifact. The use of a tripolar recording electrode (**Fig. 15.2C**) instead of a bipolar stimulating electrode is even more effective in reducing the stimulus artifacts because it eliminates a current path that would include the site of the recording electrode (*3*).

IDENTIFICATION OF THE COMPRESSING VESSEL IN OPERATIONS FOR HFS

The microvascular decompression (MVD) operation to relieve HFS is one of the few operations in which intraoperative neurophysiologic recordings can not only guide the surgeon in identifying the anatomical location of the pathology, but it can also provide evidence of a successful accomplishment of the goal of the operation.

> Hemifacial spasm can be cured by moving a blood vessel off the facial nerve (MVD operation). The offending vessel (artery or vein) is most often located near the root exit zone (REZ) of the facial nerve. To cure the disorder, the vessel(s) must be moved off the nerve, and an implant of a soft material (such as shredded Teflon) is placed between the nerve and the

vessel(s). MVD operations normally have a high cure rate (~85%) (*5, 6*). If the offending vessel is not moved off the facial nerve root, the spasm persists postoperatively, and the patient must undergo a second MVD operation. The reason for the failure of relief from the symptoms has almost always been that there was more than one vessel in contact with the facial nerve root, which was not obvious from visual inspection during the first operation. Only one vessel is usually associated with causing the spasm. Only after the "right" vessel is moved off the nerve will the patient become free of the spasm. Moving vessels other than the "right" vessel off the nerve root either had no effect on the spasm or caused only incomplete relief of the spasm. Intraoperative neurophysiologic recordings can indicate when the vessel that is associated with the abnormal muscle response is moved off the facial nerve root, and it seems as if it is the same vessel that is associated with the symptoms of HFS (spasm and synkinesis).

Introduction of intraoperative recording of the abnormal muscle response[1] in MVD operations for HFS has reduced the necessity of re-operations and improved the cure rate to more than 95% (*7*). During such operations, intraoperative neurophysiologic recordings of the abnormal muscle response can help identify the blood vessel that is involved in causing the spasm and ensure that the therapeutic goal of the operation has been achieved before the operation has been terminated.

The Abnormal Muscle Response

When a branch of the facial nerve in a person with HFS is stimulated electrically, not only do the muscles that are innervated by the branch of the facial nerve that is stimulated contract, but the muscles that are innervated by other branches of the facial nerve also contract. This abnormal muscle response (also known as the lateral spread) can thus be elicited by electrical stimulation

---

[1]The abnormal muscle response (*7–9*) is also known as the "lateral spread response" (*10*) or the "delayed muscle response."

of one branch of the facial nerve while recordings of the EMG response from muscles that are innervated by a different branch of the facial nerve are being made (*11*). For example, the abnormal muscle response can be elicited by stimulating the temporal or zygomatic branch of the facial nerve electrically while recording EMG potentials from the mentalis muscle (**Fig. 15.5**), or by stimulating the marginal mandibular branch while recording from the orbicularis oculi muscles. The abnormal muscle response seems to be specific to patients with HFS, and it can only be elicited from the side of the face where the spasm occurs.

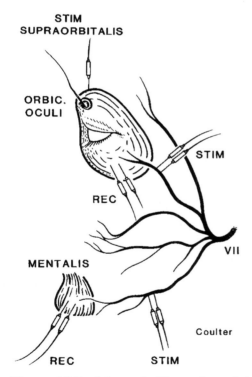

Figure 15.5: Schematic illustration of the arrangement used for stimulating one branch of the facial nerve (the marginal mandibular or zygomatic branch) and for recording EMG potentials from muscles that are innervated by a different branch for monitoring the abnormal muscle response.

The abnormal muscle response elicited by electrical stimulation of a branch of the facial nerve consists of an initial EMG component that occurs with a latency of ~10 ms, followed by a variable series of potentials (after-discharges) (**Fig. 15.6**). Such stimulation also evokes a (direct) response from the muscles that are innervated by the nerve that is stimulated.

When the blood vessel that is in close contact with the facial nerve and which is related to the patient's spasm is lifted off the nerve, the abnormal muscle response usually disappears instantaneously (*12*) (**Fig. 15.7**), but if the vessel is allowed to fall back on the nerve, the response reappears (*12*) (**Fig. 15.7**). In this patient, the abnormal muscle response remained absent after an implant (for instance, a small piece of Teflon felt) was placed between the facial nerve and the offending blood vessel, as normally occurs.

The abnormal muscle response is obviously a result of abnormal proliferation of activity from one branch of the facial nerve on the affected side to other branches of the facial nerve on the same side (crosstalk).

Evidence has been presented that the abnormal muscle response is the backfiring (exaggerated F-response) of motoneurons in the facial nucleus (8, 13–16), but there is evidence that the cause is the activation of neural plasticity (17, 18), although these motoneurons have become hyperactive and hypersensitive by unknown processes involved in the disorder (16). It is also evident that the symptoms of HFS are not caused by the close contact between the facial nerve root and a blood vessel alone, but also by one or more other factors. The location of a blood vessel on the facial nerve root is obviously necessary (but not sufficient) to maintain the hyperactivity and explains why the abnormal muscle response disappears when the blood vessel is moved off the facial nerve, but this does not mean that it is the cause of the symptoms. There is considerable evidence that activation of neural plasticity is the cause of the hyperactivity of neurons in the facial motonucleus as well as the increase in synaptic efficacy that activates connections between motoneurons, and it is the axons of

Sti Zyg. NVII

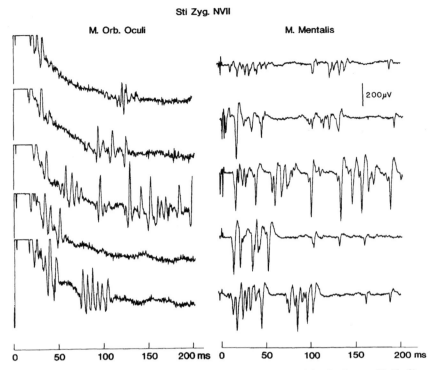

Figure 15.6: Recordings of the EMG response from the orbicularis oculi (*left*) and mentalis (*right*) muscles when the zygomatic branch of the facial nerve was stimulated electrically in a patient undergoing MVD to relieve HFS. The recordings were obtained after the patient was anesthetized, but before the operation was begun. (Reprinted from (*14*) with permission from Elsevier).

these motoneurons that form the different branches of the facial nerve. It seems obvious that the vascular contact is only one of several causes that are necessary for the symptoms to manifest.

The abnormal muscle response can be recorded while the patient is under surgical anesthesia, provided that muscle relaxants are not used. The amplitude of the abnormal muscle response is only 5–10% of that of the direct muscle response (M-response) to stimulation of the branch of the nerve that innervates the particular muscle and indicates that the abnormal muscle response activates only a small fraction of the total number of motor units. (The M-response is assumed to involve most of the motor units of the muscle when the facial nerve is stimulated at a supra-maximal strength.)

Use of the Abnormal Muscle Response for Monitoring MVD Operations for HFS. Since the abnormal muscle response disappears instantly when the offending vessel is moved off the facial nerve (*12*), monitoring the abnormal muscle response can guide the surgeon in this kind of MVD operations and help him or her achieve a better success rate (*7*).

The after-discharges that follow the initial component of the abnormal muscle response (**Fig. 15.6**) often disappear or become infrequent after the dura is opened or when the facial nerve is exposed, and usually, only the initial component (with a latency of 10 ms) remains. If the amplitude of the abnormal muscle response only decreases, but does not disappear when a vessel is moved off the facial

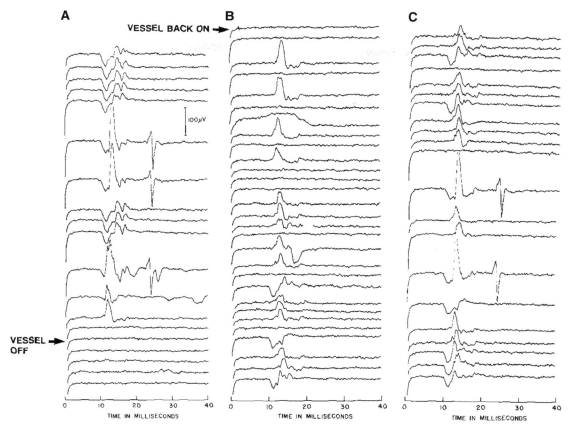

Figure 15.7: Consecutive EMG recordings from a patient undergoing MVD to relieve HFS. Each graph shows consecutive recordings (beginning at *top*) from the mentalis muscle in response to electrical stimulation of the zygomatic branch of the facial nerve. As indicated, the vessel was lifted off the facial nerve root as indicated near the *bottom* of the first column. The recordings in the middle of the right column were made when the vessel fell back on the nerve root. (Reprinted from (*12*) with the permission from Lippincott Williams & Wilkins).

nerve, it is an indication that another vessel is also affecting the facial nerve. When this other vessel is identified and moved off the facial nerve, the abnormal muscle response disappears totally.

In some patients, the abnormal muscle response may be absent when the stimulation is first switched on, but it can be activated by increasing the stimulus rate to 50 pps for a few seconds, after which the repetition rate may again be set at the customary rate of 2–5 pps (**Fig. 15.8**). Initial absence of the abnormal muscle response often occurs in patients who

have had HFS for only a short time prior to the operation. If the amplitude of the abnormal muscle response is low at the beginning of the operation, the amplitude of the response will increase after such rapid stimulation (*13*). After-discharges also often reappear, and spontaneous muscle contractions may also occur for a short time after rapid stimulation.

The amplitude of the abnormal muscle response often decreases when the arachnoidal membrane covering the lower cranial nerves is opened, and the after-discharges usually disappear at this stage of the operation (**Fig. 15.9**).

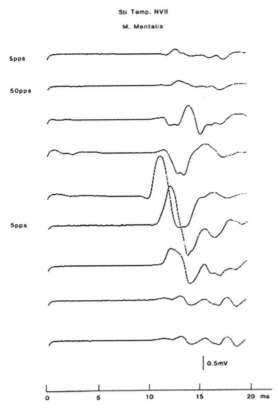

Sti Temp. NVII

M. Mentalis

5pps

50pps

5pps

0.5mV

0   5   10   15   20 ms

Figure 15.8: Recordings of the abnormal muscle response in a patient undergoing MVD operation to relieve HFS, obtained before the offending vessels were moved off the facial nerve. The effect of increasing the stimulus rate from 5 to 50 pps for a short period of stimulation on the abnormal muscle response is shown. (Reprinted from (*14*) with permission from Elsevier).

If the abnormal muscle response disappears totally when the dura or the arachnoidal membrane is opened, and if the response cannot be brought back by applying stimulation at 50 pps for a short period (**Fig. 15.8**), the offending vessel is often found to be a loose loop of an artery (either the anterior inferior cerebellar artery (AICA), the posterior inferior cerebellar artery (PICA), or a branch of either one). The disappearance of the abnormal muscle response occurs because the loop of the vessel loses contact with the nerve when the intracisternal fluid

pressure is decreased as the dura or arachnoidal membrane is opened.

In patients who have had HFS for a long time (7–15 years), muscle activity sometimes occur after the initial component of the abnormal muscle response even after the facial nerve has been exposed. In such patients, the offending vessel is often in firm contact (held in place by arachnoidal bands) with the proximal portion of the facial nerve near the brainstem. Such vessels must be dissected from the nerve in order to place an implant between the vessel and the nerve, and involves risk of injury to the facial nerve. Monitoring the function of the facial nerve to detect possible injuries to the nerve is indicated in such situations. The techniques described in Chap. 11 can be used for this purpose.

The abnormal muscle response may not disappear before small arteries or veins that are in close contact with the facial nerve are moved off the nerve root. Such vessels are often seen where the nerve root blends into the brainstem (*7, 8*). (Before the introduction of intraoperative monitoring of the abnormal muscle response, it was reported that such small vessels could cause the symptoms of HFS (*19*)). When such small vessels were moved off the nerve root or coagulated (veins), the abnormal muscle response usually disappeared, and the response could not be made to reappear by increasing the stimulus rate. Most of these patients obtained total relief from their spasms postoperatively. If the abnormal muscle response did not disappear when a blood vessel was moved off the facial nerve, the patients' spasm often remained after the operation (*7*).

The facial nerve must be stimulated at a high rate and sufficiently high stimulus intensity (at least 20 V, corresponding to 5 mA) for a few seconds before it can be concluded that the abnormal muscle response is indeed absent (*13*) (**Fig. 15.8**).

If these maneuvers cause the abnormal muscle response to reappear, even for a short period, another vessel is most likely in contact with the facial nerve, and the operation cannot be regarded to be completed before that vessel

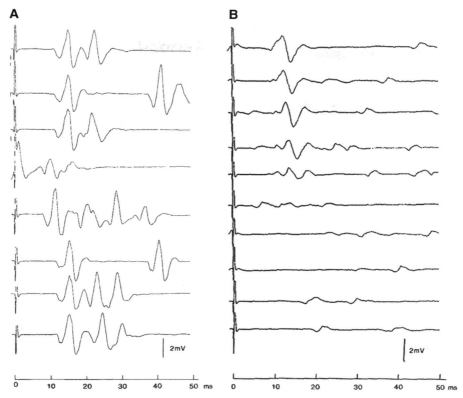

Figure 15.9: Examples of the abnormal EMG response recorded in a patient who was undergoing MVD to relieve HFS. (**A**) Recordings made before the dura was opened. The response appearing with a latency of ~10 ms is the abnormal muscle response. This is followed by variable EMG activity (after-discharges). (**B**) Recordings obtained after the dura was opened. Only the initial component of the abnormal muscle response is shown. The vessel was moved off the nerve when the recordings in the middle of this column were obtained. The bottom recordings show an absence of the abnormal muscle response. The low amplitude of the spontaneous activity seen in the recordings is indicative of slight injury to the facial nerve. (Reprinted from (7) with the permission from the Journal of Neurosurgery).

has been moved off the facial nerve. Individuals who have this kind of residual occurrence of the abnormal muscle response most likely have spasm postoperatively, but that spasm may disappear over time. If the abnormal muscle response cannot be brought back by increasing the stimulus strength and stimulus rate, there is only a very small likelihood that the patient will have residual spasm postoperatively (7).

On the basis of these findings, it seems essential that for curing HFS, blood vessels are moved off the facial nerve root to an extent that the abnormal muscle response can no longer be elicited when the stimulus rate is increased to 50 pps for a short period (7, 20). If moving one vessel off the facial nerve does not eliminate the abnormal muscle response, it is important to explore the facial nerve root further, including the surface of the brainstem where the facial nerve exits, to identify any vessel that may cause the spasm.

This technique has been used in many patients who were operated on for HFS (14), and its usefulness has been confirmed by other investigators (20) who also found that monitoring the abnormal muscle response is helpful in identifying the vessel that is causing the patient's HFS. Other investigators (*15*) have found that good outcomes may occur even when the abnormal muscle response is present at the end of the operations and thus, have questioned the value of this form of intraoperative monitoring. In some of these patients, the spasm is present at the end of the operation, but it slowly abates.

In addition to increasing the success rate of the MVD operation, the results of using the abnormal muscle response in operations on patients with HFS have provided evidence that there can be more than one vessel involved in generating the abnormal muscle response (and thus, the spasm) and also that vessels can be in close contact with the facial nerve without causing any noticeable problems. Recordings of the abnormal muscle response in operations to relieve HFS have also provided research opportunities that have contributed to both a better understanding of the pathophysiology of HFS and the understanding of other disorders that are caused by similar pathologies (*16, 18*).

Technique Used to Monitor the Abnormal Muscle Response

For monitoring purposes, it is most suitable to elicit the abnormal muscle response from the temporal branch of the facial nerve, but in patients who have had HFS for many years, stimulation of the marginal mandibular branch of the facial nerve may be used as well. EMG responses recorded from the mentalis muscle and elicited by electrical stimulation of the temporal branch of the facial nerve provide the most reproducible recording of the abnormal muscle response for the purpose of intraoperative monitoring of MVD operations for HFS.

For recording the abnormal muscle response, two fine-needle electrodes should be placed ~1 cm apart deep in the mentalis muscle (wire hooks are equally suitable). Two electrodes should be placed superficially in the orbicularis oculi muscles for recording the direct muscle response (M-response) (**Fig. 15.6**). These two pairs of recording electrodes should be connected to two differential amplifiers in order to obtain differentially recorded EMG from each muscle (**Fig. 15.10**). Electrical stimulation of the temporal branch of the facial nerve is accomplished by two similar needle (or wire hook) electrodes placed about 1 cm apart in or near the temporal branch of the facial nerve. The proper location is easily found by noting an imaginary line between the ear canal and the lateral corner of the eye and placing the stimulating electrodes about halfway between the ear and the eye on that line. The cathode (negative electrode) should be placed closest to the ear.

If the marginal mandibular nerve is to be stimulated, recordings of the abnormal muscle response should be made from muscles around the eye (orbicularis oculi muscles) (**Fig. 15.10**), and the direct muscle response (M-response) should be recorded from the mentalis muscle.

While recording of the direct muscle response (M-response) is not important to intraoperative monitoring, it makes it possible to check whether the stimulating electrodes are correctly placed in the appropriate branch of the facial nerve. Placing the stimulating electrodes correctly is facilitated by having the stimulator connected to the stimulating electrodes and the stimulation switched on (rate of 5–10 pps at about 20 V using a semi-constant voltage stimulator) while observing the face for muscle contractions when placing the electrodes. Rectangular impulses of 100–150 µs duration should be used as the stimuli. After all the electrodes are in place, the stimulus strength may be lowered to find the threshold for eliciting the abnormal muscle response. This is usually ~6 V, but can be as low as 1.5 V. During monitoring of the abnormal muscle response, a stimulus repetition rate of 2–5 pps and a stimulus level that is 20–30% above threshold will usually provide a stable abnormal muscle response.

The amplifiers for the EMG potentials should have filter settings at 10–3,000 Hz. The recorded EMG potentials may be made audible by using a device similar to that described when discussing intraoperative monitoring during removal of vestibular schwannoma (see Chap. 11) (*22, 23*).

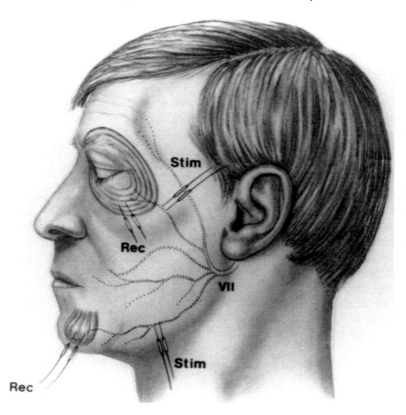

Figure 15.10: Electrode placement for monitoring the abnormal muscle response in a patient undergoing MVD to relieve HFS. (Reprinted from (*21*) with the permission from Springer).

Intraoperative monitoring of auditory function is usually performed concurrently with facial muscle contraction monitoring on patients who undergo operations for HFS. Stimulation of the facial nerve should not be a submultiple of the stimulus rate for the auditory stimulation in order to avoid interference with the recording of auditory potentials.

PHYSIOLOGIC GUIDANCE FOR THE PLACEMENT OF STIMULATING ELECTRODES AND FOR MAKING LESIONS IN THE BRAIN

Identifying specific tissue in operations where lesions are to be made in CNS structures has become an important practical use of neurophysiologic methods in the operating room. It places a particular demand regarding knowledge about anatomy and physiology of the systems in question on the physiologist who carries out such procedures. Most of the procedures are done in conscious patients, which places additional obligations on everyone who is present in the operating room.

The primary targets for lesions and implantation of stimulating electrodes (for DBS) in order to treat movement disorders and pain are the different nuclei of the basal ganglia and the thalamus. Implantation of electrodes for chronic stimulation (DBS) has replaced much of the practice of making small lesions in these structures.

Treatment of movement disorders using DBS is now in common use (*24*). Other treatments for movement disorders, such as Parkinson's disease, consist of electrical stimulation of the cerebral motor cortices (*25, 26*).

Implantation of such electrodes is a less invasive procedure than DBS of the basal ganglia, and it may provide benefit for locating the motor cortex using electrophysiologic guidance. DBS for dystonia has also been described as having a beneficial effect (27).

The use of stimulation by electrodes implanted on the cerebral cortex for promoting the expression of neural plasticity in stroke victims (28), for treatment of tinnitus (29), and for relief of pain (30) is an electrophysiologic method that is currently under development for clinical application. Implantation of electrodes for stimulation of the dorsal column of the spinal cord for pain (31, 32) and for stimulation of the vagus nerve for epilepsy and pain (33) has been in use for some years. More recently, DBS has begun to find use in the treatment of other common diseases such as depression. Stimulation of nucleus accumbens shows promise in the treatment of addiction, including eating disorders (leading to obesity).

The left vagus nerve is now the target for studies of the effect of electrical stimulation for treatment of many disorders such as pain, depression, and tinnitus.

While the anatomical location of lesions or implantation of electrodes in the basal ganglia and the thalamus is determined grossly by imaging techniques such as MRI, the exact location for lesions or for implantation of electrodes for DBS is normally made using neurophysiologic recordings as guidance (27, 34). Neurophysiologic guidance using neurophysiologic recordings is also important for the placement of auditory brainstem implants (cochlear nucleus implants) (35).

Implantation of Electrodes in the Basal Ganglia and Thalamus

The proper target for implantation of electrodes for DBS can be determined on the basis of recordings of electrical activity from cells in specific targets (36). Other groups (37) have used similar techniques for guidance of the placement of lesions in specific structures of the basal ganglia. Understanding the anatomy and physiology of the specific parts of the thalamus and the basal ganglia that are involved in pathologies (Chap. 9) is essential for the success of such procedures.

Localization of Specific Basal Ganglia Structures in Movement Disorders. For the purpose of finding the correct location for lesions or implantation of electrodes for DBS, microelectrodes are used to record responses from single nerve cells or small groups of nerve cells (multiunit recordings). The methods that are used for recordings from deep brain structures in humans for these purposes were developed by Albe-Fessard and her co-workers (38) for research purposes.

For DBS electrodes, the goal of using intraoperative neurophysiology is to find the anatomical location where implantation will provide the best therapeutic effect and the least side effect. For this purpose, microelectrodes are inserted using stereotaxic methods, and the responses are observed as the electrode is advanced through the structures that are the targets for implantations or lesions. Sometimes more than one path must be used to find the optimal location for implantation of the electrodes for permanent stimulation or for making lesions. Identification of the specific target for implantation (or lesions) is made on the basis of electrical activity recorded by microelectrodes that either record from single neural elements (mostly cell bodies) or from a small group of cells (multiunit recording). Two kinds of activity are recorded: spontaneous activity and activity elicited by specific voluntary movements that the patient is asked to perform. The target is determined on the basis of empirical data and experience since the understanding of the function of these structures and their involvement in movement disorders is still incomplete.

Microelectrodes have been used for many years in animal experiments and two types are used: glass pipettes and metal electrodes. For use in humans, metal electrodes have been used exclusively. The metal microelectrodes that are used are similar to those developed and described by David Hubel (39). The tips of such electrodes are uninsulated and have diameters of a few micrometers (μm; 1 μm = 1/1,000 of a millimeter). Some of the first uses of these kinds of electrodes in patients were for research studies of the responses from cortical cells (40) and for studies of the somatosensory part of the thalamus (41, 42). Lenz et al. (41, 42) described the construction of microelectrodes that were suitable for use in humans. The diameter of the tip of electrodes that record only from a single nerve cell should be 1–5 μm. Electrodes with larger tips (20–50 μm) will normally record from more than one cell (multiunit recordings). The electrical impedance of such electrodes is inversely proportional to the diameter of their tips and may vary from 50 kΩ for tip size in the order of 50 μm to 1 MΩ for the smallest tip size (1–3 μm), all depending on the material used and the length of the uninsulated tip. The properties of such electrodes were studied by other investigators, and these studies are the basis for the present use of such electrodes for finding targets for implantation of electrodes for DBS and for making lesions in CNS structures.

Some investigators make their own electrodes, while others use commercially available electrodes. For example, Philip Starr and his group (43) use glass-coated platinum/iridium microelectrodes that are commercially available. These electrodes have impedances between 0.4 and 1 MΩ.

Basal Ganglia Targets

Responses from Cells in the Basal Ganglia. The discharge pattern varies much from cell to cell, and it is different from nucleus to nucleus (**Figs. 15.11–15.13**). The cells from which recordings are made are often named according to their pattern of discharge, such as "burster" cells that generate bursts of activity and "pauser cells" that have tonic discharges that are

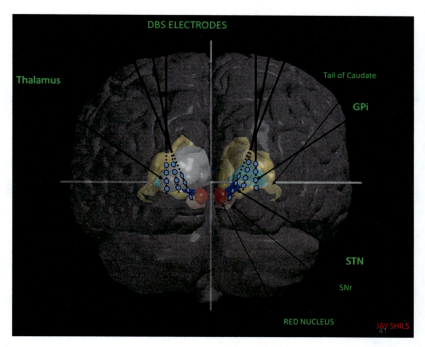

Figure 15.11: Implantation of stimulating electrodes in the basal ganglia (DBS) illustrated using an artist's rendition of the structures of the basal ganglia that are targets for lesions and implantation of electrodes for DBS with trajectories through the basal ganglia superimposed. *GPi* Globus pallidus internal, *STN* subthalamic nucleus, *SNr* Substancia nigra reticulate. (Reprinted from (*36*) with permission from Elsevier).

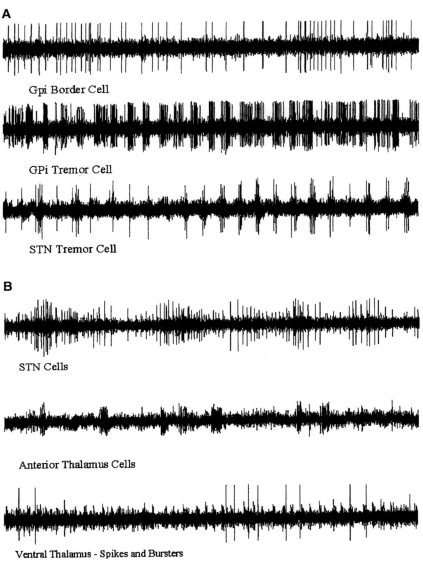

Figure 15.12: Multiunit recordings from different locations of the basal ganglia. (**A**) Typical good quality recordings from three different cells in the basal ganglia. These recordings are single cell recordings as seen from the fact that all spikes have the same amplitude. Notice that the level of the background noise is well below that of the spikes. The recording was 5 s long. (**B**) Typical multiunit recordings from three different locations in the thalamus. Individual units can be distinguished by the difference in the amplitude and the difference in the waveform, which can be detected automatically by using modern computer software. The recordings shown were 5-s epochs. (Reprinted from (*36*) with permission from Elsevier).

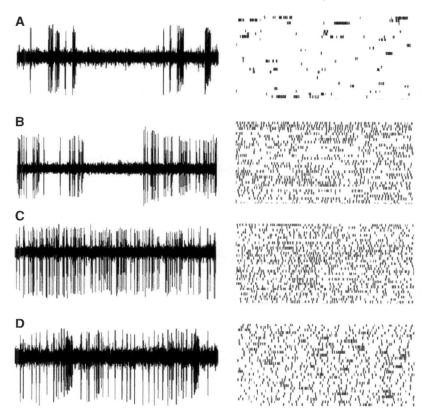

Figure 15.13: Unit recording from GPe and GPi in a patient with dystonia (1-s epochs are shown). Raster diagrams to the right: Each line represents 500 ms, and a 15-s segment of the receded activity is shown. Each vertical tick mark represents a single action potential (discharge). (**A**) Recording from a GPe burster cell. (**B**) Recording from a GPe pause cell. (**C**) Recording from a GPi cell. (**D**) Recording from "high frequency burster" cell in the GPi (Reprinted from (*43*) with the permission from the Journal of Neurosurgery).

interrupted by brief pauses in firing. Some cells will exhibit bursting activity that is superimposed on continuous activity. Different types of disorders produce specific pattern of discharges as do different cells in the different nuclei and in different parts of the nuclei. Examples of recordings of single cell activity and multiunit activity are shown in **Figs. 15.12–15.14**.

Equipment for Microelectrode Recordings. The equipment used for neurophysiologic guidance is more complex than that used for intraoperative neurophysiologic monitoring (**Fig. 15.15**). Filter setting for the amplifiers of

300 Hz–5 kHz band-pass is suitable. The recorded activity should be made audible by a loudspeaker so that everybody in the operating room can hear the activity, and be displayed on a computer screen together with statistics such as mean discharge rate and interspike interval. The software should be able to sort the different components of multiunit recordings and store data for later analysis and for use in research.

Display of Results and Quality Control. During sessions to find appropriate anatomical locations for lesions or for implantation of electrodes for DBS, the discharge properties at

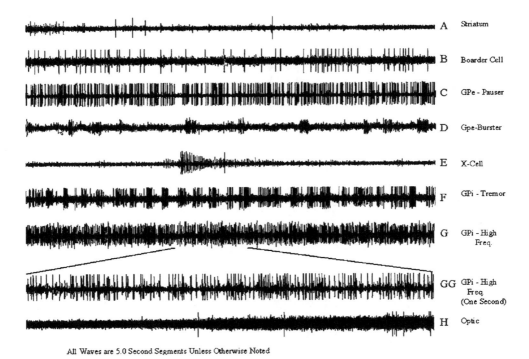

Figure 15.14: Variations in the appearance of recorded multiunit potentials from different nuclei of the basal ganglia. All recordings were 5-s epochs. (Reprinted from (*36*) with permission of Elsevier).

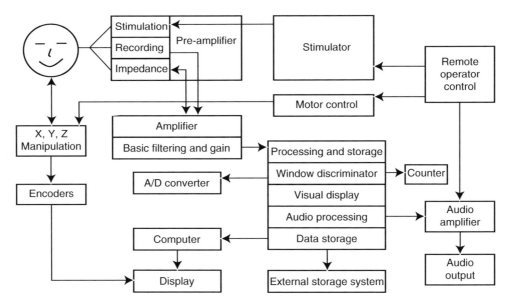

Figure 15.15: Block diagram of components of equipment involved in neurophysiologic guidance for lesions and electrode implantation such as in the basal ganglia and thalamus. (From (*36*) with permission from Elsevier).

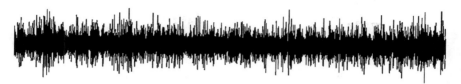

SNr Nucleus

Figure 15.16: Example of a recording of poor quality. The electrode tip was probably too large (50 μm) and its impedance (50 kΩ) was too low. The duration of the recording shown is 5 s. (Reprinted from (*36*) with permission from Elsevier).

each location should be plotted on planes that refer to relevant anatomical structures. When a location for stimulation is found, test stimulations are conducted to see if the anticipated effect is achieved, such as cessation of tremor or other abnormal muscle contractions.

Quality control is especially important for microelectrode recordings because of the high electrode impedance that makes such recordings prone to contamination with many kinds of electrical interference. Recording in conscious patients adds other sources of interference, although movement artifact should not be a problem because the patient's head is firmly secured in a head holder. Poor recordings can also result from recording far from active structures or using defective electrodes, as illustrated in **Fig. 15.16**.

The recent extensive practical use of these methods in humans has provided opportunities for research purposes. For example, much of our present knowledge about the normal and the pathologic function of the basal ganglia and parts of the thalamus have been acquired in that way. The use of these methods in clinical settings has produced a wealth of information not only about the normal functions of these structures, but also about the pathophysiology of movement disorders (*37, 41, 42, 44–49*).

MONITORING IMPLANTATION OF AUDITORY PROSTHESES

Two kinds of auditory prostheses are in routine use. Cochlear implants (*50*), the first type, are the most common. The second type, auditory

brainstem implants (ABI), stimulates the cochlear nucleus (*51*). Cochlear implants were introduced by William House (*52*), and the early implants consisted of a single electrode placed inside the cochlea and connected to electronics that converted sounds picked up by a microphone into electrical current. Modern cochlear implants consist of an array of electrodes that are implanted in the basal portion of the cochlea (*53*). Sounds reach a microphone placed near the individual's ear. A sound processor connected to the microphone generates electrical signals, and these signals are sent to the electrode array in the basal portion of the cochlea. Both adults who have acquired hearing loss and children who are born deaf are now routinely given cochlear implants.

ABI were introduced for use in individuals who have lost hearing in both ears from bilateral vestibular schwannoma (acoustic tumors), usually neurofibromatosis type 2 (NF2) (*54, 55*). More recently, it has been possible to restore hearing by the use of ABIs (cochlear nucleus implants) in individuals with disorders of the auditory nerve, such as auditory nerve aplasia or severe auditory neuropathy (*56*).

Implantation of the stimulating electrodes in the cochlea requires minimum electrophysiologic guidance, but correct placement of the implanted array of electrodes is usually checked using recordings of ABR in a similar way as that described in Chap. 7. Implantation of electrodes to stimulate the cochlear nuclei (ABI) requires testing of the position of the implanted electrode array with regard to stimulating their target neurons adequately (*35*). Intraoperative guidance in the placement of such implants has gained increasing use (*35, 57*).

Physiologic Guidance for Placement of ABI

ABI consist of an array of 8–16 electrodes placed on a plastic sheet that is placed on the surface of the cochlear nucleus (*54, 55*). The floor of the lateral recess of the fourth ventricle is the surface of the cochlear nuclei (*58*). The location for the placement of the implant is reached through the foramen of Luschka, located close to the entrance/exit of cranial nerves IX and X from the brainstem (*58*). This means that the placement of the stimulating array of electrodes on the surface of the cochlear nucleus cannot be guided visually and that electrophysiologic guidance is important. This can be accomplished by recording ABR while electrical impulses are applied to one pair after another of the implanted electrodes (*35*). The manufacturers of brainstem implants supply hardware and software that allow such testing. If some electrode pairs do not elicit a response, the implanted array of electrodes is moved and the test is repeated. This process is repeated until a satisfactory response is obtained. One of the problems in such testing is related to the stimulus artifact that is generated by the electrical stimulation, but the interference can be reduced by appropriate placement of the recording electrodes and by electronic elimination of the artifacts (*35, 57*).

GUIDANCE FOR PLACEMENT OF STIMULATING ELECTRODES IN OTHER PARTS OF THE CNS

Electrical stimulation of the dorsal column of the spinal cord has been a common procedure for many years (*30, 31*), but requirements for electrophysiologic guidance in such implantations have not yet emerged. Electrical stimulation of various parts of the cerebral cortex is beginning to gain clinical usage, and it has been shown that electrical stimulation of the motor cortex produces beneficial effects in treatment of severe pain (*30*). More recently, electrical stimulation of the somatosensory cortex has been shown to suppress some forms

of pain and also to be effective in suppressing tinnitus (*59*). Cerebral cortex implantations have been made on the basis of imaging data only. Stimulation of the auditory cortex for tinnitus (*60*) and stimulations of other parts of the cortex to enhance expression of neural plasticity for rehabilitation of stroke victims (*28*) are examples of such new usages of chronic electrical stimulation of the CNS using implanted electrodes. Methods for physiologic guidance for such implantations have not yet become established, but functional MRI (fMRI) has been used (*29*).

ANESTHESIA REQUIREMENTS

Testing of peripheral nerves is not affected by commonly used anesthetics unless muscle responses are recorded, in which case, muscle relaxants must be excluded from the anesthesia regimen. Muscle relaxants cannot be used while monitoring the abnormal muscle response in MVD operations for HFS. Even the use of a low-level, endplate-blocking agent severely hampers the monitoring of the abnormal muscle response. Therefore, when the abnormal muscle response is to be monitored, the patient should be anesthetized without the use of any endplate-blocking agent. The abnormal muscle response is only slightly affected by commonly used anesthetics. The best anesthesia regimen consists of agents such as intravenous barbiturates or Propofol, and remifentanyl (a synthetic opioid), which are used in total intravenous anesthesia, TIVA.

Electrophysiologic guidance for finding the targets in the thalamus and basal ganglia for lesions and implantation of electrodes for DBS is usually done in conscious patients, but in children it may be necessary to use some form of anesthesia. Propofol (see Chap. 16) is often used for placement of the stereotaxic frame, and terminated before recordings are completed. For children who need anesthesia during the recordings, Propofol and inhalation agents have been found to be less suitable than anesthesia maintained with ketamine and remifentanyl (*43*). Guidance of implantation of ABI uses recordings of ABR, which are insensitive to anesthetics and muscle relaxants.

REFERENCES

1. Landi A, SA Copeland, CB Wynn et al (1980) The role of somatosensory evoked potentials and nerve conduction studies in the surgical management of brachial plexus injuries. J. Bone Joint Surg. (Br.) 62B:492–6.

2. Kline DG and DJ Judice (1983) Operative management of selected brachial plexus lesions. J. Neurosurg. 58:631–49.

3. Happel L and D Kline (2002) Intraoperative Neurophysiology of the Peripheral Nervous System, in *Neurophysiology in Neurosurgery*, V Deletis and JL Shils, Editors. Academic Press: Amsterdam. 169–95.

4. Happel L and D Kline (1991) Nerve lesions in continuity, in *Operative Nerve Repair and Reconstruction,* 1st Ed., Vol 1, RH Gelberman, Editor. J.B. Lippincott: Philadelphia. 601–16.

5. Barker FG, PJ Jannetta, DJ Bissonette et al (1995) Microvascular decompression for hemifacial spasm. J. Neurosurg. 82:201–10.

6. Møller AR (1991) The cranial nerve vascular compression syndrome: I. A review of treatment. Acta Neurochir. (Wien) 113:18–23.

7. Møller AR and PJ Jannetta (1987) Monitoring facial EMG during microvascular decompression operations for hemifacial spasm. J. Neurosurg. 66:681–5.

8. Møller AR and PJ Jannetta (1984) On the origin of synkinesis in hemifacial spasm: Results of intracranial recordings. J. Neurosurg. 61:569–76.

9. Nielsen V (1984) Pathophysiological aspects of hemifacial spasm. Part I. Evidence of ectopic excitation and ephaptic transmission. Neurology 34:418–26.

10. Nielsen VK (1984) Pathophysiology of hemifacial spasm: II. Lateral spread of the supraorbital nerve reflex. Neurology 34:427–31.

11. Esslen E (1957) Der Spasmus facialis – eine Parabiosserscheinung: Elektrophysiologische Untersuchungen zum Enstehungsmechanismus des Facialisspasmus. Dtsch. Z. Nervenheilkd. 176:149–72.

12. Møller AR and PJ Jannetta (1985) Microvascular decompression in hemifacial spasm: Intraoperative electrophysiological observations. Neurosurgery 16:612–8.

13. Møller AR and PJ Jannetta (1986) Blink reflex in patients with hemifacial spasm: Observations during microvascular decompression operations. J. Neurol. Sci. 72:171–82.

14. Møller AR and PJ Jannetta (1986) Physiological abnormalities in hemifacial spasm studied during microvascular decompression operations. Exp. Neurol. 93:584–600.

15. Hatem J, M Sindou and C Vial (2001) Intraoperative monitoring of facial EMG responses during microvascular decompression for hemifacial spasm. Prognostic value for long-term outcome: A study in a 33-patient series. Br. J. Neurosurg. 15:496–9.

16. Møller AR (1993) Cranial nerve dysfunction syndromes: Pathophysiology of microvascular compression., in *Neurosurgical Topics Book 13, "Surgery of Cranial Nerves of the Posterior Fossa," Chapter 2,* DL Barrow, Editor. American Association of Neurological Surgeons: Park Ridge, IL. 105–29.

17. Møller AR (2008) Neural plasticity: For good and bad. Prog. Theor. Phys. Suppl. 173:48–65.

18. Møller AR (2006) *Neural Plasticity and Disorders of the Nervous System*. Cambridge University Press: Cambridge.

19. Jannetta PJ (1984) Hemifacial spasm caused by a venule: Case report. Neurosurgery 14:89–92.

20. Haines SJ and F Torres (1991) Intraoperative monitoring of the facial nerve during decompressive surgery for hemifacial spasm. J. Neurosurg. 74:254–7.

21. Møller AR and PJ Jannetta (1985) Synkinesis in hemifacial spasm: Results of recording intracranially from the facial nerve. Experientia 41:415–7.

22. Prass RL and H Lueders (1986) Acoustic (loudspeaker) facial electromyographic monitoring. Part I. Neurosurgery 19:392–400.

23. Møller AR and PJ Jannetta (1984) Preservation of facial function during removal of acoustic neuromas: Use of monopolar constant voltage stimulation and EMG. J. Neurosurg. 61:757–60.

24. Yu H and J Neimat (2008) The treatment of movement disorders by deep brain stimulation. Neurotherapeutics 5:26–36.

25. Arle J, D Apetauerova, J Zani et al (2008) Motor cortex stimulation in patients with

Parkinson disease: 12-month follow-up in 4 patients. J Neurosurg. 109:133–9.

26. Arle JE and J Shils (2008) Motor cortex stimulation for pain and movement disorders. Neurotherapeutics 5:37–49.

27. Tagliati M, J Shils, C Sun et al (2004) Deep brain stimulation for dystonia. Expert Rev. Med. Devices 1:33–41.

28. Brown JA, HL Lutsep, SC Cramer et al (2003) Motor cortex stimulation for enhancement of recovery after stroke: Case report. Neurol. Res. 25:815–8.

29. De Ridder D, G De Mulder, V Walsh et al (2005) Transcranial magnetic stimulation for tinnitus: A clinical and pathophysiological approach: Influence of tinnitus duration on stimulation parameter choice and maximal tinnitus suppression. Otol. Neurotol. 147:495–501.

30. Meyerson BA, U Lindblom, B Linderoth et al (1993) Motor cortex stimulation as treatment of trigeminal neuropathic pain. Acta Neurochir. Suppl. 58:105–3.

31. Meyerson BA and B Linderoth (2000) Mechanism of spinal cord stimulation in neuropathic pain. Neurol. Res. 22:285–92.

32. Yakhnitsa V, B Linderoth and BA Meyerson (1999) Spinal cord stimulation attenuates dorsal horn hyperexcitability in a rat model of mononeuropathy. Pain 79:223–33.

33. Kirchner A, F Birklein, H Stefan et al (2000) Left vagus nerve stimulation suppresses experimentally induced pain. Neurology 55:1167–71.

34. Arle JE and JL Shils (2007) Neurosurgical decision-making with IOM: DBS surgery. Neurophysiol. Clin. 37:449–55.

35. Waring MD (1995) Intraoperative electrophysiologic monitoring to assist placement of auditory brain stem implant. Ann. Otol. Rhinol. Laryngol. Suppl. 66:33–6.

36. Shils JL, M Tagliati and RL Alterman (2002) Neurophysiological monitoring during neurosurgery for movement disorders, in *Neurophysiology in Neurosurgery*, V Deletis and JL Shils, Editors. Academic Press: Amsterdam. 405–48.

37. Vitek JL, RAE Bakay, T Hashimoto et al (1998) Microelectrode-guided pallidotomy: Technical approach and application for treatment of medically intractable Parkinson's disease. J. Neurosurg. 88:1027–43.

38. Albe-Fessard D, G Sarfel, G Guiot et al (1966) Electrophysiological studies of some deep cerebral structures in man. J. Neurol. Sci. 3:37–51.

39. Hubel D, H. (1957) Tungsten microelectrode for recording from single units. Science. 125: 549–50.

40. Ojemann GA, O Creutzfeldt, E Lettich et al (1988) Neuronal activity in human lateral temporal cortex related to short-term verbal memory, naming and reading. Brain 111: 1383–403.

41. Lenz FA, JO Dostrovsky, HC Kwan et al (1988) Methods for microstimulation and recording of single neurons and evoked potentials in the human central nervous system. J. Neurosurg. 68:630–4.

42. Lenz FA, JO Dostrovsky, RR Tasker et al (1988) Single-unit analysis of the human ventral thalamic nuclear group: Somatosensory responses. J. Neurophysiol. 59:299–316.

43. Starr PA, RS Turner, G Rau et al (2004) Microelectrode-guided implantation of deep brain stimulators into the globus pallidus internus for dystonia: Techniques, electrode locations, and outcomes. Neurosurg. Focus 17:20–31.

44. Vitek JL, V Chockkan, JY Zhang et al (1999) Neuronal activity in the basal ganglia in patients with generalized dystonia and hemiballismus. Ann. Neurol. 46:22–35.

45. Lenz FA, RR Tasker, HC Kwan et al (1988) Single unit analysis of the human ventral thalamic nuclear group: Correlation of thalamic "tremor cells" with the 3–6 Hz component of parkinsonian tremor. J. Neurosci. 8:754–64.

46. Lenz FA, HC Kwan, JO Dostrovsky et al (1989) Characteristics of the bursting pattern of action potentials that occurs in the thalamus of patients with central pain. Brain Res. 496:357–60.

47. Lenz FA, R Martin, HC Kwan et al (1990) Thalamic single-unit activity occurring in patients with hemidystonia. Stereotact. Funct. Neurosurg. 54–55:159–62.

48. Lenz FA, HC Kwan, JO Dostrovsky et al (1990) Single unit analysis of the human ventral thalamic nuclear group. Activity correlated with movement. Brain 113:1795–821.

49. Lenz FA, CJ Jaeger, MS Seike et al (1999) Thalamic single neuron activity in patients with dystonia: Dystonia-related activity and somatic sensory reorganization. J. Neurophysiol. 82:2372–92.

50. Copeland BJ and HC Pillsbury (2004) Cochlear implantation for the treatment of deafness. Annu. Rev. Med. 55:157–67.

51. Toh EH and WM Luxford (2002) Cochlear and brainstem implantation. Otolaryngol. Clin. North Am. 35:325–42.
52. House WH (1976) Cochlear implants. Ann. Otol. Rhinol. Laryngol. 85 (Suppl. 27):3–91.
53. Zeng FG (2004) Trends in cochlear implants. Trends Amplif. 8:1–34.
54. Brackmann DE, WE Hitselberger, RA Nelson et al (1993) Auditory brainstem implant: 1. Issues in surgical implantation. Otolaryngol. Head Neck Surg. 108:624–33.
55. Portillo F, RA Nelson, DE Brackmann et al (1993) Auditory brain stem implant: electrical stimulation of the human cochlear nucleus. Adv. Otol. Rhinol. Laryngol. 48:248–52.
56. Colletti V, FG Fiorino, L Sacchetto et al (2001) Hearing habilitation with auditory brainstem implantation in two children with cochlear nerve aplasia. Int. J. Paediatric Otorhinolaryngol. 60:99–111.
57. Waring MD (1995) Auditory brain-stem responses evoked by electrical stimulation of the cochlear nucleus in human subjects. Electroenceph. Clin. Neurophysiol. 96:338–47.
58. Kuroki A and AR Møller (1995) Microsurgical anatomy around the foramen of Luschka with reference to intraoperative recording of auditory evoked potentials from the cochlear nuclei. J. Neurosurg. 82:933–9.
59. De Ridder D, G De Mulder, T Menovsky et al (2007) Electrical stimulation of auditory and somatosensory cortices for treatment of tinnitus and pain, in Tinnitus: Pathophysiology and Treatment, Progress in Brain Research, B Langguth et al, Editors. Elsevier: Amsterdam. 377–88.
60. De Ridder D, G De Mulder, V Walsh et al (2004) Magnetic and electrical stimulation of the auditory cortex for intractable tinnitus. J. Neurosurg. 100:560–4.

PART VI

PRACTICAL ASPECTS OF ELECTROPHYSIOLOGIC RECORDING IN THE OPERATING ROOM

Many practical aspects must be considered to achieve the goals of intraoperative neurophysiological monitoring and other uses of neurophysiological methods in the operating room. Matters such as anesthesia and the choice of equipment and its application are fundamental to success in the use of electrophysiological methods in the operating room. Chapter 16 provides basic information of common anesthesia techniques used in operations where the nervous system is involved.

Chapter 17 discusses several aspects regarding how to perform intraoperative monitoring and intraoperative neurophysiology; it describes methods to reduce the risk of mistakes, how to identify the source of electrical interference that may influence monitoring, how to reduce such electrical interference at the source, and how to reduce its effect on electrophysiological recordings in the operating room. Personnel who carry out intraoperative monitoring should understand that mistakes in the use of these methods can occur. How mistakes can be reduced as much as possible is also discussed in Chap. 17.

It is essential to successful intraoperative neurophysiology and monitoring that interference be kept at a minimum throughout the entire time of monitoring. Chapter 17 discusses how to identify the source of interference and how to reduce the amount of interference that reaches the input of the recording amplifiers from nonbiological sources in the operating room.

Correcting such problems as those caused by electrical interference is necessary for successful use of electrophysiology in an operating room that has many different sources of electrical interference. The people who use electrophysiological techniques in the operating room must, therefore, have sufficient knowledge about how electrical interference can reach the monitoring equipment and how its effect on electrophysiological recordings can be reduced so that interpretable records can be obtained promptly.

Chapter 18 provides information regarding the working of the electrophysiological equipment commonly used for electrophysiological studies in the operating room, and the different methods of analysis of neuroelectrical data that are used in the operating room are discussed. Chapter 18 provides information about how to do troubleshooting and suggests remedies for such problems.

Other practical matters such as the requirements for the stimulating and recording equipment, selection of optimal recording and stimulus parameters, and methods for processing the recorded potentials are discussed in Chap. 18, which also describes techniques for stimulation of the nervous system and techniques for data acquisition and processing of the neuroelectric potentials that are recorded in intraoperative neurophysiology and monitoring.

Objective and quantitative evaluation of the benefit from the use of intraoperative neurophysiologic monitoring is important, but few reports have been published of such studies. It is, therefore, an important task of those who use these methods in the operating room to evaluate the benefits of intraoperative neurophysiological monitoring and other electro-physiological methods in improving medical care by reducing the risk of postoperative deficits and thereby, improving the outcome of operations on the nervous system. Such results should be prepared for publication and presentation in scientific conferences. These matters are covered in Chap. 19.

16

Anesthesia and Its Constraints in Monitoring Motor and Sensory Systems

INTRODUCTION

Personnel who perform intraoperative monitoring are not involved in delivering anesthesia, but anesthesia affects the most common recordings that are made in intraoperative monitoring, and it can jeopardize intraoperative monitoring if not coordinated appropriately with the monitoring. The person who is responsible for monitoring should communicate with the anesthesiologist to obtain information regarding the type of anesthesia that is to be used, if there are changes made in the anesthesia during the operation, and, if so, what other drugs may be administered during the operation. In order to communicate and interact effectively with the anesthesia team, people who do intraoperative monitoring must have a basic understanding of anesthesia, know which agents are used, and how the different agents exert their actions. To accomplish this, the anesthesia and monitoring teams must understand each other's language. It is important that the person who is performing intraoperative neurophysiology and monitoring understands the basic principles of anesthesia.

This chapter discusses the various types of anesthesia most commonly used in connection with operations where intraoperative neurophysiologic monitoring of motor and sensory systems are made (for details about anesthesia in neurosurgery, see Cottrell J and WL Young (*1*)) (see also Sloan (*2, 3*)).

From: *Intraoperative Neurophysiological Monitoring: Third Edition*, By A.R. Møller, DOI 10.1007/978-1-4419-7436-5_16,
© Springer Science+Business Media, LLC 2011

The purpose of anesthesia is as follows:

1. To make the patient unconscious.
2. To provide freedom of pain.
3. To prevent the patient from moving.

Additional goals are to help maintain homeostasis, keep blood pressure within normal range, ensure that the patient is not harmed, and reduce the risk of recall (thus, maintaining amnesia).

To achieve these goals, general anesthesia in the Western world is largely accomplished by administering pharmacologic agents.

ANESTHESIA AGENTS

Anesthesia agents used in connection with common operations can be divided into inhalation and intravenous anesthesia types. Often a combination of these two types is used. Recently, total intravenous anesthesia (TIVA) has become in common use (2, 3).

It is possible to achieve good surgical anesthesia with just one agent such as ether that was used for many years or chloroform, a nonflammable halogenated hydrocarbon that was also used alone for many years in the early days of general anesthesia. However, it is a characteristic of modern anesthesia that two or more agents are used together to get additive (or synergistic) action for the purpose of achieving each one of the goals of anesthesia as well as to reduce the total side effects from anesthesia.

The different agents used in modern anesthesia have more or less overlapping effects. Some of the myriad of different drugs available to keep the patient unconscious also reduce pain and keep the patient immobile. Agents that have distinct actions, such as relief of pain and relaxing of muscles, are also common components of modern anesthesia. Some of those have a single action and are normally not regarded as anesthetics because they do not affect consciousness. Whatever agent is used, maintaining a stable level is important and

administration of drugs should be by continuous infusion, and bolus administration of intravenous drugs should be avoided. The effect of anesthesia on some specific kinds of monitoring using different agents has been discussed in the preceding chapters.

Inhalation Anesthesia

Inhalation anesthesia is the oldest form of general anesthesia. In its modern forms, it usually consists of at least two different agents, such as nitrous oxide and a halogenated agent, administered together with pure oxygen. The relative potency of inhalation agents is described by a measure referred to as the "minimal alveolar concentration" (MAC). One MAC is the amount of an inhalation agent that prevents 50% of patients from moving in response to skin incision.

Many different inhalation agents have been used, and many are still in use. Nitrous oxide was a constant companion to other inhalation and intravenous agents for many years, but is now less used. Evaporated fluids have been used for many years. Ether and chloroform, staples of anesthesia for many years, were succeeded by the introduction of more complex halogenated agents, many versions of which have come and gone; first halothane, then a string of similar agents such as enflurane and isoflurane. Now in use are more recent generations of these agents, such as desflurane and sevoflurane, which represent small variations in the molecular structures of these agents that are supposed to increase their anesthetic effects and reduce their side effects.

Halogenated agents such as halothane (which is used rarely now), enflurane, isoflurane, etc., will cause increased central conduction time (CCT) for somatosensory evoked potentials (SSEP) and essentially will make it impossible to elicit motor evoked potentials (MEP) by single impulse stimulation of the motor cortex [transcranial magnetic stimulation (TMS) or transcranial electrical stimulation (TES)]. This unfortunate effect is present even at low concentrations.

Intravenous Anesthesia

Some intravenous agents have almost always been used together with inhalational agents, but recently, the TIVA regimen has become increasingly more common (*2, 3*). One reason for change in regimens is that the inhalational agents, including nitrous oxide, are obstacles when electromyographic (EMG) responses are to be monitored in connection with transcranial stimulation of the motor cortex. The mechanism of action of some intravenous agents appears to be different from that of inhalational agents in such a way that it benefits monitoring of MEP (see Chap. 10).

Other Drugs

Muscle relaxants are often given to prevent the patient from moving, but such drugs prevent recording of muscle response and, therefore, cannot be used in operations where EMG potentials are to be recorded. Midazolam is a commonly used sedative agent in general anesthesia and is used as a premedication in some facilities. It is a short-acting benzodiazepine with effects similar to that of other benzodiazepines such as anxiolytics, amnestics, hypnotics, anticonvulsants, and central muscle relaxants. Drugs for control of blood pressure and heart rate may be given during an operation, but these have normally little influence on electrophysiologic recordings.

ACHIEVING THE GOALS OF ANESTHESIA

Many different kinds of drugs are, thus, used in modern anesthesia. Some are used mainly for achieving unconsciousness, and some are used for other purposes such as preventing the patient from moving. The agents that cause unconsciousness are usually the only ones that are referred to as anesthetics. The effects of different kinds of anesthetics on descending motor activity in the spinal cord (D and I waves) and on EMG potentials are described in Chap. 10.

Keeping the Patient Unconscious

Agents that cause unconsciousness (lack of awareness) are known as hypnotics or sedatives. These are what are usually regarded as anesthetic agents. Their effect is strongly related to the dosage in which they are administrated. Inhalation agents, such as halogenated agents, are typical agents that cause unconsciousness when administrated in sufficient dosages. Consciousness cannot be easily measured, but the MAC value is used as a measure of an inhalation agent's effectiveness as an anesthetic.

Barbiturates that are often used for induction of general anesthesia have similar effects as inhalation agents on evoked potentials. For example, some components of sensory evoked potentials and muscle responses to transcranial stimulation are unusually sensitive to barbiturates. The duration of action varies among the different kinds of barbiturates. The commonly used one, thiopental, is an ultra short-acting barbiturate with a duration of action of only a few minutes. For continued action, it must be infused continually.

Etomidate is another popular agent used in intravenous anesthesia. It is thought to mediate its synaptic effect on the gamma-amino butyric acid (GABA) receptors and type A (GABA$_A$) receptors. Etomidate can enhance synaptic activity at low doses, probably by inhibition of neurons that inhibit the cortical sensory pathway (hence releasing inhibition). At low doses, etomidate may cause increased amplitude of sensory evoked potentials. This effect has been used to enhance the amplitude of both sensory and motor evoked responses. It enhances sensory evoked activity at doses similar to those that produce the desired degree of sedation and loss of recall of memory when used in TIVA.

Etomidate may produce seizures in patients with epilepsy when given in low doses (0.1 mg/kg), and it may produce myoclonic activity at induction of anesthesia. The ability of etomidate to enhance neural activity or reduce the depressant effects of other drugs has been used to enhance the amplitude of both sensory and motor evoked responses (3). Some of the effects of etomidate are, thus, opposite to the action of barbiturates and benzodiazepines.

Propofol is an agent that is in increasing use because it provides excellent anesthesia and limited effect on MEP elicited by TES or TMS. Propofol is currently the most commonly used component of hypnotic/amnestics in TIVA. It is a milk-like substance, and the active drug is prepared in a soy emulsion with egg lecithin. The drug is very rapidly metabolized, and it effects synaptic conduction.

Ketamine is a valuable component of anesthetic techniques that allows the recording of responses that may be depressed by other anesthetics. Ketamine is believed to act by suppressing N-methyl-d-aspartic acid (NMDA) (glutamate) receptors and neuronal acetylcholine receptors. It decreases presynaptic release of glutamate and acts on opioid receptors. It has minimal effect on sensory evoked potentials including cortical potentials, but it increases the H-reflex. Ketamine may heighten synaptic function rather than depress it (probably through its interaction at the NMDA receptor), and it may provoke seizure activity in individuals with epilepsy, but not in individuals who do not already have epilepsy. Ketamine has minimal effects on muscle responses evoked by transcranial cortical stimulation. Because of this, a combination of ketamine and opiods has become a valuable adjunct to TIVA when recording muscle responses are to be done. The fact that ketamine can cause severe hallucinations postoperatively and may increase intracranial pressure has reduced its use in anesthesia.

Dexmeditomidine is a new drug that produces analgesia and sedation. It is a central, selective alpha-2 adrenoreceptor agonist drug that blocks pain signals in the spinal cord; it causes anxiolysis, hypnosis, and sedation.

Freedom of Pain

For achieving analgesia (pain relief), opioids have been used in anesthesia regimen together with other intravenous and inhalation agents that achieve unconsciousness (3). Opioids that are routinely used to keep the patient pain free (provide analgesia) also provide sedation, but do not cause loss of awareness to a sufficient degree. Opioids also cause relief of anxiety and loss of memory during operations (amnesia). Hence, TIVA usually includes an opioid or ketamine for analgesia and some sedative–hypnotic agents such as barbiturates (thiopental) and benzodiazepines (Midazolam).

Fentanyl, the most widely used synthetic opioid, has about 250 times the effect of morphine. Fentanyl is one of the oldest synthetic opioids but now several different agents such as alfentanil, sufentanil, and remifentanil with similar action are in use. Opioids have little or no effect on performing intraoperative neurophysiology testing and monitoring. Muscle responses evoked by transcranial cortical stimulation (electrical and magnetic) are only slightly affected by opioids. The effects of opioids can be reversed by administering naloxone, suggesting that the effect is related to µ-receptor activity.

Prevent the Patient from Moving

Anesthetics, at least those used earlier, contribute to keeping patients from moving, but specific agents that cause paralysis are included in most anesthesia regimens, at least for long operations. Muscle relaxants are part of a common anesthesia regimen – so-called balanced anesthesia (neurolept anesthesia) – that includes a strong narcotic to achieve freedom from pain, plus a muscle relaxant to keep the patient from moving, together with a relatively weak anesthetic such as nitrous oxide.

Muscle relaxants are of two types, namely, agents that block muscle endplates and agents that constantly depolarize muscle endplates. Both groups of agents prevent transmission of impulses from motor nerves to muscles. The oldest neuromuscular blocking agent is curare, but this drug has been replaced by a long series of steroid-type endplate blockers with different action durations. Curare-like substances are non-depolarizing muscle relaxants. While d-tubocuraine was used for many years, it has been followed by substances such as pancuronium (pavulon) with a duration of action of 3 h, and subsequent drugs of shorter durations of action such as atracurium (Tracrium, 30 min or less duration) and vecuronium (Norcuron, 30–40 min duration).

The most often used muscle-relaxing agent that paralyzes by depolarizing the muscle endplate is succinylcholine. The muscle-relaxing effect of succinylcholine lasts only for a very short time.

Additional Purposes of Drugs Used in Anesthesia

Benzodiazepines, notably Midazolam, are often used both in connection with inhalation anesthesia and TIVA in many kinds of operations because they provide excellent sedation and suppress memories (recall) as does thiopental. Benzodiazepines can also reduce the risk of hallucinations caused by ketamine, and they can reduce the risk of seizures.

BASIC PHYSIOLOGY OF AGENTS USED IN ANESTHESIA

Most anesthetic agents, inhalation agents, and intravenous agents, used in anesthesia have synapses as their target, and in general, they decrease synaptic efficacy by making it more difficult for incoming impulses to fire their target neurons (3). The effects accumulate in long chains of neurons. Anesthetics, therefore, have the greatest effect on structures such as the reticular formation that have long chains of neurons connected by synapses. However, the effect is not the same on all synapses, and different anesthetics agents affect different synapses differently. Different anesthetics, even from the same family of substances, have slightly different actions and distinctive side effects.

The anesthetic effect on synapses is mainly suppressive in nature (decreased efficacy), but since both excitatory and inhibitory synapses are involved, the magnitude of the effect depends on the balance between the effect on inhibitory synapses that cause increased excitation, and the

effect of excitatory synapses that cause decreased excitability. This can explain some odd consequences of the use of some anesthetics such as etomidate, which can both increase and decrease excitability.

Motor pathways that have few synapses, such as the corticospinal system, are little affected as evident from the small effect on the D wave (see Chap. 10).

Anesthetic effect on synaptic transmission can become evident in less obvious ways, such as that of suppression of muscle responses. Muscle responses depend on the excitability of the alpha motoneurons, which in turn depends on facilitatory input from the brain and to some extent from the spinal cord. The effect of different agents used in anesthesia can alter spinal reflex activity mainly through the agents' influence on the excitability of alpha motoneurons – the agents decrease the brain's facilitatory influence on the motoneurons. They can affect the H-reflex because the reflex cannot activate the alpha motoneurons unless the motoneurons receive facilitatory input from the brain. The effects of anesthetics on muscle responses is caused by an effect on structures of the brain, such as the reticular formation, that provide facilitatory input to alpha motoneurons through the descending reticulospinal tract that originates in the reticular formation that has long chains of neurons with many synapses involved.

The D wave that can be elicited by TES or TMS represents descending corticospinal activity in descending axons from the motor cortices. The D wave is not noticeably affected by anesthesia because there are no synapses involved. The I waves that can also be recorded from the corticospinal tract reflect descending activity from cells in the motor cortices and are depressed by most kinds of anesthetics because more synapses are involved in the generation of I waves than in the generation of D waves (see Chaps. 9 and 10). The I waves probably also have a facilitatory influence on alpha motoneurons, and depression of I waves may, therefore, reduce the normal facilitation of alpha motoneurons and add to the suppression of motor responses including that of spinal reflexes.

The decreased ability of alpha motoneurons to respond can be overcome by applying trains of impulses, which generate excitatory postsynaptic potentials that add through temporal summation (see Chap. 10). When the train of stimuli contains a sufficient number of impulses, it may activate the alpha neuron despite reduced facilitatory input and cause muscle contraction (provided that muscle relaxants are not included in the anesthesia).

Muscle Relaxants

It was mentioned earlier that the muscle relaxants used in surgical operations are of two main different kinds: non-depolarizing and depolarizing agents. The non-depolarizing agents are related to the arrow poison curare and bind to the nicotinic acetylcholine receptor, inhibit its binding ability, and thereby, block neuromuscular transmission. Synthetic muscle relaxants of the family of quaternary ammonium substances bind to the nicotinic acetylcholine receptor and inhibit or interfere with the binding to and the effect of acetylcholine (ACh) on the muscle endplate receptor.

The depolarizing agents, such as succinylcholine, also bind to the nicotinic acetylcholine receptor, but act in a different way. Depolarizing agents activate the receptor, resulting in muscle contractions. However, since the achieved depolarization lasts for some time, the receptors cannot be activated immediately after an initial activation, and the result is muscle relaxation.

The duration of the effect of muscle relaxants varies: the shortest is that of the depolarizing agents and that of the non-depolarizing agents varies from 10–15 min to several hours.

EFFECTS OF ANESTHESIA ON RECORDING NEUROELECTRICAL POTENTIALS

Successful neurophysiologic monitoring often depends on the avoidance of certain types of anesthetic agents: it is not possible to record EMG potentials if the patient is paralyzed.

Recording of cortical evoked potentials is affected by most of the agents commonly used in surgical anesthesia. Monitoring motor evoked responses elicited by TMS or TES of the motor cortex requires special attention to anesthesia, and the use of a special anesthesia regimen is necessary.

Recording of Sensory Evoked Potentials

Anesthetics affect some sensory evoked potentials, but not others. Therefore, the effect of anesthetics is different for different components of sensory evoked potentials such as the SSEP, as the potentials are affected by inhalation anesthetics or barbiturates to varying degrees (4). The cortical components of SSEP are affected while the subcortical components are unaffected or only minimally affected by most anesthetics. It is important to remember that the effect of any agent depends on the amount that is administrated, together with factors such as the person's age, diseases, and normal variations in the reactions to the anesthetic agents used. Therefore, the effect varies from patient to patient, with children being generally more sensitive than adults (5).

It is advantageous to reduce the use of halogenated agents and nitrous oxide in anesthesia when cortical evoked potentials are monitored. Monitoring of short-latency sensory evoked potentials is not noticeably affected by any type of inhalation anesthesia, and therefore, short-latency sensory evoked potentials should be used whenever possible for intraoperative monitoring instead of cortical evoked potentials. Auditory brainstem responses (ABR), which are short-latency evoked potentials, are practically unaffected by inhalation anesthetics and can, therefore, be recorded regardless of the anesthesia used (see Chap. 7).

The general effect of anesthetics is a lowering of the amplitude and a prolongation of the latency of an individual component of recorded sensory potentials (6) (see Chap. 6, **Fig. 6.12**).

When muscle relaxation is not used during an operation, the patient may have noticeable spontaneous muscle activity, which increases the background noise level in recordings of different kinds of neuroelectrical potentials. This is important when evoked potentials of low amplitude, such as ABR, are monitored. The resulting background noise will prolong the time over which responses must be averaged in order to obtain an interpretable recording.

Muscle activity often increases as the level of anesthesia lessens. If the muscle activity becomes strong, it may be a sign that the level of anesthesia is too low. Early information about such increases in muscle activity is naturally important to the anesthesiologist so that he/she can adjust the level of anesthesia before the patient begins to move spontaneously. In this way, electrophysiologic monitoring can often provide valuable information to the anesthesiologist, because if anesthesia becomes light, spontaneous muscle activity frequently manifests in the recording of evoked potentials from scalp electrodes a long time before any movement of the patient is noticed. In order to detect this spontaneous muscle activity, the output of the physiologic amplifier must be watched continuously.

Recording of EMG Potentials

Responses from muscles (EMG potentials or mechanical responses) cannot be recorded in the presence of muscle relaxants. It is usually necessary to use a muscle-relaxing agent for intubation either using succinylcholine or short-acting endplate blockers, such as atracurium (Tracurium[R]) or vecuronium bromide (Norcuron[R]). Using a short-acting muscle-relaxing agent for intubation will allow the monitoring of muscle potentials 30–45 min after its administration, provided that only the minimal amount of the drug is given and that it is given only once for intubation.

If a short-acting endplate blocking agent is used, it is important to be aware that the paralyzing action disappears gradually, and at a rate that differs from patient to patient. The rate at which muscle function is regained depends on the age, weight, etc., of the patient. Diseases that may be present or medications that may have been administered may affect the time it takes for a patient to regain muscle function.

During the time that the muscle-relaxing effect is decreasing, stimulation of a motor nerve with a train of electrical impulses (such as the commonly used "train of four" test) will give rise to a relatively normal muscle contraction in response to the initial electrical stimulus, but the responses to subsequent impulses are smaller than normal or will be absent.

The effect of muscle relaxants of the endplate blocking type can be shortened ("reversed") by administering agents such as neostigmine, which inhibits the breakdown of acetylcholine and v, makes better use of the acetylcholine receptor sites that are not blocked by the muscle relaxant that is used. However, a prerequisite for the use of such "reversing" agents is that a fair amount of muscle response has to be returned before the reversing agent is administered. It is also important to note that the effect of the reversing agent does not immediately return the muscle function to normal.

REFERENCES

1. Cottrell J and WL Young (2010) Cottrell and Young's Neuroanesthesia. Mosby: Philadelphia, PA.
2. Sloan TB and EJ Heyer (2002) Anesthesia for intraoperative neurophysiologic monitoring of the spinal cord. J. Clin. Neurophysiol. 19:430-43.
3. Sloan T (2002) Anesthesia and motor evoked potential monitoring, in *Neurophysiology in Neurosurgery*, V Deletis and JL Shils, Editors. Elsevier Science: Amsterdam. 451–74.
4. McPherson RW, S Bell and RJ Traystman (1986) Effects of thiopental, fentanyl, and etomidate on upper extremity somatosensory evoked potentials in humans. Anesthesiology 65:584–9.
5. Harper CM and KR Nelson (1992) Intraoperative electrophysiological monitoring in children. J. Clin. Neurophysiol. 9:342–56.
6. Samra SK (1988) Effect of isoflurane on human nerve evoked potentials, in *Neurophysiology and standards of spinal cord monitoring*, TB Ducker and RH Brown, Editors. Springer-Verlag: New York. 147–56.

17

General Considerations About Intraoperative Neurophysiology and Monitoring

INTRODUCTION

Initially, the purpose of intraoperative neurophysiological monitoring was to reduce the risks of permanent injuries to the nervous system that may cause neurologic deficits, muscles spasm, tinnitus, or pain. This is still the main purpose of using electrophysiological methods in the operating room, but now such techniques are also used for a wide range of purposes, and it has been suggested to use the name intraoperative neurophysiology for all uses of neurophysiological techniques in the operating room. These areas of intraoperative neurophysiology now include intraoperative mapping of structures such as the cerebral cortex

and the spinal cord, intraoperative diagnosis such as of peripheral nerves, specific guidance regarding microvascular decompression (MVD) operations for hemifacial spasm (HFS), and for finding the best anatomical location for implantation of electrodes for deep brain stimulation (DBS). Such tasks have become important parts of intraoperative neurophysiology.

In order to achieve the goals associated with the use of electrophysiological methods during many different kinds of operations, it is important that intraoperative neurophysiology is performed properly using adequate methods and techniques and that the acquired results are interpreted correctly. This means that the persons who are to perform the intraoperative recordings must be suitably trained and must use sound judgments in their communication with the surgeon regarding the recorded potentials and other results of intraoperative neurophysiology.

From: *Intraoperative Neurophysiological Monitoring: Third Edition*,
By A.R. Møller, DOI 10.1007/978-1-4419-7436-5_17,
© Springer Science+Business Media, LLC 2011

The most important obstacle in achieving this goal is lack of adequate education and training of the people who are responsible for acquiring and analyzing intraoperative recordings. Inadequate equipment and the risk of equipment failure or electrode failure were earlier important factors, which could jeopardize proper execution of intraoperative neurophysiology and monitoring. Today, the risk of equipment failure is very small, and technological advancements have provided far better equipment than what was available just a few years ago.

There are many similarities between intraoperative recordings and tests that are used for diagnostic purposes in the clinical neurophysiological laboratory, but there are also many differences.

Clinical set-ups for recording neuroelectric potentials are usually fixed installations, but equipment used for neurophysiological monitoring that is used in the operating room is almost always moved into the operating room for the particular operation, and cables between the equipment and the patient are placed for each individual case. This makes the risk of equipment failure greater in the operating room than in the clinical electrophysiological laboratory. While these risks of equipment failure have been greatly reduced as a result of technological advancements, the fact that equipment is still brought into the operating room for every operation involves risks of equipment failure and mistakes in setting up the equipment. This is an important difference between the clinical laboratory and the operating room that contributes to the risk of mistakes and malfunctions through cable and equipment breakdowns in intraoperative monitoring and neurophysiology.

The operating room is an electrically hostile environment, which differs from the clinical neurophysiological laboratory where recording of EMG responses and sensory evoked potentials such as auditory brainstem responses (ABR), somatosensory evoked potentials (SSEP), visual evoked potentials (VEP), and electromyographic (EMG) recordings are obtained in electrically and acoustically shielded rooms. In the operating room, many different kinds of electronic equipment are connected to the patient. In the clinic, only the equipment used for the recordings in question is usually connected to the patient. In the operating room, equipment used to monitor the patient's vital parameters and blood warmers are in direct (galvanic) contact with the patient. Many kinds of electrical equipment are operating in the immediate vicinity of the patient, such as motors that move the operating table and the operating microscope. All this equipment may operate at the same time as responses from the nervous system for monitoring purposes are recorded. Electrocoagulation, drilling of bone, etc. are other activities that typically interfere with intraoperative neurophysiological recordings.

Human mistakes or the results of inadequate training are now the greatest risk of human errors in communication of the results of intraoperative neurophysiology. Similar causes affect other activities in the operating room.

Other common obstacles to successful monitoring are poor quality of the recorded events, which may depend on the patient's preoperative diseases, but it often is caused through human errors made by the intraoperative neurophysiologist and is often caused by inadequate skills and training. If the recorded responses are obscured by noise, the recordings cannot be interpreted, or if electrodes lose contact with the patient, it makes it impossible to perform adequate neurophysiology. Mistakes, such as incorrect placement of electrodes for recording and stimulation or setting up the equipment incorrectly, can invalidate the results of monitoring. Such problems can usually be traced to human shortfall. Intraoperative neurophysiology or monitoring that is not completed correctly may be worse than no monitoring or intraoperative neurophysiology at all because its results may be misleading.

Another important difference between the operating room and the clinical electrophysiology laboratory is that in the clinic it is common that a technician who is trained in performing the tests does the actual recordings, which are then interpreted by a different person. In the operating room, the results must be communicated to the surgeon immediately. To be of any value, it must be communicated in a form that makes sense to the surgeon. In the clinic, delays in interpretations are acceptable and "second opinions" can be obtained. This means that in most situations, the person who does intraoperative monitoring must also be able to describe the results for the surgeon in a form that makes the information meaningful to the surgeon. There are few opportunities for getting second opinions regarding results of intraoperative monitoring, and there are few opportunities to correct mistakes that are made, and these factors increase the demands regarding skills and judgments of the persons who do intraoperative monitoring.

In some settings, a person with experience in interpretation of results of monitoring may be available for interpretation, but that person often serves more than one operating room and may not be available at critical times. Since matters that need expert opinions often occur without warning, it will often be the person who does the monitoring who must describe such critical events to the surgeon. This places extensive requirements regarding basic knowledge about anatomy and physiology, and it requires training and experience of intraoperative neurophysiological recordings of anyone who does intraoperative monitoring and intraoperative neurophysiology.

Shortage of personnel and the desire to reduce cost has promoted introduction of remote monitoring where a person can view and comment on recordings made in several operating rooms without being present in the operating room. The opinions about the adequacy of such procedures vary.

Intraoperative monitoring is carried out differently in different institutions, and there are major differences between how it is carried out in different countries.

MISTAKES AND ERRORS

Mistakes and errors are natural phenomena that can only be avoided by making it physically impossible to make them. That means that mistakes may be regarded as a law of nature that, unlike man-made laws, cannot be broken. This is also often referred to as Murphy's Law and states, "If something can go wrong, it will do so." It may happen as frequently as one in ten or as infrequently as one in a thousand or one in a million, but anything that can go wrong, will do so sooner or later.

How Can Mistakes Be Avoided?

Mistakes can only be avoided by making them impossible. One example of how a specific mistake can be avoided by making it physically impossible comes from recording of ABR (see Chap. 7). Such potentials are evoked by (click) sounds that are delivered by an earphone placed in the ear. If the purpose is to monitor the function of the auditory nerve in operations in the cerebellopontine angle (CPA), the sound should be delivered to the ear on the side of the operation. If earphones for monitoring ABR in such operations are placed in both ears, there will always be a certain risk that the ear on the unoperated side is selected for stimulation by mistake. Such a mistake may be made when connecting the earphone to the stimulator or by mistakenly switching the stimulus to the wrong ear during the operation. The mistake is not obvious from observing the recorded ABR, because the waveforms of the ABR recorded from both sides are similar in most people, regardless of which ear they were elicited from. Such a mistake will make it impossible to detect any change in the function of the auditory nerve on the operated side. The recordings obtained to contralateral stimulation will not show any change if the auditory nerve is injured, not even if it was severed. It will make monitoring useless in detecting injuries to the auditory nerve for which it was intended. This means that such monitoring is worse than no monitoring at all because it provides a false sense of security to the surgeon.

This is a typical example of how false-negative responses can occur (no change in the recorded potentials is noted, despite the fact that an injury has occurred). It may cause the patient to lose hearing on the operated ear permanently without being detected during the operation. The mistake could have been prevented if the operated ear was the sole ear to have been equipped with an earphone so that it would have been physically impossible to stimulate the wrong ear. Therefore, an earphone should never be placed in the ear on the unoperated side unless it is strongly indicated to do so for monitoring reasons.

Similar reasoning applies to other areas of intraoperative neurophysiology and monitoring. For example, when monitoring SSEP in an operation from one side of the spinal cord, the stimulating electrodes should only be placed on peripheral nerves on the same side as the operation. If placed on both sides, there is a risk that the SSEP that are being observed are being elicited from the unoperated side, because the stimulus has been mistakenly applied to the peripheral nerve on the wrong side of the body. There is some justification in stimulating also the unoperated side because it can serve as a control where the recordings can indicate general changes such as in the patient's body temperature, blood pressure, and oxygenation.

Stimulating nervous tissue with dangerously high currents is another mistake that can have catastrophic consequences, but which can be avoided by making it physically impossible to apply dangerously high stimulus currents. Limiting the output of the stimulator so that it cannot produce stimuli that are dangerously high is the best way to avoid dangerously high stimulus currents. Such precaution is not often taken because the limits for dangerously high stimulus current are different for different types of stimulation, such as stimulation of peripheral nerves compared to stimulation in the brain.

How to Reduce the Risk of Mistakes?

If it is not possible to make mistakes impossible, measures should be taken to make it as *unlikely* as possible that mistakes occur. In many situations of everyday life, it is customary to tolerate some degrees of risks in the form of accidents, natural disasters, etc. This is because it is either not possible to find a way to eliminate accidents or the cost of preventing accidents has been judged to outweigh the gain from the action in question.

There are many ways that mistakes in connection with intraoperative neurophysiological monitoring can be reduced. Following a checklist for setting up equipment, placement of electrodes, checking items (including spare ones) to bring to the operating room, etc., can reduce the risk of forgetting essential elements and setting parameters for stimulation and recording incorrectly. Adhering to the same specific routines whenever possible can also help reduce the risk of making mistakes. Doing the monitoring the same way in similar operations every time instead of keeping altering procedures makes it less likely that a mistake is made.

When many electrodes are to be placed on a patient, mistakes may be made if the electrodes are all applied to the patient and then after that, all electrodes are connected to the electrode box at one time. The risk of making mistakes in connecting the electrodes is much smaller if each electrode is connected one at a time to the electrode box after it is placed on the patient and before the next electrode is applied to the patient.

The "KISS" Principle (Keep It Simple and Stupid) of Intraoperative Neurophysiology. The risk that something will go wrong is likely to increase with increasing complexity of the equipment and the complexity of the methods used for intraoperative neurophysiology and monitoring. A complex computer system that is difficult to set up, with menus with many options, increases the risks of making mistakes. An overly-complex procedure for equipment operation may also waste time. It is indeed possible to balance your checkbook using a supercomputer, but it is not the most practical option. It is also possible to use complex equipment for the rather uncomplicated tasks of collecting neurophysiological data.

Recording evoked potentials on many channels rarely provides more useful information than what can be obtained by using a few carefully selected recording channels, but it does add to the complexity of recording. This means that in intraoperative neurophysiology and monitoring, it is important to observe the "KISS" Principle – Keep It Simple and Stupid, or "keep it simple, stupid". Following the "KISS" principle can save much aggravation and also reduce the risks of minor and major disasters. It may be more difficult to design a simple system than a complex system, but it certainly is rewarded (Leonardo de Vinci: "simplicity is the ultimate sophistication").

Importance of Thinking Ahead. Possible problems to expect in an operation should be considered before the operation starts, so that the person who does the intraoperative neurophysiology and monitoring is prepared to handle at least the most common problems. Naturally, the highest quality electronic equipment will provide the most reliable service, and equipment failure is in fact now very rare, but it is important that backup electronic equipment, especially spare electrodes and connectors, are available for use within a very short time. Having spare cables and electrodes available in the operating room is important, and it is wise to have redundant electrodes placed on the patient particularly in areas prone to manipulation during the operation. Attending to every possible detail will be rewarded with fewer problems and better quality of the monitoring. A checklist can help achieve that end because it helps keep a person from forgetting important matters. Always thinking ahead and considering possible sources of problems are helpful in handling problems that can occur in intraoperative monitoring and neurophysiology.

Advantage of Using a Checklist. The airline industry has been extremely successful in reducing the risks of accidents and mishaps. One reason for the high degree of safety is the airline's meticulous adherence to praxis that is known to involve minimal risks. When boarding a commercial airplane, one will often see the captain (and probably the first officer, who sits on the right side of the cockpit) ticking off a checklist. This occurs for short trips as well as for long trips, it occurs for large airlines as well as for small airlines and a similar procedure is followed by private pilots. The same should be the case for intraoperative neurophysiology. Just because a person knows how to do a specific job (monitoring or surgery, for that matter) does not mean he/she should not use a checklist. Airline pilots do not use checklists because the captain does not know how to fly the airplane. The purpose of the checklist is to avoid forgetting something (that he/she knows about).

The same rationale applies for intraoperative neurophysiology and monitoring. A checklist helps with remembering all small details, some of which could easily be forgotten even if the person who does the monitoring is very experienced. Just because someone may know his or her job well does not mean that a checklist is not helpful.

Unexpected Events. Most problems that occur in connection with intraoperative neurophysiology happen when not expected. The sudden appearance of electrical interference is a common example of an event that may interrupt monitoring because it obscures the recorded potentials. It will result in the neurophysiologist stopping data collection. If intraoperative neurophysiology is going to be successful, it is necessary to identify the sources and the nature of such suddenly appearing interference within a very short time. The nature or the waveform of interference often indicates the origin and the cause of the interference. It is, therefore, important that the neurophysiologist observe not only the averaged potentials that are recorded, but also observe the recorded potentials directly, and that he/she be able to diagnose the problem and identify its source on the basis of appearance of the waveform of the interference. For example, it is important to distinguish between external electrical interference and interference that is of a biological origin, such as muscle activity.

It is important to know what to do when the unexpected occurs. Again, the airlines are a model. The crew has available a series of checklists that cover actions to take in case of equipment failure or other emergencies. Much could be gained if similar help was available in intraoperative monitoring and neurophysiology, and for that matter, in surgery in general.

Equipment   Malfunction. Equipment malfunction is becoming more and more rare, but if it does happen, it either must be remedied within a very short time or the operation will continue without the aid of neurophysiology. Thorough knowledge about the equipment and its function is invaluable for troubleshooting and restoration of normal function. Most problems with modern computer equipment are software related, and the user must understand the function (and common malfunctions) of the software used in the equipment. A great source of "malfunction" is operator error caused by insufficient knowledge about how to use the equipment and especially its software. Basic knowledge about computer problems is important; for example, rebooting the computer can often solve malfunctions caused by software glitches.

Absence of Response. Simple tests can reduce the risk of getting no response or an unanticipated response. For example, the risk that no sound is being delivered by the earphone when monitoring the auditory system because of failure of the sound generator, or more likely, a cable, or by earphone malfunction can be reduced by having the sound switched on and having the person who is placing the earphone in the patient's ear listen to the earphone immediately before it is placed in the patient's ear. It will ensure that the earphone is delivering a sound at least in the beginning of the operation.

There is often a period where monitoring is not needed. Continuing monitoring during that time, and collecting and storing the acquired data makes it possible to detect malfunctions

that may occur during that time. If monitoring is stopped and something happens during that idle time it may not be possible to resume monitoring when needed, and it may be difficult to find out what has happened.

A common cause of the absence of evoked responses is that the patient suffers from a disorder that affects evoked responses. Hearing loss or peripheral nerve neuropathy are common causes of the absence of evoked responses. Preoperative tests can avoid such surprises. If not available, collection of the evoked potentials that are to be monitored should be started as soon as possible and not be delayed until the monitoring is required. When monitoring is started early, it leaves time to check equipment and electrode placement, perhaps selecting a better electrode placement. For example, when lower limb SSEP are monitored, the best placement of the stimulating electrodes is the posterior tibial nerve on the foot. As an alternative, stimulation of the common peroneal nerve at the knee (a shorter peripheral nerve) may be attempted if the patient has severe peripheral nerve neuropathy because the neuropathy is likely to affect the most distal parts of a nerve pathway to the greatest extent.

Unexpected absence of a muscle response to electrical stimulation of a nerve is often caused by the anesthesia team paralyzing the patient. Other causes for a lack of a muscle response include failure to stimulate the nerve adequately. Failure to obtain a muscle response in response to cortical stimulation is often caused by using too much of the anesthetic or by inadequately selecting the anesthetics used for anesthetizing the patient (see Chaps. 10 and 16).

In situations where it is difficult to obtain good recordings of SSEP, placement of the recording electrodes are important (see below and Chap. 6), as is reduction of interference (see below).

Communication Is Important

The neurophysiologist who is responsible for performing intraoperative neurophysiology should communicate frequently with the surgeon, but it is also important to communicate with the anesthesiology team regarding the anesthesia used and regarding the patient's vital signs. Such communication is also often beneficial to the anesthesiologist. For instance, an increase in the spontaneous muscle activity that may be due to a decrease in the level of anesthesia is often noticeable in electrophysiologic recordings long before the level of anesthesia has dropped so much that the patient moves. Relaying information about electrophysiologic recorded muscle activity to the anesthesiologist may avoid the anesthesia becoming so low that the patient moves spontaneously. Such information is, therefore, valuable to the anesthesiologist as well as to the surgeon.

ELECTRICAL AND MAGNETIC INTERFERENCE IN THE OPERATING ROOM

The quality of recorded potentials from the nervous system and muscles depends on the level of electrical and other kinds of interference. As mentioned above, there are several kinds of interference in the operating room that can jeopardize intraoperative neurophysiology and monitoring. One kind of interference is caused by electrical currents from other equipment or from the power line that reach the amplifiers used in monitoring. Another source of interference in the operating room are magnetic fields that induce electrical current in electrode wires and thereby, reach the input of amplifiers that are used for monitoring. Biological noise, such as that from muscles and the ongoing EEG, can also interfere with electrophysiological recordings and can even obscure the recorded electrical potentials such as sensory evoked potentials.

Electrical interference from outside and from the body of the patient can never be totally eliminated, but it can be reduced, and often it can be reduced to a level where the recorded potentials can be interpreted directly, or if the amplitude of the potentials is small, after signal averaging and appropriate filtering.

Electrical equipment in the operating room that operates simultaneously with the equipment used for intraoperative neurophysiology may emit many kinds of electrical interference. The most common interference is the signal that originates from the power line (a frequency of 60 Hz in North America and 50 Hz in Europe), but many types of electronic equipment that are in routine use in the operating room emit many other kinds of signals that may interfere with recording of neuroelectrical potentials.

Magnetic interference is mainly caused by equipment that contains transformers, which generate a magnetic field related to the power line frequency. Deflection coils in old types of video monitors can emit a magnetic field that can generate high-frequency interference.

Several sources of interference emit electrical signals that are periodic in nature, and these sources cause special problems in connection with the recording of evoked potentials where signal averaging is used (see Chap. 18).

Some kinds of interference may not manifest in the beginning of an operation, but appear suddenly later. A prerequisite for reducing the emission of such electrical interference signals is to be able to identify the source of the interference. An example is blood warmers that are often switched on after an operation is started.

Identifying the Sources of Electrical and Magnetic Interference

There are many ways to identify sources of magnetic and electrical interference. One way is to switch off suspected equipment and see if the interference disappears. This may be used before an operation, but it is normally not an option during an operation. A closer examination of the operating room when it is not in use is an efficient way to identify sources of interference because equipment can then be moved and switched on and off freely.

A survey should be performed in all operating rooms to identify possible sources of interference prior to attempting to do intraoperative neurophysiological monitoring in a location that is not known to the person who performs monitoring. Equipment in the operating room that emits signals that may interfere with the electrophysiologic recordings should be identified and actions taken to eliminate or reduce the interference.

Examining the Operating Room for Sources of Electrical Interference. Electrical interference may reach the amplifiers used to record electrical potentials from the nervous system through galvanic connections to the source of interference such as through direct connections or through fluid lines. The most common route is, however, through the air by capacitive coupling. Identification of the sources for the kinds of interference that appear in the form of electric fields can be made by using the amplifiers and computer display that is normally used for monitoring neuroelectrical potentials intraoperatively. With a wire connected to one of the two differential inputs of an amplifier to act as an antenna (see **Fig. 17.1**), the electrical fields of signals that are present near the antenna will appear on the display. The other input to the amplifier should be grounded, and a resistor (of about 100 kOhm, see **Fig. 17.1**) is placed between the ground and the input to which the "antenna" is connected. As the antenna is brought closer to the equipment that is "leaking" an electric signal, the amplitude of the signal that is picked up by the antenna will increase and that can be observed on the computer display of the output from the amplifier.

The sources of interference that are conducted to the amplifiers through galvanic coupling to the amplifiers and indirectly through the patient are more difficult to locate. One common source of such problems is the way in which equipment and the patient are grounded.

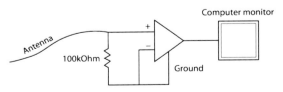

Figure 17.1: Using a standard physiologic amplifier to identify sources of electrical interference.

Most electrical equipment is encased in a metal box that is connected to a ground lead, for the purpose of electrical safety. A piece of equipment that is not properly grounded is not only a safety hazard, but improperly grounded equipment is also a source of interference for electrophysiologic recordings because the casing no longer acts as an electrical shield. Locating such equipment can easily be made by the methods described above (**Fig. 17.1**). The function of the equipment itself is usually not affected if the ground wire becomes disconnected, and accidental disconnection of the safety ground lead will, therefore, normally go unnoticed. The only indication of such a loss may be increased interference in intraoperative electrophysiological recordings.

Another way to identify equipment that emits interference signals is to use a volunteer placed in the same position on the operating table as a patient who is to be operated upon. With electrodes placed on the volunteer and connected to the input of the physiologic amplifiers, no electrical interference should be noted when all other equipment in the operating room is switched off. Equipment that will be used by the anesthesia team and others during the operation can then be switched on one at a time while observing the display of the output of the physiologic amplifier for interference.

If interference is present after all equipment other than that used for monitoring has been switched off, it must be generated either by the recording equipment itself or by the electrical installation in the room such as cables in the floor and walls, and the lighting in the operating room. Power lines in the floor or ceiling are common sources of such "hidden" interference. The frequency of such interference signals is most likely that of the power line, and the setup shown in **Fig. 17.1** can be used to find the location of such sources of interference. Operating tables that are electrically controlled are also frequent sources of interference.

Interference signals can be conducted galvanically to the recording equipment through, for example, intravenous lines, which are frequent routes for interference signals. The

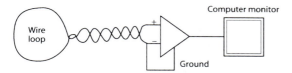

Figure 17.2: Arrangement for identifying a source of magnetic interference.

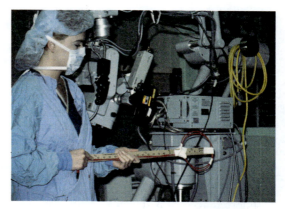

Figure 17.3: Use of a simple wire loop to find the source of magnetic interference (it was the light source for a microscope).

normal operating room situation involves fluid lines that are in contact with the patient and that situation cannot easily be simulated with a volunteer patient. There are also other situations in an actual operation that are not easily simulated in an idle operating room. For example, during an operation, changes may be made in the way that the anesthesia equipment is connected to the patient, and such changes may cause interference with recordings of the neuroelectrical potentials that are to be monitored.

Examining the operating room for magnetic interference. The sources of magnetic interference can be identified in a way similar to that described above for electrical interference with the difference that a wire in the form of a loop is connected to the two input terminals of the amplifier (**Fig. 17.2**). Note that one of the inputs should be grounded. A magnetic field will induce an electrical current in the wire loop. When the loop is moved closer to the source of a strong magnetic field, the amplitude of the waveform seen on the display will increase.

The source of a magnetic field that may generate electrical currents in the electrode leads (and thereby, act as electrical interference) can be identified by searching the area around the operating table with such a loop (**Fig. 17.3**). The orientation of the loop is important for detecting the magnetic field, and the wire loop should, therefore, be rotated to keep it optimally positioned with regard to the orientation of the magnetic field. If there is doubt about which device is generating the interference, switching off each of the suspected devices one at a time can identify the equipment that is the source of interference.

If the waveform (and frequency) of the signal that is picked up by the test loop is the same as that of the interference observed when recording from a patient then that specific piece of equipment is most likely magnetic interference, and the source of the observed interference is the location where the signals picked up by the loop are strongest.

Transformers, such as the power transformers that are a part of most electronic equipment, may generate magnetic fields. Powerful light sources in operating microscopes are examples of equipment that may generate similar magnetic fields, which can act as interference in neurophysiological recordings. The deflection coils in old types of display monitors can generate strong, high-frequency magnetic fields that can act as interference, but which can easily be identified by the arrangement in **Fig. 17.3**.

The Signature of Different Interference Signals

The waveform of the interference signals often provides important information about the identity of the source of the interference signals and how they have entered the recording system; factors that are important to the elimination of the interference. The most important signature for identifying the source of interference is its frequency. Interference signals that have the frequency of the power line must be generated by the power line in one or another way.

The waveform of the current that the power line delivers is usually nearly sinusoidal, but in electrophysiologic recordings interference from the power line does not always appear as a sinusoidal waveform. Magnetically conducted power line interference is often rich in higher harmonics, which is a great help in identifying the source of the interference, but unfortunately, it also makes the interference more troublesome because these harmonics of the power line frequency may overlap with the frequency range of recorded neuroelectrical potentials.

Interference from the power line can also appear as a sinusoid with a series of sharp spikes superimposed, either with the same frequency as the power line signal (60 or 50 Hz) or with a frequency twice of that of the power line signal. Such spikes usually originate from equipment with power regulators that chop the waveform of the power. Inexpensive equipment is the worst offender and blood warmers are notorious in this respect.

Many kinds of digital equipment generate interference signals. The frequencies of the signals generated are different from that of the power line. Digital control equipment, such as found in blood warmers, infusion pumps, computers, or other digital equipment, often radiates electric signals of much higher frequencies than the power line and contribute to the interference in addition to interference of the power line frequency. Some digital equipment generates impulses that occur randomly or in ways that depend on the operation of the equipment.

Determining the exact frequency and nature of an interference signal is valuable in identifying the source of the interference. If the interference waveform is complex, a spectrum analysis of the recorded interference potentials may help in identifying the source of the interference (see Chap. 18).

How Can Interference Signals Reach Physiological Recording Equipment?

The ways electrical and magnetic interference can interfere with recording of neuroelectrical potentials are different. Electrical signals from the environment and from the body itself can act as interference signals directly, through different routes. Magnetic fields as such cannot affect recording of electrical signals, but the electrical current induced by the magnetic field can act as interference.

Electrical Interference. It is important to consider that electrical interference is only a problem when it reaches the recording equipment. Electrical interference can reach the recording equipment in two different ways: as electrical fields that are conducted through capacitance coupling ("through the air") or through electrically conductive media (galvanic conduction) such as ground leads or fluid lines. Interference signals can also be conducted through the patient or directly to the recording equipment. There are basically five different ways that electric signals can enter the recording equipment and interfere with recorded potentials:

1. Electrical fields can be picked up by unshielded electrode leads (capacitance coupling) from nearby interference sources.
2. Electrical signals can be injected into the recording system by a common path, such as ground loops (galvanic coupling).
3. Electrical current can be galvanically conducted to the patient via other recording or stimulating electrodes that are placed on the patient (such as anesthesia monitoring equipment), by infusion lines or devices that are in galvanic contact with the patient such as head holders.
4. Electrical interference can be picked up by capacitance coupling to the patient such as from heating pads or motor driven operating tables.
5. Interference signals can leak directly into the physiologic amplifiers via the power line.

Perhaps the most common path for electrical interference to reach the input of physiological amplifiers is through the electrode wires. It is also the easiest problem to remedy. Twisting or braiding the wires and keeping them short and placed away from equipment that generates interferences are effective ways of reducing that kind of interference.

Typical examples of galvanically conducted interference is interference generated by blood warmers and infusion pumps in which electrical current from the electronic circuits in these devices is conducted to the patient through the fluid that is infused. Intravenous infusion lines and arterial lines all carry electrically conductive fluids, and therefore, electrical signals that these lines may pick up will be conducted directly to the patient. These signals may then reach the input of the amplifiers that are used for intraoperative neurophysiological monitoring through the recording electrodes that are placed in various locations on the body of the patient. Since bags with infusion solutions are often hanging high above the patient, they will act as effective "antennas" that can pick up various types of interference, and this interference is then injected directly into the patient (via the electrically conductive fluid infusion), and it can then reach the recording amplifiers through the electrodes that are placed on the patient.

Infusion lines often pass through electronic devices, such as intravenous pumps or blood warmers that can act as sources of interference. Intravenous infusion pumps have electronic control circuits that may generate high-frequency electrical signals that may be conducted to the patient via the electrically conducting fluid of these lines. The common power line often powers blood warmers and may cause severe interference with electrophysiologic recordings because these signals are transferred to the patient via the conductive fluid in the infusion lines. Blood warmers are notorious in causing electrical interference; the models used in the operating room are often selected because they were the least expensive, and the inexpensive power regulators in such equipment can cause severe interference. Such interference may not be apparent in the beginning of an operation, but may "appear suddenly" during the operation as circumstances change and new infusion bags are added or when blood warmers are switched on.

Devices that are connected electrically to the patient can also cause interference with recorded neuroelectrical potentials. The interference from different equipment other than that used for intraoperative neurophysiological monitoring may be worse if such equipment is connected to a different power source (different isolation transformer) than the one used for the equipment used for neurophysiological monitoring. All equipment that is in galvanic contact with the patient should, therefore, get power from outlets that are supplied by the same isolation transformer. It is not always easy to find out what supplies the different power outlets. It may be easier just to try different outlets if that is the suspected cause of the interference.

Electrical stimulation of muscles on the hand for testing the level of paralysis by the anesthesia team can cause sudden electrical interference with recorded neuroelectrical potentials.

Electrical signals may also be conducted to the patient through head holders and other devices that are in direct (galvanic) contact with the patient. The head holder is in contact with the operating table that may be grounded for safety reasons, but the safety ground may provide a ground loop that can cause interference with the frequency of the power line.

Items other than those that are directly connected to the patient, such as heating blankets that are connected to the power line, may also create electrical interference with intraoperative recordings of neuroelectrical potentials. Electrically controlled operating tables are another frequent source of electrical interference. Although equipment that is connected directly (galvanic connection) to the patient may be more likely to cause interference, these other devices may radiate enough electrical signals to interfere with recording of neuroelectrical potentials.

The cables that connect the electrode box with the main amplifiers can also pick up electrical and magnetic interference. However, technological advances have made that less likely in two different ways that benefit from the possibility to have amplifiers and analog to digital converters built into the electrode box. One of these methods makes use of fiber optic cables between such advanced "electrode boxes" and the recording equipment. Another makes use of USB connection to the electrode box. The USB connection also provides all power needed for the amplifiers and analog/digital converters that are located in the "electrode box". Fiber optic cables or USB cables are not sensitive to electrical or magnetic interference that may occur in the operating room.

Magnetic fields may also induce electric currents in cables that connect the electrode box to the amplifier, but again, technological advances have now made this less likely because most modern equipment now has the analog–digital converter located in the "electrode box". The digital signals transmitted to the computer are essentially resistant to magnetic interference. Fiber optic lines that are used to transmit digital signals from the electrode box to the amplifiers are not affected by magnetic (and electrical) interference.

How to Reduce the Effect of Interference

There are two main ways to reduce the effect of electrical and magnetic interference, namely, to reduce the emission of the interference signal and to reduce the ability of the recording systems to pick up the interference. When a source of interference has been identified, its effect on recordings can be minimized or eliminated by reducing the emission of the interference signal at its source and by hindering the interference signal from entering the amplifiers.

As a last resort, when these two possibilities have been exhausted, special processing of the recorded electrical potentials from the nervous system is used to reduce the effect of interference on interpretation of the biological signals that are recorded (processing of recorded potentials will be discussed in Chap. 18). Selecting optimal recording parameters, optimal signal processing methods, and optimal stimulus parameters can also reduce the effect of interference.

Electrical Interference. The first action to be taken in efforts to reduce the effect of electrical interference is to identify the source of the interference. With that knowledge, the

emission of the interference signals can in many cases be eliminated or reduced. When interference with electrophysiological recordings is caused by unshielded or faulty equipment, the remedy is to repair or replace the equipment. If interference is emitted by unshielded equipment, the best way to reduce the interference is to move the offending equipment as far away from the patient and the leads of the recording electrodes as possible. If the interference is severe, such equipment should be replaced by equipment that causes less interference. It is usually inexpensive equipment that causes the worst interference, and frequently, interference problems are solved by replacing such equipment with equipment of better quality. (Such replacements can often be justified not only by the fact that interference is reduced or eliminated, but also because the equipment's performance often improves as well.)

If it is not possible to reduce the emission of electrical interference, methods to prevent the unwanted signals from reaching amplifiers should be employed for reducing the interference. Twisting or braiding the electrode wires that are connected to the input of a differential amplifier is perhaps the most effective way to reduce interference that is picked up by the electrode wires from electric fields. This method is effective because the two leads that serve as inputs to a differential amplifier will transmit approximately the same amount of interference. Differential amplifiers are only sensitive to the difference between the potentials that reach the two inputs, and therefore, the amount of the interference that appears at the output will be greatly reduced by twisting or braiding electrode wires. If the electrode wires are widely separated, they will pick up different amounts of interference that will cause a large output of the amplifiers. Using the shortest possible electrode leads is another effective means to reduce the amount of electrical interference that electrode leads can pick up.

The electrode impedance should be kept as low as possible because the leads to electrodes that have high impedance pick up more interference than leads to low impedance electrodes. If platinum reusable needle electrodes are used, they must be treated correctly by soaking the electrodes in a chlorine solution to remove the coating of proteins that otherwise will increase their impedance. Such treatment (unlike autoclaving) will also remove all kinds of pathogenic organisms including viruses and agents that are believed to cause degenerative brain disorders such as Creutzfeldt–Jakob disease. Disposable electrodes should naturally be used if at all possible. The use of wire hook electrodes when possible is preferred. Such electrodes are disposable and provide stable recordings for long times. The performance of surface electrodes that are now routinely used in the clinic has improved much and such electrodes are now a useful alternative to needle electrodes and wire hook electrodes.

Reduction of interference is more difficult when intraoperative neurophysiological monitoring includes recording from parts of the body other than the head. When the two recording electrodes that are connected to a differential amplifier are placed far apart, they will pick up more interference than when placed close together. The placement of the grounding electrode may not be of much help in reducing the amount of interference signals.

If some equipment conduct interference signals directly into the amplifiers, or by being in contact with the patient, other methods must be used for reducing the interference. Grounding equipment has often been regarded as the solution to reducing interference from the power line. While it is true that a lack of a ground or faulty grounding of equipment can cause severe electrical interference, it is also true that too many ground connections can increase interference. Multiple grounds can create what is known as "ground loops," a condition in which electric current circulates between the various pieces of equipment and the patient. In many cases, the most effective remedy for reducing electrical interference consists of revising the entire grounding system and connecting all the ground wires from all the equipment to one common point. This, however, is not always

possible because most equipment is already grounded internally by a safety ground through the connection to the power line.

It is also common practice to place a ground connection on the patient, but in fact, it is often advantageous to remove ground leads to the patient because the patient may already be grounded through other equipment, such as the equipment used by the anesthesia team. Generally, modern amplifiers have made the grounding problems less of a problem.

Modern operating rooms are usually equipped with power regulators and isolation transformers that have leakage detectors. Such devices are useful, and they no doubt increase safety in the operating room, but they can also increase the power line impedance. If a piece of equipment that draws heavy current in only certain phases of the power waveform is connected to the same isolation transformer as the electrophysiologic recording equipment, severe interference may result. The obvious remedy is to connect the particular piece of equipment to a different isolation transformer or, even better, to replace the equipment that is causing the distortion of the waveform of the electrical power with better equipment that does not have such adverse properties.

Magnetic Interference. It is generally more difficult to reduce interference caused by a magnetic field than that caused by electrical fields. Alternating magnetic fields induce electric currents in any electrically conducting medium. The most effective way of minimizing that kind of interference, is to keep electrode leads straight and short because loops of a wire pick up magnetic fields to a greater extent than a short and straight wire (although magnetic fields can induce electrical currents even in straight wires). The electric current that a magnetic field induces in a straight wire depends on the wire's orientation within the magnetic field, and it is, therefore, worthwhile to change the orientation of electrode wires while observing the interference on the computer display (that shows the output of the recording amplifiers) to find an optimal orientation of the electrode leads. Twisting (or braiding) the electrode leads is helpful in reducing interference from magnetic fields because it results in the magnetic field inducing nearly the same current in each one of the leads that are connected to the input of a differential amplifier.

ELECTRICAL SAFETY IN THE OPERATING ROOM

Exposure to electrical current in the operating room can place patients and the personnel who work in the operating room at risk from electrical shock, which can cause heart arrest and cause injuries in the form of burns of the skin and other tissue or by affecting the nervous system.

Patient Safety

The greatest risk to the personnel in the operating rooms from electric shocks comes from the electric power line. This is also a risk to patients, but there are additional electrical risks for patients to consider. Operating room equipment should not expose the patient to dangerous electrical current via recording and stimulating electrodes that are applied for monitoring purposes. This is particularly important when recording directly from surgically exposed portions of the nervous system during many types of operations.

Equipment used in the operating room must comply with the highest standards of electrical safety. Electrical stimulation of nerves and CNS structures that are used in intraoperative neurophysiological monitoring poses certain risks. Whenever electric current is used to stimulate peripheral nerves, the spinal cord, or the brain, there is a risk that the current will cause neural injury if the stimulus strength exceeds a certain level. Applying excessive electrical current to the CNS can have many different effects depending on the location of the application of the current. As mentioned above, the only way to avoid this risk is to arrange the electrical stimulation so that it is physically impossible to exceed the stimulus strength that may cause injury. If a cur-

rent that is higher than the safe limit for stimulation can be selected from the stimulator, then there is always a risk that stimuli of an unsafe level may be applied through operator error. This risk can be reduced (but not avoided) by appropriate training of those who operate the equipment. A clear display of what stimulus current (or voltage) is in use is important for reducing the risks of mistakes.

Anesthetized or unconscious patients do not react to dangerous situations and cannot protect themselves from stimulation that may imply a risk of injury. Appropriate safety precautions must, therefore, be the responsibility of the people who work in the operating room.

Excessive stimulation of motor nerves can cause extremely strong contractions that can injure muscles. Normally, neural safety mechanisms in the spinal cord prevent that from happening by inhibiting the alpha motoneurons, but these safety mechanisms are not active when a motor nerve is stimulated electrically. Passing electrical current through the heart can cause ventricular fibrillations or cardiac arrest.

Excessive electrical current applied to the skin through surface or needle electrodes can cause local irritation or injuries in the form of burns. Stimulation with direct current (DC) is the most dangerous and should never be used for stimulation in anesthetized patients. The injury by electrical current is caused mainly by heat, which is proportional to the product of the squared value of the current (I) and tissue resistance (R) through which it flows ($I^2 \times R$), and the amount of time the current is applied. The surface area of the electrode is important; a smaller surface area means higher risk of burns with the same current. Needle or wire electrodes, therefore, involve a greater risk of burns than surface electrodes.

Probably the most common cause of burns to the skin of anesthetized patients is due to ineffective return leads (pads, usually placed on the thigh) from electrocautery equipment. Burns can be caused at the site of neurophysiological recording electrodes that are placed on the skin because the recording electrodes provide a path to ground for the high-frequency current used in the electrocautery when the normal electrocautery return is blocked or interrupted to the electrocautery pad.

Amplifiers pose a potential risk of applying electrical current to the patient through recording electrodes. Some preamplifiers have optic isolation units that isolate the preamplifiers from the other parts of the amplifiers. The other conceivable safety risk is that the supply voltage of the first stage of the amplifier can be delivered to the patient through the recording electrodes. This can happen if a short circuit in the preamplifier occurs. This can be prevented by solid-state devices placed at the input of the amplifiers that increase the impedance if the input current should exceed a certain (small) value. The limit of current is usually 5 μA, and such devices cause the currents that exceed that limit to practically disconnect the patient from the amplifier.

The increasing use of transcranial electric stimulation using stimulus strength of as much as 1,000 V poses safety questions (1). The strong contraction of muscles on the head (mastication muscles) that are caused by such electrical stimulation can cause tongue and lip lacerations, and it can even produce jaw fractures (1). Transcranial electric stimulation and transcranial magnetic stimulation have been suspected to cause seizures, but that suspicion seems unwarranted except in patients with seizure disorders. It seems unlikely that excessive transcranial electric stimulation could cause brain damage (1).

Safety to Personnel Working in the Operating Room

In the U.S.A, equipment that is to be used in the operating room must be approved by the Food and Drug Administration (FDA), and routine tests must be performed at regular time intervals to ensure that the safety of the equipment is maintained during the equipment's lifetime. This interval can be defined by the equipment manufacturer, but must not exceed one year. All tested equipment must be labeled with a clearly visible expiration date. These

safety standards have the form of recommendations, but some countries regulate this matter through the hospital accreditation process.

Isolation transformers that are commonly installed in operating rooms isolate the power supply from the primary hospital power supply circuits, and often, each operating room has its own isolation transformer and thus, a floating power supply. Line isolation monitors are used to detect the degree of isolation quality and sound an alarm in case the leakage current exceeds a certain amount. Leakage current is the sum of currents flowing from all equipment in the operating room to the ground. In the case of excessive leakage currents, these monitors will interrupt the power supply. The amount of accepted leakage current has been established by various safety organizations[2]).

Commonly accepted rules state that accessible conductive parts that are connected together must not have a potential difference of more than 100 mV. All accessible conductive parts in operating rooms must be grounded. All electrical power supply outlets must be tested regularly for loose connections and interruption of the safety ground connection.

Leakage current may be limited differently for different kinds of equipment. Equipment belonging to class I is protected by grounding of accessible conductive parts and enclosures, while class II equipment is protected by the use of double or reinforced insulation. Class III equipment comprises devices that have internal power supplies (batteries) with voltages not exceeding 60 V DC or 24 V AC.

The role of cable stray capacitance in causing leakage is defined by $C=S/d$, where d=dielectric constant and has a fixed value, S=cable surface area ($S=2rl$, where r=cable radius, l=cable length). Since cable stray capacitance depends on cable length and its distance from the grounded surfaces, it is important to use cables as short as possible and place them as far as possible from the ground. Because its impedance decreases with increased frequency ($Xc=1/2fC$), high-frequency current sources cause more leakage than low-frequency sources (2).

OTHER RISKS FROM WORKING IN THE OPERATING ROOM

Risks of contracting infectious diseases from patients that are being operated upon is a prominent risk in working in the operating room. The most common risk is probably contracting hepatitis C. All people working in the operating room should be immunized for hepatitis B (as there is currently no vaccine for hepatitis C). There are other diseases that can be transferred from a patient to the personnel from contact with body fluids. The risk is greatest for those who have contact with blood and other body fluids of patients that can transfer pathogens through needles or through small wounds. These kinds of risks mostly affect the anesthesia personnel, surgeons, and nurses. The biggest risk for those who do intraoperative monitoring to contract infectious diseases from patients is through handling of needle electrodes.

The use of reusable electrodes is problematic for these and other reasons. Removing such electrodes from the patient involves risks for the person who is to remove them, and handling such electrodes for sterilization, disposal, etc., also involves risks. As surgical instruments, needle electrodes can transfer pathogens for diseases such as Creutzfeldt–Jakob disease whose pathogens can survive normal autoclaving – only treatment with products containing chlorine (bleach, sodium hypochlorite) can ensure that such pathogens are eliminated. The use of disposable wire hook electrodes mostly solves such problems except in the process of disposing of these electrodes, which must be made without anyone getting into contact with such electrodes while they are being removed from the patient.

REFERENCES

1. MacDonald DB (2002) Safety of intraoperative transcranial electrical stimulation motor evoked potential monitoring. J. Clin. Neurophysiol. 19:416–29.
2. Išgum V and V Deletis, (2004) Electrical Safety in the Operating Theatre, in *Neurophysiology in Neurosurgery*, V Deletis and JL Shils, Editors. 2004, Academic Press: Amsterdam.

18

Equipment, Recording Techniques, and Data Analysis and Stimulation

INTRODUCTION

In the early days of intraoperative monitoring, either custom-made equipment or equipment taken from the clinical testing laboratory of the neurophysiological animal laboratories was used in the operating room. Now, there is specialized equipment commercially available for nearly all needs of intraoperative monitoring. This means

From: *Intraoperative Neurophysiological Monitoring: Third Edition*
By A.R. Møller, DOI 10.1007/978-1-4419-7436-5_18,
© Springer Science+Business Media, LLC 2011

that the persons who perform monitoring and intraoperative neurophysiology do not need to know as much about recording and stimulating equipment as they once did. However, knowledge about the basic function of the equipment that is used for intraoperative monitoring enables optimal use of the equipment and is important for troubleshooting. The equipment now commonly utilized for intraoperative neurophysiology is capable of appropriate signal processing, has several ways of filtering the recorded responses, and has many options for displaying the potentials recorded. The user must have sufficient knowledge, however, about the basis for filtering and signal averaging to use these methods in optimal ways.

The easy access to advanced digital techniques has increased the number of options for setting parameters for recording and stimulating equipment. Most modern equipment allows both stimulus and recording parameters to be controlled through computer commands. To make the best choice of settings, the person who uses such equipment must know the optimal settings for the tasks to be performed. For example, he or she must know which parameter to choose in order to obtain an interpretable recording of evoked potentials in as short a time as possible.

When evoked potentials are monitored, it is the change in the intraoperatively recorded response from the patient's baseline recording that is important. Because data must be interpreted immediately after being collected, special features are required of the equipment that is used for intraoperative neurophysiology. Thus, the hardware and software employed should permit instantaneous display of a current recording superimposed on a baseline recording, and it should provide online quality control of the recorded potentials.

Complete failure of good quality equipment designed for use in the operating room occurs rarely, but a malfunction of the equipment during intraoperative monitoring has serious consequences because it makes it impossible to continue monitoring if the malfunction cannot be corrected within a short time.

EQUIPMENT

Commercially available equipment can perform most tasks required for monitoring and other physiological recordings in the operating room. Several companies now have equipment available that can record and process many channels of recordings such as EMG, multimodality evoked potentials, and EEG simultaneously. Most commercial equipment contains everything that is needed in one unit – stimulators, amplifiers, signal averagers, display units, and equipment for storing the results. Even such equipment as high-voltage stimulators for transcranial stimulation of the motor system are now available as an integral part of equipment designed for use in the operating room.

Equipment that is designed to meet the need to monitor more than one modality of recorded potentials simultaneously is now widely available. Equipment that is designed especially to assist the person who is doing the monitoring as much as possible by aiding in the interpretation of the recordings will most likely also become more common if monitoring professionals make their needs known. Ideally, such equipment would be user-friendly and present recorded potentials of all types in the most interpretable form for each modality, and such equipment would automate such functions as the detection of changes in the latencies of selected components of the recorded potentials.

Failures of good quality modern equipment used for intraoperative monitoring now occur rarely. The cables that connect the equipment to the patient are now the weakest part of equipment used in the operating room. Cables are subjected to mechanical stress in the operating room and may become wet. Software glitches, although also rare, may occur.

Equipment used for intraoperative electrophysiological recordings and stimulation (amplifiers, stimulators, and computers) – just as other equipment used in the operating room – should, therefore, be selected not only on the basis of how well it performs the function for which it was designed, but also on the basis of its durability, reliability, and electrical safety features. Because the specifications of equipment do not usually include information about properties that make it fail less often than other equipment, it is tempting to select equipment based on the cost alone.

Almost all commercially available equipment now uses readily available personal computers for processing of recorded data, controlling stimulations, and for providing displays and storage of recorded potentials. Only amplifiers and stimulators are now made specifically for intraoperative neurophysiologic monitoring. In addition, these computers also perform administrative chores such as inclusion of comments made during operations and report generation.

The miniaturization of electronic equipment has made equipment for intraoperative monitoring much smaller during the past few years, which is important when applied to crowded operating rooms. It has also enabled some other advantages such as the possibilities to place the amplifiers and analog to digital converters close to the patient and transfer the data in digital form to the computer.

There is now equipment available that houses the preamplifiers and analog to digital converters in a small box that can conveniently be placed near the patient. It communicates with the computer through a USB line from which it also gets its power. Digital data transmission has a high degree of resistance to electrical and magnetic interference, which was a problem when recorded potentials were conducted as analog signals to the central equipment. Some equipment makers provide fiber optic cables between the preamplifier and the main amplifier, which reduces the electrical noise pick-up.

Requirements of Equipment for Intraoperative Monitoring

Much of the present commercially available equipment is considerably more complex than necessary and often has options that are not used. This complexity complicates its use and may increase the possibility of making mistakes. Some equipment features complex displays and many options, but may lack some important basic functions. The availability of inexpensive computing power of modern equipment could be better employed to improve signal processing than to make fancy displays and unnecessary options. For example, the option to continuously observe the output of the physiological amplifiers used in recording of evoked potentials seems to have disappeared

from modern equipment. When using averaging, the raw output from the amplifiers should be displayed continuously for observing interference and interpreting of what kind of interference has occurred. That function was earlier served by an oscilloscope, but now crowded computer displays often lack the possibility to display the output of the physiological amplifiers, and only through separate command can the directly recorded potentials be viewed. The extra time needed to view directly recorded potentials makes it difficult to react quickly to suddenly occurring interference.

Equipment manufacturers have been slow to incorporate features such as software for "finite impulse response zero-phase digital filtering." Such filtering by computer software provides more options than analog filters, and it does not shift the components of a record in time. Most important, perhaps, it does not cause stimulus artifacts to be spread out in time where they can interfere with the recorded response (see page 353).

However, the digital filters that are supplied with most of the commercially available equipment for use in the operating room are just emulations of analog (electronic) filters. Such filters do not have the advantages that can be achieved from digital filtering (such as finite impulse response and zero-phase shifts).

The availability of ample computing power and memory now allows for general use of optimal techniques for signal averaging and aids in interpreting recorded evoked potentials such as automatic display of latencies of peaks and valleys in sensory evoked potentials and other recorded potentials. However, such features are not incorporated in most of the commercial equipment now offered for use in monitoring and for intraoperative neurophysiology. Other features that would be useful are noise-based averaging (page 360) and efficient routines for quality control of recorded potentials. Such routines could be incorporated to a greater extent in the equipment without adding noticeably to the cost or sacrificing its user-friendliness.

To increase user-friendliness, it should be possible to set defaults regarding recording and stimulus parameters, one for each modality of sensory evoked potentials, MEP, etc.

Amplifiers

Most manufacturers of intraoperative monitoring equipment provide good quality differential amplifiers that are suitable for recording of a variety of different neuroelectrical potentials. The amplifiers have built-in filters to attenuate both low-frequency components (high-pass filters) and high-frequency components (low-pass filters). The filter settings as well as the amplification are usually digitally controlled. Often the most commonly used settings are factory set as default options.

Common-Mode Rejection. A differential amplifier is presumed to sense only the difference in the potentials that appear at its two inputs, so that if identical signals appear at the two inputs of a differential amplifier, there should ideally be no output from the amplifier. Cancellation of identical signals that are applied to both inputs is known as the common-mode rejection ratio (CMRR). Manufacturers now offer amplifiers with common-mode rejection of 90 dB (decibels). That means that the output would be 1,000,000,000 times lower when the same electrical potential was applied to both inputs than the output would be if the signal was applied to only one of the amplifier's two inputs. The CMRR given by manufacturers refers to an ideal situation that is rarely attainable. The CMRR depends on the symmetry of the two electrodes that are connected to the amplifiers. Perfect symmetry can rarely be achieved when amplifiers are used to record biological potentials from electrodes placed on the skin or on neural tissue. Thus, the practical obtainable CMRR is lower than that given in the specifications for any amplifier.

Another important feature of amplifiers, namely, their input impedance was a concern in earlier times. However, modern amplifiers have very high input impedances, of as much as 1,000 MΩ, which has eliminated that concern for all practical purposes of work in the operating room.

All of these properties that are mentioned above only apply for input signals with amplitudes below certain values. If the input signal exceeds the value at which the amplifiers become overloaded, the amplifier's input impedances and CMRR will be affected in a major way.

Maximal Output. All amplifiers have a maximal output voltage and when that output has been exceeded, the amplifier cannot properly amplify the signals that are applied to the two input terminals of a differential amplifier. The maximal output voltage varies among different types of amplifiers, but it is usually between 5 V and 15 V. When, for instance, the amplification is set at 10,000×, input signals with an amplitude of 0.5 mV will result in an output signal of 5 V. If the maximal output of the particular amplifier is 5 V with that level of amplification set, any input signal above 0.5 mV will overload the amplifier, and the output will be distorted. Ideally, the amplifier will resume its normal operation when the amplitude of the input signal decreases below 0.5 mV, but this is rarely the case. If an amplifier has been subjected to an input voltage that is much higher than that which gives the amplifier's maximal output (in this case, 0.5 mV), most amplifiers become blocked for a brief time after being overloaded and will not amplify the input signal properly. The resulting output signal may be distorted. In intraoperative monitoring, amplifier overload can result from stimulus artifacts, interference from the electrocoagulator, or strong intermittent electrical interference.

Overloading of a physiologic amplifier is more likely to occur when high amplification is used. One way to minimize the risk of an amplifier becoming overloading is to use a lower amplification. It is all too common to use an amplification setting that is too high. When signal averaging is used, the amplification can be reduced considerably from that which has been traditionally used (e.g. 100,000X) without noticeable problems because the process of signal averaging in itself increases the dynamic range of signal acquisition.

When signal averaging is used, the problems associated with amplifier overload can be remedied by using computer programs that identify when overloading occurs and stop signal averaging for a certain time after overloading ceases in addition to the actual period where overloading produces a distorted output from the amplifiers. This is discussed in more detail later in this chapter (page 359).

Low-Pass and High-Pass Filters. Two kinds of filters are used in the equipment used for intraoperative monitoring. One type is the analog (electronic) filter and the other is the digital filter (discussed on page 347). All physiological amplifiers have built-in analog filters of two kinds, high-pass and low-pass filters. High-pass filters attenuate low frequencies ("pass" high frequencies). Low-pass filters attenuate high frequencies ("pass" low frequencies). (This terminology that emanates from electrical engineering seems slightly illogical, and some descriptions of filters and their specifications call low-pass filters "high filters" while high-pass filters are called "low filters". While this may seem more logical, the engineering terminology for filters is used in this book.)

There are also filters that attenuate a narrow band of frequencies (notch filters).

Analog filters, low- and high-pass filters, are described by their cut-off frequency which is usually defined as the frequency at which the attenuation reaches 3 dB[1], but some manufacturers instead list the frequency at which the attenuation reaches 6 dB. Cut-off frequencies for low- and high-pass filters are usually variable and set by the user, often digitally by computer commands.

The attenuation of signals outside the pass band of analog filters increases gradually as the frequency deviates more and more from the cut-off frequency of the filter. The slope of the attenuation that is usually given in dB/octave is different for different types of filters, and the user

usually cannot change the slope because it is related to the type of filter that is used. The attenuation of a low-pass filter may increase at a rate of 6, 12, 18, or 24 dB/octave above the cut-off frequency, depending on the type of filter (one octave corresponds to an increase, or decrease, in frequency by a factor of 2). The attenuation for a high-pass filter increases as the frequency is lowered below the filter's cut-off frequency at rates of 6, 12, 18, or 24 dB/octave. The specifications for filters in monitoring equipment often omit the rate of attenuation and give only the cut-off frequency. Information about the slope of the attenuation of the filters that are in the amplifiers is important because the rate of attenuation not only determines the efficiency of the filter in attenuating signals outside their pass band, but also determines the amount of phase shift to which the signal is subjected by the filter. The phase shift of filters used in processing of recorded potentials may cause a shift of different components of a signal differently. A filter's phase shift can, therefore, cause distortion of the waveform of recorded potentials.

Low-pass filters that are built into amplifiers and attenuate high frequencies before the signal is converted to digital form have their greatest importance in preventing aliasing (see page 361) and should be set according to that task. High-pass filters placed before analog to digital conversion have their greatest importance in removing slow (low frequency) interference that could otherwise overload the amplifier.

Since high-pass filters are more likely to cause distortion of recorded potentials than low-pass filters, it is preferable to use high-pass filters with 6-dB/octave slopes of attenuation, but filters with 12-dB/octave slopes are acceptable. Low-pass filters should have slopes of at least 18 dB/octave and preferably 24 dB/octave because of the need of attenuating high-frequency interference signals (see page 361).

---

[1]The decibel scale is a logarithmic measure of ratios, such as the ratio between the amplitude of the output and that of the input; thus, it is a measure of attenuation or amplification. For voltage ratios, it is defined as $20 \log_{10} E_o/E_i$, where E_i is the input voltage and E_o is the output voltage, an attenuation of 3 dB means that the output is 0.707 times the input, a 6 dB attenuation means that the output voltage is half of the input, a 10 dB attenuation means that the output is 0.3 of the input, a 20 dB attenuation means that the output is 0.1 of the input, and so on.

The main need of filtering for the purpose of preparing the recorded signals for interpretation should be served by digital filters that operate on the digitized signals (see page 360) because digital filters are superior to analog filters in many respects. The effects of filtering are discussed in more detail later in this chapter (page 356) along with the use of digital filters and digital filtering are discussed.

Notch Filters (Line Frequency Rejection Filters). Some amplifiers have notch filters that are intended for reducing interference from the power line (60 or 50 Hz). However, the use of notch filters is strongly discouraged when recording neuroelectric potentials. Notch filters can cause a sharp stimulus artifact to appear as a damped oscillation that can interfere with the biologic potentials that follow and which may be interpreted as part of the recorded bioelectric potentials because the waveform is reproducible. Thus, as a general rule, notch filters should never be used in intraoperative neurophysiological monitoring where stimulus artifacts are present or when the recorded potentials contain sharp waves.

Electrical Stimulators

The electric stimulators used to stimulate neural tissue in connection with neurophysiological recordings usually deliver rectangular impulses. The amplitude (voltage or current), duration, and the repetition rate of the delivered impulses are usually variable within a wide range.

It should be possible to choose between constant-voltage and constant-current output of the stimulator (see Chap. 4), and the stimulus level (voltage or current) should be clearly displayed to reduce the risk of mistakenly setting the stimulus at a level that may cause injury.

There should also be a way to (physically) limit the possibility of a stimulator delivering a current that is in excess of what is regarded to be safe. Stimulators that can deliver a continuous direct current (or voltage) should never be used in the operating room for reasons of safety. Inexpensive disposable stimulators, some of which deliver DC current, may be effective in

stimulating a nerve, but such stimulation may also injure the nerve. Such stimulators should not be used in intraoperative assessment of the function of nerves and CNS (central nervous system) structures.

A stimulator should be able to generate impulses at a rate in the range of 0.5 and 250 pulses per second (pps). The duration of the delivered impulses should also be variable, from approximately 0.05 to 5 ms, and it should be easy to invert the stimulus polarity. The stimulus rate should be chosen so that it is not a submultiple of the frequency of a periodic interference signal, such as the power line frequency, because the periodic signal would then be included in the signal average. Even better, it should be possible to modulate the stimulus rate randomly in order to reduce the effect of interference from periodic signals when signal averaging is employed (see page 358). Modern stimulators are computer-controlled and some have the option to make the repetition rate vary randomly within a small range.

Stimulators used in connection with intraoperative neurophysiological monitoring should have the capability to deliver trains of impulses.

Stimulators that are used in intraoperative monitoring must have a stimulation isolation unit that causes the output current to be delivered between the two output leads without producing any appreciable current flow between the output leads and the ground. Such isolation units are absolutely essential, for both reducing stimulus artifacts and for patient safety.

Special high-voltage stimulators that can deliver impulses in excess of 1,000 V to be used for TES of the motor cortex are available, and some general equipment for intraoperative monitoring has this feature built in.

Constant-Current Versus Constant-Voltage Stimulation. Stimulators can either deliver a constant (or nearly constant) voltage or a constant current. Which one of these two options is optimal for use depends on the individual circumstances. Because it is the amount of electric current that flows through the neural tissue that determines the degree of stimulation, it would be ideal that a stimulator delivers a current to the neural tissue that is independent of changes in external circumstances, such as electrode impedance and shunting of current around the neural tissue by fluid and other tissues (**Fig. 18.1**).

Constant-current stimulators are suitable when the electrode impedance may change because constant-current stimulators deliver the same current independent of the electrode impedance. Using a constant-current stimulator, therefore, prevents changes in the delivered stimulus current when the electrode impedance changes. When electrodes placed on the skin are used to deliver electrical stimulation to a peripheral nerve, the electrode impedance will often change spontaneously, and thus, a constant-current stimulator would be the best choice. This is why it is common to use constant-current stimulators in clinical studies where peripheral nerves are often stimulated by using surface electrodes.

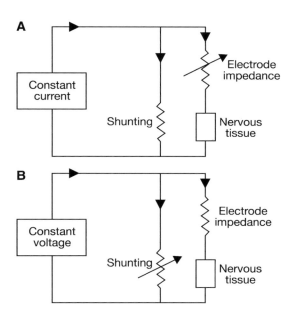

Figure 18.1: Illustration of how change in electrode impedance and shunting can affect the stimulus current that is delivered to a nerve. (**A**) Using a constant-current stimulator. (**B**) Using a constant-voltage stimulator.

Some of the stimulus current flows through nonneural tissue located adjacent to the nerve that is to be stimulated and shunts current around the nerve. The shunting of current does not vary very much when stimulating peripheral nerves either with surface electrodes or needle electrodes and, therefore, the shunting of stimulus current is not a major concern when stimulating peripheral nerves using electrodes placed on the skin.

When stimulating structures in the brain and the spinal cord, however, the situation is different because some fraction of the current applied will be shunted away by the fluid that surrounds the structures that are to be stimulated. The amount of current that is shunted away from the target tissues will vary from time to time (*1, 2*) (**Fig. 18.1**). At one moment, the field may be flooded by cerebrospinal fluid (CSF) and at another moment, the fluid will move away and the area will be relatively dry. Such change in the degree of wetness causes a varying degree of shunting of stimulus current that is applied for the purpose of stimulating a nerve or other nerve tissue, and consequently, changes will occur in the current passing through nervous tissue.

If a constant voltage is applied to the stimulating electrode in the brain or spinal cord, the change in the shunting of current due to the change in condition of the area from wet to dry will not affect the current delivered to a certain volume of tissue and thus, provides a rather stable delivery of a stimulation of a nerve that is located in such an environment. The current that flows through a nerve that is located close to a stimulating electrode would be determined only by the electrode impedance and that of the tissue.

Stimulation with constant current, on the other hand, would result in large variations in the current that passes through the tissue that is to be stimulated (*1, 3, 4*) (**Fig. 18.1**).

However, since constant-current stimulators have been so frequently used in clinical studies, it was controversial to suggest that the use of stimulators of the constant-voltage type might be more suited for monitoring of, for example, the facial nerve in operations in the cerebellopontine angle (1, 2).

Many modern stimulators can be set to deliver either a (semi) constant voltage or a constant current. In order to deliver a constant voltage, the internal impedance of a stimulator must be zero, which is never the case. Instead, all stimulators have a certain internal impedance and deliver a semiconstant voltage.

A stimulator that delivers a semiconstant voltage with an inner impedance of 1 kΩ, together with an electrode impedance of about 3 kΩ (total inner impedance about 4 kΩ), is suitable for stimulating nerves and other neural tissue where the shunting of current varies. With such a stimulator, the current that passes through any part of the tissue changes very little when the electrical shunting of the stimulus current changes, and the same setting of the output of the stimulator can be used when the operative field is wet as well as when it is relatively dry.

It has been suggested that the problems with variations in shunting of stimulus current using a constant-current stimulator could be solved by using a stimulating electrode insulated except at its tip ("flush-tip" stimulating electrode) (5). While this may be true, it seems more logical to use stimulators that deliver a constant voltage for stimulating in a surgical field where the degree of wetness (and thus, shunting of stimulus current) varies over time.

The choice of the type of stimulator – constant-voltage or constant-current – that is most suitable thus depends on whether it is the electrode impedance that varies or the shunting of the stimulus current that is likely to vary most. (These matters are also discussed in connection with monitoring cranial motor nerves and pedicle screws, see Chaps. 7 and 10).

Output Limitations of Electrical Stimulators. Electrical stimulators of the constant-current type have limitations as to the load under which they can deliver a specific current. Again, recalling Ohm's law (voltage is the product of current and impedance), it

becomes evident that if a constant-current stimulator is set to deliver 1 mA of current and the electrode impedance is 10 kΩ (10,000 Ω), the required voltage will be 10 V, which is within the limits of most stimulators. Many stimulators can also deliver 10 mA at that impedance (10 kΩ), which will require a voltage of 100 V. However, if a current of 20 mA is required, and the electrode impedance is 10 kΩ, many conventional stimulators will fail because a voltage of 200 V is required to drive 20 mA through such a load.

Constant-voltage stimulators have similar limitations regarding the current they can deliver into low-impedance loads. Thus, if a constant-voltage stimulator is set to deliver 5 V to an impedance (the sum of electrode and tissue impedance) of 5 kΩ, it would only require a current of 1 mA, which is well within the range of almost all stimulators. Many stimulators set to deliver 50 V with an electrode impedance of 1 kΩ can also provide the required current (50 mA). However, if the voltage were set at 100 V with the same electrode impedance, it would require 100 mA to be delivered, which may be outside the limit of some stimulators.

Performance outside these limits is required for TES in connection with monitoring of motors systems (see page 209). Stimulators for this purpose require the ability to deliver voltages as high as 1,500 V in connection with electrode impedances of as low as 100 Ω. This amount of voltage is only needed for transcranial electrical stimulation of the motor cortex and was earlier only met by special stimulators. Now, some standard intraoperative monitoring equipment include a unit that can supply high-voltage electrical stimulation for TES and such stimulators can deliver the required current into the load of a few hundred Ohms.

Stimulating Electrodes. Needle (and wire hook) or surface electrodes are suitable for stimulating peripheral nerves. The same type of needle electrodes as used for recording potentials can also be used for stimulation, but surface electrodes such as children-size EKG pads can also be used for stimulating peripheral nerves and dermatomes. Large surface electrodes may stimulate structures other than those anticipated being stimulated. Modern self-adhesive stimulating electrodes are also suitable.

Needle and wire hook electrodes do not have these disadvantages, and they can be placed very close to a peripheral nerve, thus effectively stimulating a specific nerve without stimulating other structures. When stimulating electrodes are placed on motor nerves (or mixed nerves), it is helpful to have the stimulation switched on at the time the electrodes are applied because muscle contractions caused by the stimulation can be observed which can help position stimulating electrodes close to the respective nerve (naturally this is provided that the patient is not paralyzed when the electrodes are being placed).

Probing the surgical field can be used to find the location of a motor nerve in the brain. For that type of electrical stimulation, a monopolar handheld stimulating electrode is used (1). An all-metal hypodermic needle is used as a return electrode.

> Some investigators have described surgical dissection instruments that also function as stimulating electrodes (6) when connected to a stimulator. The purpose of designing such instruments was to be able to warn the surgeon when dissecting near a motor nerve.

The stimulating electrode should be connected to a stimulator via an appropriate interface (stimulus isolation unit) placed outside the sterile field in a way similar to that described for the electrode box used for recording electrodes. Similar arrangements should be made for electrical stimulation of the spinal cord, spinal nerves, or surgically exposed peripheral nerves.

Magnetic Stimulation

Magnetic stimulation can be used to stimulate the cerebral cortex (TMS) and peripheral nerves, but this type of stimulation is mostly used in the clinic. Magnetic stimulation makes use of brief impulses of a strong magnetic field that is generated by a coil through which a large electrical current is passed. It is not the magnetic field that activates neural tissue, but instead, it is the electrical current that the magnetic field induced in brain tissue (see **Fig. 10.1**). Changes in the magnetic field induce electrical currents in a wire or other electrical conductors, such as brain or spinal cord tissue, which are good electrical conductors. Magnetic stimulation has had some use in stimulation of the motor cortex for monitoring motor systems (see Chap. 10), but now the most common way of stimulating the motor cortex is by electrical stimulation (TES).

Sound Generators

Sound generators used in connection with recording ABR (and CAP from the auditory nerve and the auditory nervous system) in the operating room should be able to deliver rectangular impulses to an earphone to produce click sounds. The duration of these impulses is usually fixed at 100 μs, which is the standard duration used for most intraoperative monitoring as well as for clinical ABR testing. However, this is not the optimal duration and 75 μs or 150 μs would be more suitable (7). The polarity of the clicks should be easily reversible to produce rarefaction or condensation clicks. The use of clicks with alternating polarity (to reduce stimulus artifacts) should not be used because condensation and rarefaction clicks often elicit responses that are different. Stimulus artifacts can be reduced by other means (see Chap. 18).

The rate at which stimuli are presented should be variable from 5 pps to 80 pps, with the most important range being 30 pps–50 pps. It should be possible to modulate the rate of the impulses delivered to the earphone so that the rate varies 5–10% randomly. This will reduce the effect of interference signals that are periodic in nature. If this option is not available, the repetition rates should be variable in small steps so that a repetition rate can be selected that is not a submultiple of the frequency of electrical interference that may be present. The output of an audio-stimulator should be variable in 5 dB steps, to make it possible to change the intensity of the sound stimulation. The sound delivered should be calibrated in dB hearing level (HL).

Most audio-stimulators are designed for use in connection with a specific type of earphone, but they should be sufficiently versatile so that other types of earphones can also be used. However, if earphones are chosen that are different from those supplied with the specific audio-stimulator being used, then it is necessary to calibrate the sound (see Chap. 7).

Earphones that connect to the patient's ear through a (plastic) tube with a length of 20–30 cm are commonly supplied together with intraoperative monitoring equipment. The sound that reaches the ears is delayed from the time the electrical signal is generated to its arrival at the earphone because of the travel time of the sound in the tube (the delay is approximately 1 ms for a tube of 34 cm length). That delay increases the separation of stimulus artifact and response.

Inexpensive miniature insert earphones (Chap. 7) have been in use for many years for generating clicks and other auditory stimuli for monitoring the auditory system, and such earphones still offer an alternative to the much more expensive insert earphones, and they, in fact, provide a better quality of the sound than insert earphones sold together with monitoring equipment.

Light Stimulators

Light stimulators have been described that make use of light-emitting diodes bonded to contact lenses (8), but this type of device is not commercially available. The light-emitting diodes that are either bonded to contact lenses or placed in goggles can be driven by a common electrical stimulator that can deliver pulses of approximately 100 mA. If a constant-voltage stimulator is used, a suitable resistor (of about 1,000 Ω) must be placed in series with the light-emitting diodes to limit the current. The duration of the current pulse should be variable between 1 and 50 ms at a repetition rate of 1–5 pps, thus

well within the range of the requirements that were described above for electrical stimulators.

Fiber optic cables have been used to conduct white light of high intensity to the eye in anesthetized patients. High-intensity light stimulators for use in the operating room have been described (9).

Audio-Amplifiers and Loudspeakers

It is often of great value to have the recorded potentials made audible so that the surgeon can "hear" the potentials (1, 10, 11), and most equipment that is commercially available for intraoperative monitoring has an audio amplifier and loudspeaker built in for that purpose.

Computer Systems

Currently, computer systems are often based on personal computers using one of Microsoft's operating systems. Since the hardware of most personal computers has sufficient computational and storage capacity for intraoperative monitoring and other physiology tasks, the focus should be on the available software when selecting systems for use in intraoperative neurophysiological monitoring. Often manufactures are tempted to include many more options than suitable or necessary for use in intraoperative monitoring. The computer system should allow digital filtering (using zero-phase, finite impulse response filters), artifact rejection, quality control, etc., in connection with signal averaging. It should be possible to easily review current settings (amplification, filter cut-off frequencies, stimulus parameters, etc.) to reduce the risk of errors. The computer programs should allow the user to establish defaults for different types of monitoring such as ABR, SSEP, MEP, etc., so that it is not necessary to set these parameters manually every time monitoring is begun. User-friendliness should be a high priority for selecting equipment for use in the operating room.

Display Units. The display is an important part of a monitoring system. It should be easy to change and should have the ability to show the recorded potentials in different ways. It is important that the display unit is sufficiently large and that it has fine resolution. The display unit should be able to display at least eight channels (most modern equipment can display 16 channels and some can display 32 channels) simultaneously. The averaged waveform of sensory evoked potentials, as well as other types of potentials, and a baseline should be displayed simultaneously. Most manufacturers provide different modes of displays such as single traces of averaged potentials, "water fall" displays (Stack), and various forms of trend displays. However, the most useful form of display of evoked potentials is a simple display of the current recording superimposed on the baseline recording. This provides immediate and clear information about changes in the recorded potentials. The "waterfall" displays are suitable for record keeping and documentation purposes such as in a final report by showing the history of changes in recorded potentials, but these kinds of records are of less value for use in the operating room.

The possibility to display different modalities of recorded potentials is important, but there is also a risk of information overload by crowded displays. Many equipment makers also offer displays of the surgeon's view through a microscope, which is useful to keep the person who does monitoring aware of what happens in the surgical field. A separate display unit for that purpose is perhaps more suitable than having it together with traces of recorded potentials. One equipment manufacturer now offers a possibility to display recorded responses on the operating microscope so that the surgeon sees the recorded potentials overlaid on the view of the surgical field.

It is important to display the recorded signals directly. This is true even when the recorded potentials are not of sufficient amplitude to be discerned without signal averaging. A direct display of the raw output of the amplifiers is important for diagnosing the interference that may occur at any time during monitoring and identifying the source of electrical or other kinds of interference. Switching between displaying averaged responses and the direct output

of the physiologic amplifiers should be simple, requiring only a minimal number of keystrokes, or even better, the directly recoded potentials should be shown continuously in a separate window. When displaying only the averaged potentials, the only indication of interference is that all responses are rejected, and that is not useful information for identification of the source of the interference.

When automatic scaling of the amplitude of the displayed potentials is used, the value of the amplitude should be displayed numerically or by a vertical scale on the recorded potentials.

RECORDING TECHNIQUES

Three main kinds of potentials are recorded in the operating room, namely, responses from muscles (EMG potentials) and near-field and far-field potentials from the nervous system. Recordings of electrical potentials from nerves, the CNS, and muscles are basic parts of intraoperative neurophysiological recordings in the operating room. Techniques for recording these different kinds of potentials have both commonalities and differences and depend on from which structures they record. A fourth kind of neuroelectrical potentials, action potentials recorded from single nerve fibers or cell bodies (unit potentials) and from clusters of nerve cells (multiunit recordings), has become of importance recently for guidance in making lesions in the CNS and for implantation of electrodes for deep brain stimulation (DBS).

Recording of Far-Field Evoked Potentials

Far-field sensory evoked potentials such as ABR, SSEP, and VEP are recorded from electrodes placed on the body surface (the scalp). The electrodes used for such recordings can be needle or wire hook electrodes or surface electrodes. The recording electrodes can be arranged so that both of the electrodes that are connected to a differential amplifier record the same kind of potentials or arranged so that one electrode does not record the evoked potentials in question (acting as a noncephalic reference electrode).

The amplitude of far-field sensory evoked potentials is mostly less than 1 μV. Even under the best possible recording conditions with a minimal amount of electrical interference, the amplitude of these potentials is smaller than the background spontaneous activity from the brain (EEG). It is, therefore, necessary to use signal-averaging techniques to obtain records that are interpretable (see Chap. 18).

It is always an advantage to get as large evoked potentials as possible. There are several factors that determine the amplitude of evoked potentials as discussed in Chap. 7 regarding ABR recordings and in Chap. 6 regarding SSEP. The amplitude of the recorded evoked potentials depends on the stimulus parameters used and on the placement of the recording electrodes. Most sources of evoked potentials behave as if they were generated by a dipole. Such (fictive) dipoles have different orientations for the different components of most evoked potentials. Recording electrodes should be placed in accordance with orientations of these dipoles, as was discussed in connection with recordings of ABR (see page 128).

Recording of Near-Field Evoked Potentials from Muscles and Nerves and from the CNS

Near-field potentials can be recorded by placing surface electrodes on the skin over muscles or nerves, or by using needle electrodes or wire hook electrodes percutaneously in the structures (muscles or nerves) from which recordings are to be made. Recordings of evoked near-field responses from structures of the brain and spinal cord can only be made after surgical exposure of these structures. Intraoperative recordings of near-field responses are commonly made from the auditory nerve, cochlear nucleus, spinal cord, and the cerebral cortex.

Since near-field potentials have much larger amplitudes than far-field evoked potentials, recordings of such potentials often do not require signal averaging to make the responses interpretable. Such recordings can, therefore, be interpreted immediately after they are acquired, and they can usually be observed directly on a computer screen after being amplified or after averaging only a few responses. Recordings of near-field potentials, therefore, offer nearly instantaneous monitoring of the function of specific neural systems.

Recordings of unit or multiunit potentials from the structures belonging to the basal ganglia and the thalamus by microelectrodes may be regarded as special forms of near-field potential recordings. Such recordings are used to guide placement of lesions or implantation of stimulating electrodes (DBS) and are now a part of intraoperative neurophysiological recordings that are carried out through stereotactic access to these structures. These potentials are observed by displaying them on a computer screen as well as by making them audible (see Chap. 15).

Using EMG recordings to detect muscle contractions is far superior to visual observation of muscle contractions. Although several devices have been described to detect facial muscle contractions using various kinds of mechanotransducers designed for use in connection with monitoring of the facial nerve (12, 13), recording EMG potentials is the most suitable method for detecting contractions of specific muscles. This technique was first developed for monitoring the facial nerve (1, 4, 8, 14), but it is applicable to other muscles of the head and of the body (see Chaps. 10 and 11).

Bipolar or Monopolar Recordings. Near-field potentials can be recorded either by monopolar recording electrodes or bipolar recording electrodes. Monopolar recording electrodes are easier to place on the structure from which recording is to be made, but have less spatial specificity than bipolar recording electrodes (see Chap. 3).

SIGNAL PROCESSING AND DATA ANALYSIS

The purpose of signal processing in connection with intraoperative monitoring and intraoperative neurophysiology is to make signals easier to interpret. Only under the most favorable recording conditions can some far-field evoked potentials such as SSEP be observed without signal averaging (*15*). The amplitudes of some far-field sensory evoked potentials are too small to be discernable in the background noise consisting of ongoing brain activity (EEG) and from electrical and magnetic interference from sources outside the patient. The most used form of signal processing that can make far-field SSEP become visible and allow for interpretation is signal averaging. Filtering is also an important form of signal processing that can enhance certain features of recorded potentials that are important and suppress features that are not important, making interpretation easier and more accurate.

Signal Averaging of Evoked Potentials

The use of signal averaging to enhance evoked potentials that appear in a background noise (unwanted signals) is based on three assumptions:

1. The potentials evoked by individual stimuli have the same waveform.
2. The individual components of the response appear with the same time delay (latency) after the stimulus is delivered.
3. The waveform of the noise does not have a fixed-time relationship with the stimulation.

When the signal fulfills the above three criteria and the background noise consists of random noise, the ratio between the response and the background noise (signal-to-noise ratio, SNR) is improved by a factor that is the square root of the number of responses that are added together. Adding four responses thus results in a twofold improvement in the SNR. In the same way, it is necessary to increase the number of responses that are added from 1,000 to 4,000 in order to achieve a twofold increase in the SNR obtained by averaging 1,000 responses. If the purpose is to increase the SNR by a factor of two when 4,000 responses have been averaged, 16,000 responses must be added instead.

This means that if the amplitude of the signal is only slightly smaller than that of the noise, a relatively small number of responses need to be added in order to achieve a considerable improvement of the SNR, but when the amplitude of the signal is small compared with the noise, it will take many added responses to obtain the same degree of improvement in the SNR. Thus, when the amplitude of the signal is small compared with that of the noise, signal averaging becomes a slow process to improve the SNR and other means should be explored such as reduction of the noise or better placement of the recording electrodes to get larger amplitudes of the evoked potentials.

The improvement of the SNR by a factor that is the square root of the number of responses that are added together is only achieved when the background noise is random noise and when all responses are identical. However, because none of the three criteria mentioned above is completely fulfilled under practical circumstances, the improvement in the SNR through signal averaging of neuroelectrical potentials is always less than the optimal improvement.

Effect of Periodic Interference Signals. Situations where the interference is periodic or semiperiodic are especially difficult to manage when signal averaging is used. Electrical and magnetic signals generated by various pieces of electrical equipment constitute the most severe problems in intraoperative monitoring because these signals are often periodic in nature. When recordings are made from the scalp, spontaneous brain activity (EEG) is a substantial source of background noise. While these signals are quasiperiodic in nature, they do give similar problems as electrical and magnetic interference signals.

The effects on the averaged responses of the interference that is periodic or semiperiodic in nature can be completely different from those seen when the noise has a random or nearly random character. While the effects of random noise can be reduced by the signal averaging technique, as described above, a similar reduction in the interference from periodic signals can only be realized if certain conditions are fulfilled. Thus, if the frequency of one such interference signal is a multiple or submultiple of the repetition rate of the stimulus, the interference signals will add in very much the same way as the stimulus-related responses when the responses are averaged; this means that periodic interference signals may appear in the averaged response with an amplitude that is not much less than it is without averaging. This in turn means that periodic interference signals can totally obscure the response. Because signal averaging does not enhance the responses in the noise in such a case, it does not help to add more responses, and other actions must be taken to enhance the responses.

Thus, the problem with periodic noise occurs when its frequency is the same or a multiple or submultiple of that of the stimulus presentation. It is not possible to change the frequency of the noise, but changing the frequency of the stimulus frequency can have the same effect. The effect of periodic interference signals can, thus, be reduced by setting the stimulus repetition rate so that it is not a multiple or submultiple of the frequency of the interference, a process that requires that the repetition rate can be changed in small steps.

The best way, however, to reduce the effects of periodic interference signals is to modulate the stimulus repetition rate with a random signal. This has a similar effect as changing a periodic interference to a nonperiodic interference. About 5–15% random variation in the stimulus repetition rate is likely to reduce problems with periodic interference substantially without having any significant influence on the response. The author used this technique for many years, but it has not yet come into general widespread use in commercially available equipment.

In addition, the amount of periodic or semiperiodic signals that reach the recording system should be reduced as much as possible as discussed in Chap. 17.

Artifact Rejection. When signal averaging is used in connection with recording of evoked potentials, the effect of intermittent interference, the amplitude of which is much larger than those of the recorded potentials, can be eliminated using artifact rejection. Artifact rejection works by excluding recordings in which the amplitude exceeds a certain value. This means that the recorded potentials that follow a stimulus should first be examined (by a computer program) with regard to the amplitude of any component that occurs within the recording time window before they are included in the averaged response. Commercially available signal averaging equipment for recording sensory evoked potentials has the capabilities needed for such artifact rejection.

Some equipment allows the user to set the signal amplitude that triggers artifact rejection, and it should be set so that all responses that contain intermittent interference are rejected, while all other responses are included in the average. If the threshold for the artifact rejection is set too low, then too many responses will be rejected, and the time it takes to obtain an interpretable recording will be unnecessarily prolonged. If the threshold for rejection is set too high, interference may be included in the averaged response.

Some equipment does not allow the user to set the artifact rejection level; instead the level is set at the maximal output (or slightly less) of the amplifier. This is unfortunate because artifacts then will cause the output of the amplifier to exceed its maximal output and become overloaded by all artifacts that are rejected from being included in the average response. Overloading will affect the function of the amplifier for a certain time, and it may affect the responses following the artifact because of the time it takes for the amplifier to recover. To remedy this problem, the amplification must be set at a (low) value so that most kinds of artifacts do not overload the amplifiers. This requires that it is possible for the user to set the rejection level. Some kinds of artifacts, such as those from electrocoagulation, will, under all practical circumstances, overload the amplifiers and appropriate precautions must be taken so that amplifier blockage does not affect the averaged responses (see below).

If the artifact rejection is activated by periodic interference signals, it will enhance the appearance of the periodic interference in the averaged response. Continuous interference, such as from the power line frequency (60 Hz in North America and 50 Hz in Europe), should never be allowed to activate artifact rejection. If the observation window is shorter than one period of the interference, artifact rejection of such interference may result in a part of the interference wave to be included in the averaged response and that generates an odd looking artifact in the averaged response that could be mistaken for a part of the response.

When the background noise contains low-frequency components or slow baseline changes, these low-frequency components may activate artifact rejection. Artifact rejection that occurs in synchrony with the low-frequency components may result in the averaged recording appearing as a slanted line on which the responses are superimposed. However, a simple computer program (digital high-pass filtering) can restore the response to a straight horizontal line. If the recorded potential appears on a curved line, as may also happen when the interference is a low-frequency signal, the best remedy is to use a zero-phase finite impulse response digital high-pass filter to remove such a baseline shift.

Some (most) equipment examines the entire record for artifacts. However, it would be advantageous to be able to exclude the earliest part of a record that may contain a stimulus artifact from examination of artifacts. This possibility is useful in connection with recordings of responses to electrical stimulation where a large stimulus artifact occurs before the response appears. The equipment should, therefore, permit the user to select a fraction of the total analysis time window in which the artifact rejection routine checks the amplitude.

Reducing Effects of Amplifier Blockage. The technique for eliminating transient interference from averages of evoked potentials by artifact rejection works well as long as the amplification that is used is low enough so that

the amplifier does not become blocked by these transients as mentioned above. However, if the transients (including large stimulus artifacts) have a large enough amplitude to block the amplifiers, the amplifiers may fail to work properly when the interference stops and averaging is resumed (overloading of amplifiers was discussed on page 348, 366).

Interference due to electrocoagulation is an example of interference that often causes blockage of the amplifiers that are being used to record the evoked potentials. Such blocking may last for several seconds after cessation of the electrocoagulation depending on the type of amplifier used and depending on the amplification that is used. This means that the output of the amplifiers can be nearly zero or that the amplification may be lower than normal for several seconds after cessation of electrocoagulation. Many amplifiers generate different types of noise signals as a result of such overloading, and most amplifiers will not operate properly for some time after they begin to recover from overloading. If the output is zero (no amplification), the recording will not be rejected if rejection is based on the amplitude of the signal exceeding a certain value. Because the averaged response is the sum of all recordings that are not rejected divided by the number of recordings, accepting "empty" recordings will result in a lowering of the amplitude of the averaged response. During the recovery period of the amplifiers, the signal may be amplified, but it is often distorted and the amplification is not optimal.

These adverse effects of amplifier blockage can be remedied by having the computer that performs the averaging continue to reject responses for a certain time (usually a few seconds) while the amplifier is recovering following cessation of electrocoagulation. This means that the computer program must be able to identify when amplifiers have been blocked for a certain time compared with what is caused by a single transient. In fact, more sophisticated computer programs can recognize exactly when the amplifiers have fully recovered after being overloaded because they are able to identify normal noise background. Such computer programs will allow only the recordings that have normal noise background to be included in the averaged response.

Ways to Optimize Signal Averaging. Artifact rejection in connection with signal averaging, as just described, totally eliminates responses that contain too much noise from being included in the average. Other and more sophisticated methods than artifact rejection have been designed to improve the efficiency of signal averaging. Noise that interferes with recording evoked potentials often varies over time and one method, known as weighted averaging (*16, 17*), increases the efficiency of signal averaging by giving the different responses different weight when added, depending on their content of noise.

If all responses with such varying background noise are added together in the conventional way using an ordinary averaging technique, adding more responses may in fact decrease the quality (SNR) of the averaged response. This paradox may occur because the responses that are added later contain more noise than those that were added earlier. The problem can be reduced by assigning weighting factors to the individual responses, with the values of these weighting factors being dependent on the amount of background noise. Thus, recordings that contain more noise will add less to the resulting average than recordings that contain less noise. Responses that contain a great deal of noise (but less than that needed to trigger the artifact rejection routine) are given less weight than recordings that contain less noise (Bayesian statistics; see (*17, 18*) sorted averages (*19*)). This assignment of different weights to each response, depending on the noise content before the responses are added, can increase the efficiency of signal averaging when the level of the background noise varies over time (*16, 18*).

Averaging Slowly Varying Evoked Potentials. When signal averaging is used to enhance signals that are buried in noise, it must be remembered that the validity of this technique is based on the assumptions that the waveform of the signals does not change during the period over which averaging is performed and that the time relationship to the stimulus is unchanged during the period over which responses are collected. However, evoked potentials that are recorded during operations often change slowly over time because the potentials are affected by surgical manipulations. The task of monitoring is to detect such changes and advise the surgeon accordingly. But since these potentials change over time, the averaged response (the arithmetic mean of these changing potentials over a period of time) will be different from the waveforms of the individual responses that were collected; further, the amplitude of the averaged response will be smaller than it would have been if the responses that were collected were identical. This is particularly important to bear in mind when many responses are averaged over long time periods, and the problem is particularly noticeable when ABR are recorded under unfavorable conditions (low amplitude and large amount of interference) where collection of enough responses may take 1 min or more.

Reducing the time over which the responses are averaged can reduce this problem. Filtering of the recorded signal can reduce the number of recordings that must be summed in order to obtain an interpretable record. The time for obtaining an interpretable record can be reduced substantially by using optimal filtering such as zero-phase digital filtering. It is naturally important to use optimal recording conditions with optimal placement of recording electrodes, optimal stimulation, and reduction of interference as much as possible (discussed in Chaps. 6 and 7).

Quality Control of Evoked Potentials. When signal averaging is used to recover signals buried in noise, the neurophysiologist must ascertain if the averaged waveform is the signal (evoked potential) and not just filtered noise. The replication of averaged recordings is the standard clinical way of verifying that an averaged response is a valid physiological response and not just noise that happens to look like a response. Since the time it takes to obtain an interpretable recording is important in intraoperative monitoring, this method is disadvantageous because it increases the time it takes to obtain an interpretable record. When aggressive filtering is performed after signal averaging, the waveform of filtered noise may many times resemble evoked potentials making it even more important to have means to ensure that the displayed potentials are an evoked response rather than just filtered noise.

One method to obtain a measure of the reliability of an averaged response compares an averaged response with a similar average in which every other recording is inverted (± average) (18, 20, 21). Adding and subtracting every other response cancels any signal that is identical, and thus any evoked potential will be canceled by this procedure. This method provides quantitative measures of the validity of recorded potentials such as far-field evoked potentials without requiring replication of the record. It makes use of the assumption that recorded evoked potentials to every stimulus are identical, whereas the superimposed noise varies from time to time. The ratio between the root mean square (RMS) value of the ordinary average and that of the ±average becomes a measure of the amount of noise that the averaged response contains. If the response is an authentic evoked potential (thus, different from noise), this ratio will increase as more and more responses are added.

This method for quality control does not prolong the time it takes to obtain an interpretable recording because the ±average can be obtained simultaneously with ordinary averaging. Other ways of achieving quality control make use of the ratio of variance (the RMS value is the square root of the variance; hence, the RMS values are equivalent to the square root of the values used by Wong and Bickford (21)). Other methods for quality control of evoked potentials have been described, and some of these are implemented in some of the

commercially available equipment for use in the operating room.

How to Reduce the Effect of Electrical Interference

Chapter 17 discussed how to identify sources of electrical interference and how to reduce the amount of electrical interference that reaches the input of the recording amplifies. It is not always possible to eliminate electrical interference to an extent that that it does not interfere noticeably with recorded neuroelectric potentials. Here we will discuss how to reduce the effect of interference that reaches the recording system.

Interference signals often contain noticeable energy at much higher frequencies than the neuroelectric potentials. Appropriate filtering should make it possible to reduce such high-frequency interference, the spectrum of which is outside that of the neuroelectric potentials that are recorded in connection with intraoperative monitoring and other neurophysiological recordings. However, this may only be possible if the filtering is done before the signals are sampled and digitized. After sampling, aliasing can transpose high-frequency signals into the low-frequency range of neuroelectric potentials and thus, make such high-frequency noise interfere with responses at much lower frequencies. Aliasing occurs when the sampling rate is too low or when high-frequency components are not attenuated sufficiently before sampling and digitizing. Therefore, aliasing is more important with regard to electrical interference than to the recorded neuroelectric potentials, as mentioned briefly above.

The problem of aliasing is probably greatest in connection with averaging of evoked potentials, but can be a problem in connection with any recorded potentials because practically all modern equipment for intraoperative monitoring digitizes recorded potentials from the nervous system before they are displayed or processed.

An example of interference signals that was picked up by recording electrodes and which contained components of much higher frequencies than the recorded neuroelectric potentials is shown in **Fig. 18.2**. The spectrum of the

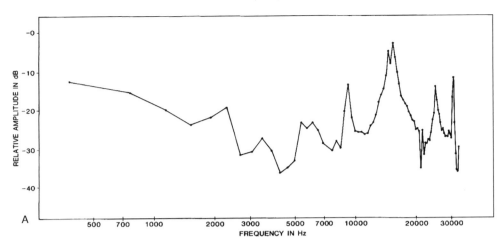

Figure 18.2: The spectrum of typical interference picked up by electrodes placed on the vertex and earlobe for differential recording of ABR in a patient undergoing an operation to relieve hemifacial spasm. The sampling rate was 100 kHz. (Reprinted from (27)).

signals was recorded from electrodes placed on the vertex and the earlobe in a patient undergoing an operation where the auditory nerve was at risk.

As seen from **Fig. 18.2**, sharp peaks of high amplitudes appear in the spectrum at frequencies of 9.8 kHz, 16 kHz, 25.7 kHz, and 31.6 kHz. The amplitude of the 16-kHz component was approximately 10 μV peak-to-peak at the input of the amplifier. Tests using a wire loop (Figs. 17.2 and 17.3) done after the operation with all equipment on showed evidence of magnetic fields at 16-kHz and we drew the conclusion that the 16 kHz interference signal that appears as a peak in the spectrum of interference seen in **Fig. 18.2** was generated the same magnetic field as detected by the wire loop. The wire loop test showed that the interference came from a video monitor. Similar tests indicated that the 25-kHz signal seen in the spectrogram in **Fig. 18.2** was generated by the blood pressure monitoring equipment, and the cable to a disposable pressure transducer radiated the signal mainly as a magnetic field. Again, these are examples only. Other kinds of equipment may generate interference signals that are different and which have other spectra.

The interference shown in **Fig. 18.2** was thus generated by specific equipment used in an operating room. Since equipment that is used in the operating room changes with technological developments, similar signals may not be present in an operating room at a given time, but the spectrogram may serve as an example of interference that may be present in an operating room.

The large high-frequency signals in this particular interference have their energy outside the spectrum of the biological signals that are of interest in connection with intraoperative neurophysiological monitoring, but they may exert their effect as interference signals because aliasing may transpose the signals to lower parts of the spectrum after sampling and digitizing and these transposed signals may, therefore, interfere with the recorded neuroelectrical potentials. Aliasing may occur if high-frequency signals are not sufficiently attenuated by a low-pass filter before being sampled and digitized or because the sampling rate used is too low.

What Is Aliasing and How to Avoid It

Display, storage, and processing of recorded signals are performed after the signals are converted to a string of numbers (digitized). For that, the signals are sampled in time and that is where aliasing can occur. Aliasing describes what happens when a signal that contains energy at frequencies higher than one-half the sampling rate is digitized (the Nyquist frequency). When signals that contain energy above the Nyquist frequency are digitized, the digital version of the signals becomes folded around the Nyquist frequency and spectral components above the Nyquist frequency are transposed into lower frequencies.

The use of low-pass filters to reduce the risk of aliasing of high-frequency signals before sampling and conversion to digital form was discussed earlier in this chapter (page 349). The risk that high-frequency signals are transposed to lower frequency ranges is a noticeable risk regarding interference signals encountered in the operating room, which often contain energy at much higher frequencies than the neuroelectric potentials that are recorded.

> The Nyquist Theorem tells us that we can sample and digitize frequency components correctly up to one-half the sampling frequency and preserve the signal faithfully as a digital record. The sampling frequency, therefore, determines the highest frequency component that can be handled correctly. Thus, if a sampling frequency of 25 kHz (sampling interval of 40 µs) is chosen, only signals with frequencies below 12.5 kHz will be correctly reproduced in the digitized waveform. Signals with frequencies higher than half the sampling rate (known as the Nyquist frequency) will be "folded" around the Nyquist frequency after sampling and thus, appear as components with a lower frequency in the digitized record. The signal, the spectrum of which is displayed in **Fig. 18.2**, was sampled at 100 kHz, thus a Nyquist frequency of 50 kHz.

Signals that are to be converted into digital form must, therefore, not contain (noticeable) energy at frequencies above the Nyquist frequency. In practice, the sampling rate has to be kept somewhat higher than twice the upper frequency limit of interest, and the input signal must be properly filtered to sufficiently reduce the content of signals at frequencies higher than half the sampling rate.

High-frequency components must, therefore, be attenuated by suitable (analog) low-pass filtering before they are sampled and digitized. This is why electronic (analog) low-pass filters are necessary in all equipment that collect and process potentials recorded from the nervous system. It is in this connection that the slope of the low-pass filter used becomes important.

The effect of using different sampling frequencies is illustrated in **Fig. 18.3**, which shows how correct sampling of a sinusoidal signal can reproduce the signal correctly, while sampling at too few points (**Fig. 18.3B**) can distort the signal and create signals with frequencies that do not exist in the original signal before sampling has been performed.

In the example in **Fig. 18.3A**, a sinusoidal signal with the frequency of 2.2 kHz is sampled at an 8 kHz sampling rate, and it is correctly reproduced in the digitized form as a 2.2 kHz sinusoid. When a 7 kHz sinusoid is sampled in the same way (at a sampling rate of 8 kHz), a 1 kHz sinusoidal wave is created instead of the 7 kHz signal (**Fig. 18.3B**). Sampling a 7 kHz sine wave at an 8 kHz sampling rate violates the sampling theorem. This means that the 7 kHz signal that was sampled does not appear as a 7 kHz signal in the digitized form, but rather as a 1 kHz signal (8–7 kHz = 1 kHz).

However, it is rare that biological potentials from the nervous system contain energy at 7 kHz. It is much more likely that such high-frequency components are interference signals as seen in **Fig. 18.2**. Interference signals may have significant energy at such high frequencies.

Thus, it is obvious that low-frequency components can arise from aliasing of high-frequency interference components that are not sufficiently attenuated by the analog filters before the signal is sampled and converted to digital form. The low-pass filters that are usually built into physiological amplifiers, such as those commonly used to record evoked potentials, often have a slope of only 12 or even only 6 dB/octave. A low-pass filter with a slope of 6 dB/

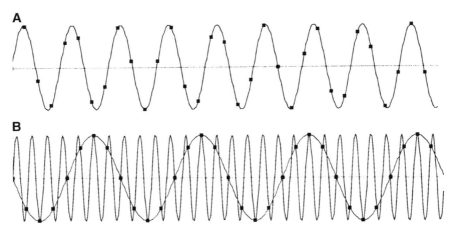

Figure 18.3: A sinusoidal signal at different frequencies that is sampled at 8 kHz (125 μs interval) (Nyquist frequency of 4 kHz). (**A**) A 2.2 kHz sine wave, sampled at 8 kHz. The sampling points are indicated by squares. (**B**) A 7 kHz sine wave, sampled at 8 kHz. The superimposed sine wave shows the 1 kHz wave that results from aliasing. From: Applet demonstration.

octave and set at a cut-off frequency of 3 kHz will only have an attenuation of 20 dB at 30 kHz and 14 dB at 15 kHz, which means an attenuation of only five times. This degree of attenuation is often insufficient to attenuate the high-frequency interference signals that can occur in the operating room to a degree that the aliased components do not interfere with recording of neuroelectrical potentials.

A change in the slope of the attenuation of the low-pass filters in the amplifiers with a cut-off frequency of 3 kHz used to amplify evoked potentials from 6 dB/octave to 24 dB/octave increased the attenuation to 40 dB at 13.6 kHz, which means that a 13.6-kHz signal is attenuated by a factor of about 100 (and signals at frequencies above 13.6 kHz are attenuated more).

The same results as those obtained by this extra filtering could have been achieved by using a sampling rate of 100 kHz and an observation window of 1,024 data points, instead of 256, and then using digital filtering of the averaged response to remove the high-frequency components. This, however, increases the size of the computer file of the recorded data and requires more computer power for processing the data, because a larger number of samples are generated

in each recording. With the advances of more powerful computers with large memory sizes, this should no longer be a concern.

Thus, the effect of aliasing on high-frequency interference can be reduced either by adequate filtering of the signal before it is sampled or by increasing the sampling rate. The choice of which one of these two options to use depends on the availability of suitable analog filters and on the computer power that is available. If faster computers are available, increasing the sampling rate for solving the problems associated with interference from high-frequency signals may be preferred over analog filtering.

In summary, aliasing is avoided (or reduced) by using a sufficiently high sampling frequency and adequately low-pass filtering the signal that is to be sampled and digitized so that components of the signal that have energy above the Nyquist frequency are sufficiently attenuated. Unfortunately, modern equipment for intraoperative monitoring rarely allows the user to select the sampling frequency (or even know what it is), and when low-pass filters are concerned, usually only the cut-off frequencies are given in the specifications, which omit important information about the slope of the attenuation of the filters.

Filtering of Digitized Signals

Digitized signals can be filtered using computer programs (software), while analog filtering must be performed by electronic devices (analog filters). The type of filtering discussed above was analog filtering, which had to be made before the sampling and digitizing to reduce the effect of aliasing. While digital filtering is the most suitable way of filtering evoked potentials and other neuroelectric recordings for obtaining an interpretable record, analog filtering is necessary before digitizing.

Digital filters that operate on digital signals have many advantages over analog filtering of the analog signal. In connection with signal averaging, the averaged response is filtered, rather than the signal before it is averaged. Because the averaging process is a linear process that consists of a summation of responses, filtering after averaging is equivalent to filtering before averaging, except that the artifact rejection will not be affected by the filtering and may, therefore, work differently, depending on whether the filtering is performed before or after averaging.

Digital filters are computer programs that can filter signals in a similar way as analog filters can filter analog signals, thus digital filters can be designed to emulate analog filters, but digital filters can also be designed to perform filtering that cannot be made by analog filters and such filters offer several advantages over analog filters. Digital filters that are implemented in commercially available equipment for intraoperative monitoring are often designed to emulate ordinary analog filters such as Butterworth filters having low-pass, high-pass, or band-pass characteristics.

Most analog filters shift components of recorded potentials – such as peaks and valleys – in time by an amount that depends on the spectrum of the individual peaks in relation to the filter's cut-off frequency and the type of filter that is used. This severely limits the use of analog filters for aggressive filtering of recordings of evoked potentials where interpretation depends on the ability to determine the absolute values of the latencies of different peaks, such as is the case in the clinic. The reason that ordinary analog filters shift the different components of a signal differently is that the phase shift that they introduce is not a linear function of frequency (22, 23).

Common analog high-pass filters can also cause severe distortion of the waveform and even cause waveform peaks to appear inverted (24). If the phase shift was a linear function of frequency, the shift in time would be the same for all components of a signal's waveform, such as the ABR or the SSEP, and the shift in time could, therefore, be easily compensated for by adding a certain value to the observed latency time of the various peaks. However, such filters are more difficult to design than conventional analog filters (25). The only analog filter that has a phase shift that is a linear function of frequency is the Bessel filter, which is rarely used (25).

The errors introduced by phase shifts are largest when analog high-pass filters that have a steep slope of attenuation are used, but low-pass filters also have phase shifts that can cause peaks of a response to shift in time.

While analog filters must obey laws of physics, which implies that they can only operate on the past history of a signal, digital filters can operate on signals as they might appear in the future. Digital filters can be designed to attenuate signals according to their spectrum (high- and low-pass filters) that have exactly the same attenuation of signals above or below a certain frequency as ordinary analog filters, but without a phase shift ("zero-phase digital filters"). However, there are many other advantages that can be gained by proper design of digital filters. Digital filters can be designed to operate on the waveform of a signal, and they can enhance specific components of the waveform of a signal and attenuate components of the response that are not important for its interpretation.

Proper selection of filtering techniques can enhance particular features of the response that are of interest, such as the peaks in the ABR or SSEP, thereby making it easier to interpret the recordings (see Chaps. 6 and 7). This is important when evoked potentials are used as a diagnostic aid in the clinic, but it may be even more important for obtaining an interpretable recording in the operating room where interference may be greater and where it is important to be able to interpret the recording with fewer averaged responses because of the necessity to obtain an interpretable record in as short a time as possible.

When evoked potentials are filtered to suppress noise (improve the SNR), the goal is usually to avoid, as much as possible, attenuating the spectrum of the response while attenuating the energy that is outside the spectrum of the signal as much as possible. However, the assumption that the entire spectrum of evoked potentials must be preserved in order to obtain an interpretable record is not always valid: often only parts of the spectrum of the evoked responses are important for interpreting potentials such as ABR, SSEP, and VEP. For instance, it is easy to show that the low-frequency components of the ABR do not contribute to the identification of the peaks of the response. Evoked potentials such as the ABR are often rich in low-frequency components, and reducing the low-frequency components of the recorded responses makes it easier to identify the peaks.

Filtering may affect the recorded response unfavorably. For example, as mentioned above, the use of analog filters can shift components in time and thereby, affect the measurement of the latency of individual components of the responses. Even worse, analog filters can prolong a sharp, initial stimulus artifact so that it obscures parts of the response.

Digital filters can be implemented in different ways. If implemented in the time domain using convolution between the (digitized) signal and a weighting function (equivalent to a filter's finite duration impulse response), no spread of energy beyond the duration of their impulse response will occur independently of how large the amplitudes of a component (such as a stimulus artifact) of the signals that are being filtered are.

Filtering in the Time Domain. Analog filtering is done in the frequency domain and the characteristics of such filters are described as their attenuation as a function of the frequency of the signals that they filter. The filtering that is performed by analog filters can be emulated on computers and the filtering can be done either in the frequency domain or the time domain.

There are several advantages to filtering in the time domain and describing the filter function by its weighting function (corresponding to an analog filter's impulse response) rather than by its frequency transfer function (*26*). The arithmetic operation of filtering in the time domain consists of convolving the signal that is to be filtered with a weighting function. The "signal" is a digital file. Filtering in the time domain may use more computing power than filtering in the frequency domain, but the abundance of generally available computing power in modern equipment makes the difference in computational requirements for time domain filtering compared with frequency domain filtering irrelevant.

Stimulus artifacts are often troublesome despite the fact that they occur earlier in a record of evoked potentials than the components of the recorded potentials that are of interest. Conventional high-pass filtering or low-pass filtering can cause the stimulus artifact (especially in such recordings as ABR and SSEP) to interfere with the actual response because the artifact is prolonged by filtering (and by overloading of the amplifier, see page 348). This "smearing" in time of transients, such as stimulus artifacts, occurs in connection with the use of analog filters or digital filters that are emulations of high- and low-pass analog filters. However, the prolongation of the stimulus artifact can be limited by using finite impulse response digital filters. Because of their limited impulse response, such filters cause a limited spread of transient components such as stimulus artifacts. Using such filters implemented in the time domain will limit the duration of a transient such as a stimulus artifact to the duration of the filter's weighting function because such filters have zero transmission for any event after a (short) time that is equal to the width of the filter's impulse response.

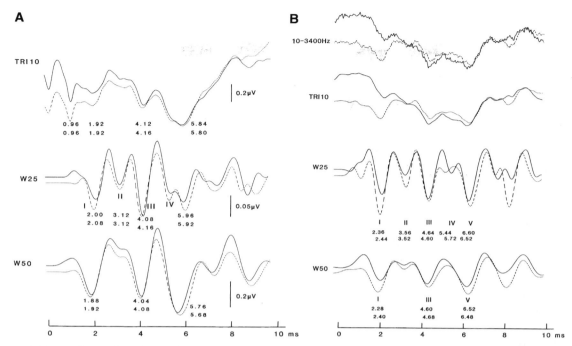

Figure 18.4: The effect of digital filtering using the same filters as illustrated in Chap. 7, **Fig. 7.4**, but obtained in the operating room from a patient undergoing an MVD operation of CNVIII. These graphs show the same response filtered with different zero-phase finite impulse response digital filters. The responses were filtered by an analog filter (top tracing) before analog-digital conversion and averaging was done. The averaged responses were filtered with three different digital filters (TRI 10, W25, and W50). The weighting functions for the three different digital filters are shown in **Fig. 18.5**. The latency values of the vertex positive peaks were printed using "hands-off" computer programs that automatically identified the peaks and printed their latencies. (Reprinted from: (*27*)).

Such zero-phase finite impulse digital filters can perform the same attenuation of spectral components as analog filters and without causing any shift in the location of the components of recorded potentials (*22, 26*).

Practical Use of Digital Filters in Intraoperative Monitoring. The efficiency of filtering with different zero-phase finite impulse response digital filters in enhancing the peaks of ABR recordings is demonstrated in Fig. 18.4, which shows ABR obtained in a patient undergoing a neurosurgical operation. (The effect of similar kinds of filtering of ABR obtained in the laboratory in an individual with normal hearing was shown in Chap. 7).

A filter that has a triangular weighting function (TRI 10 in **Fig. 18.5**) only smoothes the ABR curve. The ABR filtered by the two other filters, W25 and W50, have characteristics that allow the peaks of the ABR to appear more clearly, and computer programs can identify the peaks and print the latencies "hands off" (**Fig. 18.4**). These two filters have weighting functions that resembled truncated sinc functions $(\sin(x)/x)$ (**Fig. 18.5**). The W50 filter reproduces peaks I, III, and V of the ABR, but does not usually reproduce peak II and peak IV. The filter that is suitable for use in clinical testing (W25) (*28*) has a narrower weighting function than the W50 filter, and it is seen to reproduce all of the peaks in the ABR

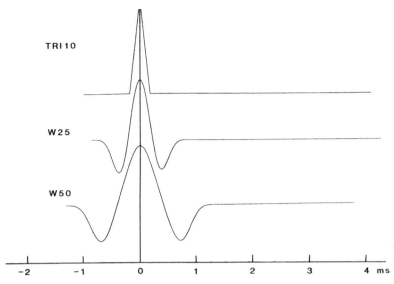

Figure 18.5: Weighting functions of three zero-phase digital filters with finite impulse response. The time scale assumes a sampling interval of 40 μs. (Reprinted from (*27*)).

(**Fig. 18.4**). The greater noise suppression by the W50 filter makes that filter more suitable for use in intraoperative monitoring of ABR.

The shapes of the frequency transfer function of the three filters (**Fig. 18.6**), the weighting functions of which are shown in **Fig. 18.5**, are different from that of common analog band-pass filters. Only the filter with the triangular weighting function (TRI 10) has a transfer function that is similar to an analog low-pass filter and reproduces signals with no attenuation up to a certain frequency, above which it attenuates the signal to a degree that increases with increasing frequency. The W25 and W50 filters attenuate both low- and high-frequency spectral components of the signal, but they do not produce a response with a flat portion as found in commonly used analog filters. The shapes of the frequency transfer functions of these two filters (**Fig. 18.6**), thus differ from those of the analog low- and high-pass filters.

The digital filters discussed above have no phase shift – the peaks in a record that are filtered by these filters appear precisely at the same location as before filtering; however, if similar filtering had been accomplished by using analog (electronic) filters, the latencies of

the peaks would have been shifted in time and with a different amount for different settings of the cut-off frequencies of the analog filters.

Because the digital filters illustrated above attenuate the background noise in addition to enhancing specific features of the signal that is filtered, two advantages have been gained:

1. A clearer waveform is produced, making more accurate interpretation possible.
2. A reduction in noise is produced, with the obvious consequence that fewer responses need to be averaged in order to obtain an interpretable recording, and consequently, an interpretable record can be obtained in a shorter time.

These advantages are illustrated in the example ABR obtained during a neurosurgical operation shown in **Fig. 18.7**. While the unfiltered averaged responses are noisy to an extent that makes it impossible to identify any of the peaks except peak V, peaks I, II, and III appear clearly after filtering with the W50 digital filter.

It would be difficult to determine the latencies of any of the peaks of the ABR in **Fig. 18.8** from examining the raw recordings. Low-pass

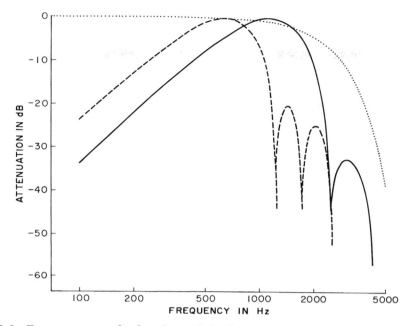

Figure 18.6: Frequency transfer functions of the three digital filters, the weighting functions of which are seen in **Fig. 18.5**: TRI 10, *dotted lines*; W25, *solid lines*; W50, *dashed lines*. The frequency scale corresponds to a sampling rate of 25 kHz. (Reprinted from (*27*)).

filtering using the triangular weighting function improves the recording to a point where it may be possible to identify peak V, but not without some difficulty. However, after filtering with the W50 digital filter (**Fig. 18.8**), the record shows a clearly identifiable and reproducible peak V, and possibly also a peak III. The resulting filtered recording demonstrates that digital filtering can improve the quality of the averaged responses of ABR of low amplitude and strong interference.

It is important to emphasize that the weighting functions of finite impulse zero-phase digital filters, such as those just described, do not have time as their horizontal axis, as does the impulse response of an analog (electronic) filter. Rather, the weighting functions of digital filters have the number of samples as the horizontal axis. Thus, the time axis depends on the sampling interval that is used: the weighting function of the triangular filter shown in **Fig. 18.5** is eight samples wide, which means that it is 0.8 ms wide when a 100 μs sampling

interval is used, but it is 0.32 ms wide when a 40 μs sampling interval is used, as is the case when recording ABR.

More Complex Filtering. Several "intelligent" ways to filter evoked potentials and extract information from potentials obscured by noise that is not stationary random noise have been proposed and tested (*17, 29, 30*). When the spectrum of the signal (for instance, evoked potentials) and that of the unwanted background noise are both known, it is possible to design a filter that will separate the signal from the noise in an optimal way so that it provides the greatest possible reduction in the mean square difference (error) between the response and the true response. The mathematical basis for this is known as "Wiener filtering" (*30, 31*), and it presumes that the signal (such as evoked potentials) does not vary during the observation time and that the noise is a stationary broadband noise. The method further requires that the spectrum of the signal (such as an evoked potential without noise) and that of the background noise are known. However, this kind of complex

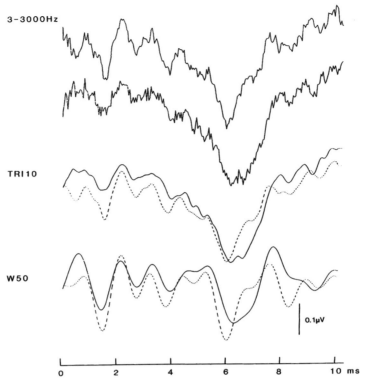

Figure 18.7: Recording of ABR from an electrode placed on the vertex using a noncephalic reference obtained from a patient during an operation to relieve hemifacial spasm. The two upper curves are repetitions of summations of 2,048 responses using a filter setting of 3–3,000 Hz (6 dB/octave). The curves labeled TRI 10 are the same recordings (the repetition is shown by the *dashed line*), but after low-pass filtering with the TRI10 filter. The curves labeled W50 show the same recording, but after digital band-pass filtering with the W50 filter (the weighting functions of the digital filters are shown in **Fig. 18.5**). The sampling rate was 25 kHz and each record consists of 256 data points. (Reprinted from (*27*)).

processing of evoked potentials is not commonly incorporated in commercially available equipment for intraoperative monitoring.

Other more sophisticated systems for filtering evoked potentials make use of two-dimensional filtering based on Fourier analysis of the raw responses computed along the time axis as well as along the cross-trial sequence axis. Such filtering has been proven effective in processing of evoked potentials (*17*) by a method similar to that used for image processing (*32*). One of the great advantages of these methods is that they can be used when the evoked potentials change during the recording period. The feasibility of such processing was demonstrated

many years ago when the main limitation was the availability of sufficient computing power (*17*). With the present state of computers, such analyses could be made using standard personal computers.

More complex methods for enhancing signals in noise using adaptive filtering have been described recently (*33*). The results using an "adaptive signal enhancer" in connection with averaging of SSEP were described by Lam et al. (2004) (*34*). Although there has been little practical experience in the use of such signal processing, it seems to be powerful and may represent one very efficient way to quickly obtain interpretable responses.

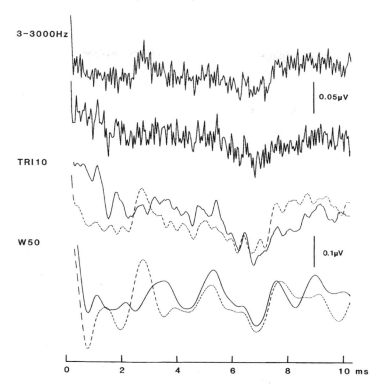

Figure 18.8: Similar recordings of ABR as in **Figs. 18.4, 18.6,** and **18.7,** but from a patient who had a low amplitude of the ABR in addition to the presence of severe interference. The two top curves are consecutive recordings showing the average of 2,048 responses each. These two recordings appear as *solid and dashed lines* in the digitally filtered responses (TRI 10 and W50 filters) in the two lower pairs of curves. The sampling rate was 25 kHz and each record consists of 256 data points. (Reprinted from (*27*)).

Reducing Stimulus Artifacts

When an electrical stimulus is used to elicit the response that is to be monitored, some of the stimulus current may spread to the sites of the recording electrodes and thereby, be amplified in a way similar to that of the response. This type of interference is known as the stimulus artifact. The electrical signals that are used to drive an earphone to generate an acoustic stimulus can act in a similar way and cause stimulus artifacts to appear in the recorded signal. Magnetic types of acoustic transducers (such as earphones of older design) generate a magnetic field that may also give rise to a stimulus artifact because the magnetic

field can create electric currents in the electrode leads. Unshielded earphone leads may cause interference from the electrical signal used to drive the earphone if the leads are unshielded and placed close to the recording electrode leads.

The largest and most troublesome stimulus artifacts usually appear in connection with electrical stimulation. Since the duration of the electrical impulses used to drive transducers (100 μs) such as earphones is as short as the duration of the electrical impulses used to stimulate nerves (50–200 μs), the stimulus artifact does not overlap in time with the response, and the stimulus artifact itself should, therefore, not interfere with the response. The stimulus artifacts only become a problem when they are smeared out in time (prolonged) by the action of the amplifiers and filters so that they interfere with the recorded potentials. In some instances, the interference from the stimulus artifact may be so severe that it totally obscures the response.

The most common reason for prolongation of stimulus artifacts is filtering especially by the use of analog filters or digital filters that are emulations of analog filters, but amplifiers may prolong the stimulus artifact if the stimulus artifact overloads the amplifiers.

One way to reduce the effect of a stimulus artifact is, therefore, to prevent the stimulus artifact from overloading the amplifier and from entering the filters used. As mentioned above, the use of finite impulse response digital filters can limit the "smearing" of stimulus artifacts by digital filters.

When recording is to be made close to the site of stimulation, as is the case when measuring the nerve conduction time of an exposed nerve, the bipolar recording technique and bipolar stimulation should be used. For electrical stimulation, choosing optimal position for the stimulating electrode and using low amplification to avoid overload of amplifiers are especially important measures to reduce stimulus artifacts. Even more effective in reducing the stimulus artifact is the use of a tripolar electrode (35, 36) (Chap. 15).

When signal averaging is used, alternating the polarity of the stimulus is widely used when recording auditory evoked potentials (alternating rarefaction and condensation clicks); however, this technique should be used cautiously, because the stimulus of one polarity may elicit responses that are different from the responses elicited with the inverted polarity. This difference is particularly pronounced in patients with high-frequency hearing loss, such as that commonly seen in elderly patients. Electrically evoked responses from nerves are also dependent on the polarity of the stimulation, and alternating the polarity of the stimuli is, therefore, not advisable.

Stimulus artifacts can be removed digitally from a digitized record before the signal is filtered. This way to eliminate stimulus artifacts was used in the illustrations in **Figs. 18.4**, **18.6**, and **18.7**. When this technique is used in connection with digital filters that have finite impulse responses and which are implemented in the time domain rather than in the frequency domain, it is unnecessary to use shielded earphones when recording ABR intraoperatively, and this combination has considerably reduced the effects of the stimulus artifact on responses that are elicited by electrical stimulation.

In summary for averaged evoked potentials, selecting the proper type of filtering (finite impulse zero-phase digital filters) and removing the stimulus artifact from the averaged signal using computer programs before it is subjected to digital filtering are measures that normally can reduce the appearance of stimulus artifacts to acceptable levels.

REFERENCES

1. Møller AR and PJ Jannetta (1984) Preservation of facial function during removal of acoustic neuromas: Use of monopolar constant voltage stimulation and EMG. J. Neurosurg. 61:757–60.
2. Yingling C (1994) Intraoperative monitoring in skull base surgery, in *Neurotology*, RK Jackler and DE Brackmann, Editors. Mosby: St. Louis. 967–1002.
3. Stecker MM (2004) Nerve stimulation with an electrode of finite size: Differences between constant current and constant voltage stimulation. Comput. Biol. Med. 34:51–94.
4. Yingling C and J Gardi (1992) Intraoperative monitoring of facial and cochlear nerves during acoustic neuroma surgery. Otolaryngol. Clin. North Am. 25:413–48.
5. Prass R and H Lueders (1985) Constant-current versus constant-voltage stimulation. J. Neurosurg. 62(4):622–3.
6. Kartush J and K Bouchard (1992) Intraoperative facial monitoring. Otology, neurotology, and skull base surgery, in *Neuromonitoring in Otology and Head and Neck Surgery*, J Kartush

and K Bouchard, Editors. Raven Press: New York. 99–120.

7. Møller AR (2006) Hearing: Anatomy, Physiology, and Disorders of the Auditory System, 2nd Ed. Amsterdam: Academic Press.

8. Møller AR (1987) Electrophysiological monitoring of cranial nerves in operations in the skull base, in *Tumors of the Cranial Base: Diagnosis and Treatment*, LN Sekhar and VL Schramm Jr., Editors. Futura Publishing Co.: Mt. Kisco, New York. 123–32.

9. Pratt H, WH Martin, N Bleich et al (1994) A high-intensity, goggle-mounted flash stimulator for short-latency visual evoked potentials. Electroencephalogr. Clin. Neurophysiol. 92:469–72.

10. Prass RL, SE Kinney, RW Hardy et al (1987) Acoustic (loudspeaker) facial electromyographic monitoring: Part II. Use of evoked EMG activity during acoustic neuroma resection. Otolaryngol. Head Neck Surg. 97:541–51.

11. Prass RL and H Lueders (1986) Acoustic (loudspeaker) facial electromyographic monitoring. Part I. Neurosurgery 19(3):392–400.

12. Jako G (1965) Facial nerve monitor. Trans. Am. Acad. Ophthalmol. Otolaryngol. 69:340–2.

13. Sugita K and S Kobayashi (1982) Technical and instrumental improvements in the surgical treatment of acoustic neurinomas. J. Neurosurg. 57(6):747–52.

14. Lanser M, R Jackler and C Yingling (1992) Regional monitoring of the lower (ninth through twelfth) cranial nerves, in *Intraoperative Monitoring in Otology and Head and Neck Surgery*, J Kartush and K Bouchard, Editors. Raven Press: New York. 131–50.

15. MacDonald D (2001) Indiividually optimizing posterior tibial somatosensory evoked potential P37 scalp derivations for intraoperative monitoring. J. Clin. Neurophysiol. 18:364–71.

16. Hoke M, B Ross, R Wickesberg et al (1984) Weighted averaging: Theory and application to electrical response audiometry. Electroencephalogr. Clin. Neurophysiol. 57:484–9.

17. Sgro J, R Emerson and T Pedley (1989) Methods for steadily updating the averaged responses during neuromonitoring, in *Neuromonitoring in Surgery*, J Desmedt, Editor. Elsevier Science Publishers: Amsterdam. 49–60.

18. Elberling C (1984) Quality estimation of averaged auditory brainstem responses. Scand. Audiol. 13:187–97.

19. Muhler R and H von Specht (1999) Sorted averaging: Principle and application to auditory brainstem responses. Scand. Audiol. 28:145–9.

20. Schimmel H (1967) The (+/−) reference: Accuracy of estimated mean components in average response studies. Science 157:92–4.

21. Wong PKH and RG Bickford (1980) Brain stem auditory potentials: The use of noise estimate. Electroencephalogr. Clin. Neurophysiol. 50:25–34.

22. Doyle DJ and ML Hyde (1981) Analogue and digital filtering of auditory brainstem responses. Scand. Audiol. 10(2):81–9.

23. Boston JR and PJ Ainslie (1980) Effects of analog and digital filtering on brain stem auditory evoked potentials. Electroencephalogr. Clin. Neurophysiol. 48:361–4.

24. Janssen R, VA Benignus, LM Grimes et al (1986) Unrecognized errors due to analog filtering of brain-stem auditory evoked responses. Electroencephalogr. Clin. Neurophysiol. 65:203–11.

25. Doyle DJ and ML Hyde (1981) Bessel filtering of brain stem auditory evoked potentials. Electroencephalogr. Clin. Neurophysiol. 51:446–8.

26. Møller AR (1988) Use of zero-phase digital filters to enhance brainstem auditory evoked potentials (BAEPs). Electroencephalogr. Clin. Neurophysiol. 71:226–32.

27. Møller AR (1988) Evoked potentials in intraoperative monitoring. Baltimore: Williams and Wilkins.

28. Møller MB and AR Møller (1983) Brainstem auditory evoked potentials in patients with cerebellopontine angle tumors. Ann. Otol. Rhinol. Laryngol. 92:645–50.

29. Boston JR and AR Møller (1985) Brainstem auditory evoked potentials. Crit. Rev. Biomed. Eng. 13(2):97–123.

30. Walter DO (1969) A posterior "Wiener filtering" of average evoked responses. Electroencephalogr. Clin. Neurophysiol. 27:61–70.

31. Doyle DJ (1975) Some comments on the use of Wiener filtering for the estimation of evoked potentials. Electroencephalogr. Clin. Neurophysiol. 38:533–4.

32. Gonzalez RC (1977) Digital image processing. Boston MA: Addison-Wesley Publishing Co.

33. Lin BS, FC Chong and F Lai (2005) Adaptive filtering of evoked potentials using higher-order adaptive signal enhancer with genetic-type vari-

able step-size prefilter. Med. Biol. Eng. Comput. 43:638–47.

34. Lam BS, Y Hu, WW Lu et al (2004) Validation of an adaptive signal enhancer in intraoperative somatosensory evoked potentials monitoring. J. Clin. Neurophysiol. 21:409–17.

35. Happel L and D Kline (2002) Intraoperative Neurophysiology of the Peripheral Nervous System, in *Neurophysiology in Neurosurgery*, V Deletis and JL Shils, Editors. Academic Press: Amsterdam. 169–95.

36. Happel L and D Kline (1991) Nerve lesions in continuity, in *Operative nerve repair and reconstruction 1st ed vol 1*, RH Gelberman, Editor. J.B. Lippincott: Philadelphia. 601–16.

19

Evaluating the Benefits of Intraoperative Neurophysiological Monitoring

INTRODUCTION

The benefits from monitoring that are aimed at reducing postoperative neurological deficits should be evaluated on their abilities to reduce the risk of iatrogenic injuries to the nervous system in patients who are operated upon and to improve the quality of medical care in general, as well as on their ability to provide economic savings in the service of evidence based medicine.[1] Intraoperative monitoring of the facial nerve has been regarded as a standard of care in connection with surgical removal of vestibular schwannoma for many years (1). Investigators (Sala et al. 2002 (2)) have con-cluded that published studies provide sufficient evidence to recommend intraoperative monitoring as a standard of care in many kinds of surgical operations. After they surveyed various studies in the literature on outcome and complications, these authors recommend that monitoring be performed in operations on supratentorial CNS structures (tumors, aneurysms, etc.), brain stem tumors, intramedullary spinal cord tumors, conus and cauda equina tumors, rhizotomy for relief of spasticity and spina bifida with tethered cord.

Somatosensory evoked potential (SSEP) monitoring is generally regarded beneficial in intraoperative assessment of the functional

---

[1]Evidence based medicine: process and use of relevant information from peer-reviewed clinical and epidemiologic research to address a specific clinical issue, and thereby weighing the attendant risks and benefits of diagnostic tests and therapeutic measures; literature to address a specific clinical problem; the application of simple rules of science and common sense to determine the validity of the information; and the application of the information to the clinical problem (Stedman's Electronic Medical Dictionary).

From: *Intraoperative Neurophysiological Monitoring: Third Edition,*
By A.R. Møller, DOI 10.1007/978-1-4419-7436-5_19,
© Springer Science+Business Media, LLC 2011

integrity of sensory pathways including peripheral nerves, the dorsal column, and the somatosensory cortex. Since SSEP cannot provide reliable information on the functional integrity of the motor system, these authors (Sala et al. 2002, (2)) also conclude that monitoring of MEP is an important part to assess the functional integrity of descending motor pathways in the brain, the brain stem and, especially, the spinal cord.

While recording auditory brainstem responses (ABR) has for many years been regarded the standard technique for neurophysiologic monitoring in operations in the cerebellopontine angle and the posterior fossa, it is also valuable in monitoring general functions of the brainstem (3). Many surgeons believe that mapping techniques, such as of the surface of the cortex for determining the location of the central sulcus and that of the cranial motor nerves VII, IX–X, and XII when they come close to the floor of the fourth ventricle, are of great value in identification of "safe entry zones" into the brain stem. However, other techniques, although safe and feasible, have not gained similar acceptance.

The advantage of many techniques in improving outcome and/or decreasing the risk of complications has not been recognized using established quantitative statistical methods of study. The success and the feasibility of the use of spinal MEP have been studied in a survey (4) recommending the use of SSEP and MEP together in operations where there was risk of spinal cord injury. Auditory evoked potentials (ABR and CAP from CN VIII and the cochlear nucleus) have been found to reduce the occurrence of postoperative hearing loss in studies using historical data (5). The use of MEP has been studied in retrospective reviews by several authors who found that SSEP and MEP were effective in detecting changes in functions during operations (6, 7). However, little quantitative data are available regarding the efficacy of MEP in reducing the risk of postoperative complications.

The advantage of using neurophysiological methods for intraoperative guidance and diagnosis has been established for operations to repair peripheral nerve injuries (8). Various studies have shown that neurophysiological recordings improve the outcome for microvascular decompression (MVD) operations for hemifacial spasm (HFS) (9, 10), while a few surgeons have questioned the value of this method of electrophysiological guidance in such operations (11). Many surgeons feel that operations involving placement of electrodes for deep brain stimulation (DBS) should only be carried out with neurophysiological guidance (12), but some studies have failed to find noticeable advantages regarding accuracy in placement (and thus, better outcome) or in reduced complications or side effects (13).

REDUCING THE RISK OF POSTOPERATIVE DEFICITS BY THE USE OF INTRAOPERATIVE MONITORING

The benefit from the use of intraoperative neurophysiological monitoring and intraoperative neurophysiology regarding reductions of the risk of postoperative neurological deficits is important for two reasons: benefit to the patient (improvement of medical care) and economic benefits for the health care provider.

Various organizations have issued guidelines for the use of intraoperative neurophysiologic monitoring:

The Therapeutics and Technology Subcommittee of the American Academy of Neurology has concluded that the following are useful and non-investigational.

1. EEG, compressed spectral array, and SSEP in carotid endarterectomy (CEA) and brain surgeries that potentially compromise cerebral blood flow.
2. ABR and cranial nerve monitoring in surgeries performed in the region of the brainstem or inner ear.
3. SSEP monitoring performed for surgical procedures potentially involving ischemia or mechanical trauma of the spinal cord (14).

Earlier, the National Institutes of Health Consensus Development Conference (held December 11–13, 1991) (*91*) stated in a "Consensus Statement," "There is a consensus that intraoperative real-time neurophysiological monitoring improves the surgical management of vestibular schwannoma, including the preservation of facial nerve function and possibly improves hearing preservation by the use of intraoperative auditory brainstem response monitoring." "Intraoperative monitoring of cranial nerves V, VI, IX, X, and XI also has been described, but the full benefits of this monitoring remains to be determined." In the "Conclusion and Recommendation" of this report it is stated: "The benefit of routine intraoperative monitoring of the facial nerve has been clearly established. This technique should be included in surgical therapy of vestibular schwannoma. Routine monitoring of other cranial nerves should be considered" (Consensus Statement 1991, page 19) (*1*).

There is also a need for taking an economic point of view into account when evaluating the use of electrophysiological methods in the operating room because a reduction of potential complications reduces associated costs of medical care. The benefits from the use of neurophysiological monitoring in the operating room also have another impact on surgeons and hospitals in that these benefits make some procedures feasible that otherwise were not regarded as safe or feasible. The ability of intraoperative monitoring to reduce the stress on the surgeon should also be regarded as a noteworthy benefit and often produces a reduction in the time necessary for an operation.

Justification for the use of intraoperative neurophysiological monitoring should rely on quantitative evaluation of the reduction of the risk of postoperative neurological deficits (evidence based medicine[1]). It is, therefore, an important task for those who do intraoperative monitoring and intraoperative neurophysiology to document the advantages of monitoring. Evaluation of these benefits depends on reliable information about the efficacy of intraoperative monitoring in reducing such risks.

So far, few of these benefits from intraoperative monitoring have been verified in statistical studies. Quantitative information regarding the intrinsic benefit of intraoperative monitoring is also important for the purpose of deciding which kinds of operations should be monitored.

It is not possible to evaluate the benefit of intraoperative neurophysiological monitoring using the conventional double blind technique. Instead, a comparison with historical data has been made, but that method is fraught with error. One noticeable source of error is the lack of reliable data regarding postoperative deficits in general. Surgeons are usually reluctant to publish their statistics regarding postoperative neurological deficits that can be related to surgical operations. Another uncertainty in evaluating the role of intraoperative monitoring in reducing the risk of complications is related to improved surgical techniques that also have reduced the occurrences of postoperative deficits.

Studies that have used historical data in assessing the frequency of postoperative deficits before and after the introduction of intraoperative monitoring have been reported (*5, 15–17*). Such studies, however, have been criticized, and it has been claimed that they provide an overestimation of the role of intraoperative monitoring in reducing postoperative neurological deficits because other developments and improvements in surgical techniques have also contributed to the observed improvement regarding the occurrence of postoperative neurological deficits.

Benefits from monitoring auditory evoked potentials in operations where the auditory nerve has been at risk have been reported by many investigators (*5, 18, 19*), but some investigators have questioned the benefits from such monitoring in specific operations (*20*).

Other uses of monitoring of sensory evoked potentials have been reported regarding operations such as carotid endarterectomy (CEA) surgery (*21, 22*). Perhaps the best known benefits of monitoring are from operations to correct spinal deformities (*23, 24*) and other operations affecting the spinal cord using SSEP and motor evoked potential monitoring (*7, 25–30*). Such operations had a low rate of postoperative neurological deficits before introduction of monitoring, but the deficits in question (paraplegia) were devastating. For example, a reduction from 1% of severe deficits without monitoring to 0.5% with monitoring would be an important improvement in alleviating human suffering. In fact, the reduction was probably much greater.

This amount of reduction would provide an enormous cost saving, which could justify intraoperative monitoring on a purely economic basis even when based on the most conservative estimates of the costs related to postoperative deficits. The reduction in human suffering, not only regarding the individual patients, but also for their relatives, is of course far more important than economic savings, but much more difficult to estimate and to quantify. Likewise, the use of intraoperative monitoring has been found to reduce iatrogenic injuries in connection with insertion of pedicle screws. It has been shown that pure economic reasons would justify the use of intraoperative neurophysiological monitoring in connection with placement of pedicle screws (*16*).

The ability to save the function of the facial nerve in operations for removal of vestibular schwannoma is probably one of the most dramatic improvements from the introduction of intraoperative neurophysiological monitoring (see Chap. 11) although no attempts to place economic values on saving facial function have been published. Studies of the use of facial nerve monitoring in middle ear surgery, primary and revision surgeries have shown a significant reduction of iatrogenic facial nerve injuries in such operations (*31*). Similar studies regarding facial nerve monitoring in parotid gland surgery were less convincing regarding benefits from monitoring (*32*).

It has been shown that intraoperative SSEP recordings have good predictive value regarding postoperative absence of deficits in skull base operations (100%), but less effective value predicting postoperative deficits (90%) (*33*). Other studies agree that intraoperative monitoring of SSEP and ABR can reduce the risk of iatrogenic injuries (*34, 35*), whereas monitoring of VEP seems less efficient in reducing iatrogenic injuries (*36*), although new techniques may have made such monitoring more effective (*37*).

Intraoperative guidance of the surgeon has been demonstrated to increase the outcome of specific operations such as MVD operations for HFS (*10*) and repair of peripheral nerves (*8, 38*). More recently, electrophysiological methods for guidance of electrode implantation for DBS or lesions in the basal ganglia and thalamus have gained acceptance (*39*), and there are reports of an increase in the precision of such procedures (*40*), although some investigators have failed to find such advantages (*13*).

Despite lack of hard evidence regarding the benefit of intraoperative neurophysiological monitoring, many kinds of intraoperative monitoring are regarded to be of sufficient value that they are requested systematically by many surgeons. Surgeons who have experienced the benefits from intraoperative neurophysiological monitoring are often reluctant to deprive their patients of intraoperative monitoring because they believe such monitoring to be beneficial to their patients, which excludes the use of studies where patients are randomly assigned for monitoring.

Evaluation of Postoperative Neurological Deficits

A prerequisite for being able to evaluate the neurological deficits that may have been acquired during an operation is that adequate preoperative and postoperative testing were carried out regarding the parts of the nervous system that are relevant for intraoperative monitoring. For example, complete hearing tests, which should include pure tone audiograms and speech discrimination scores using recorded test words (not "live voice"), should be performed both before and after operations in which there is a risk of injury to the auditory nerve. The evaluation of deficits should use change in speech discrimination scores rather than changes in pure tone audiograms (see Chap. 7).

Evaluations of facial function have improved with the development of a standard grading scale (41),[2] but such evaluations still rely on a physician's examination of the patient and can never be totally objective. More objective tests of facial function have been described (42, 43) utilizing measurements of the excursions (movements) of selected points on the face using computer programs that display the outlined face of the patient and measure the excursions as the patient performs voluntary face movements. The results derived from both sides of the patient's face are then compared to information obtained before the operation. Such objective methods to evaluate neurological deficits are only available for a few kinds of operations.

Assessment of many other kinds of neurological functions still relies on subjective evaluation. For example, to a great extent, evaluation of the function of eye muscles even when evaluated by specialists in this area relies on subjective judgments.

Even the most thorough examination and evaluation of postoperative deficits rarely reflect the handicap to which the person is subjected. For example, hearing tests rarely involve evaluation of tinnitus, and many times do not include speech discrimination tests. The results of commonly used vestibular tests poorly correlate with the patient's deficit. Examination of motor deficits that are conducted after an operation involving the spinal cord is mostly concerned with distal limb function, thus involving the corticospinal system only (lateral system, see Chaps. 9 and 10), while much less attention is paid to the medial system that controls the proximal limb muscles and trunk muscles. One reason for the lack of attention paid to the medial system may be that the patients are observed postoperatively while in bed, and the focus is on deficits in the use of hands and feet.

Quality of life issues are almost never assessed in studies of complications in surgical procedures, although it has been shown that decreased quality of life is a rather common complication to operations that involve the CNS even when there are no objective signs of complications (44, 45). Closely related to quality of life issues are chronic pain and severe tinnitus. These two disorders can totally ruin a person's life, but cannot be verified by objective tests.

The implication for a patient of chronic postoperative pain or severe tinnitus cannot be assessed by a physician's examination of the patient. Postoperative evaluations should be performed by professionals who are trained to perform the evaluations, and the surgeon who operated on the patient or any member of the surgical team should not do the examination and evaluation of postoperative deficits.

Cost-Benefit Analysis of Reduction in Iatrogenic Injuries Through Monitoring

Only a few kinds of operations have been analyzed regarding the economic feasibility of intraoperative monitoring. Difficulties in estimating the reduction in the likelihood of acquiring a postoperative neurological deficit through the use of intraoperative monitoring and difficulties in estimating the economic implications of neurological deficits (16) are two factors that hamper cost-benefit analysis of intraoperative monitoring (34, 35).

The cost-benefit ratio has been evaluated in only a few kinds of operations. In operations on the middle ear, studies have shown that facial nerve monitoring, primary and revision surgeries, is economically beneficial (31). Similar results were obtained regarding monitoring in

---

[2]The decibel scale is a logarithmic measure of ratios, such as the ratio between the amplitude of the output and that of the input; thus, it is a measure of attenuation or amplification. For voltage ratios it is defined as $20 \log_{10} E_o/E_i$, where E_i is the input voltage and E_o is the output voltage, an attenuation of 3 dB means that the output is 0.707 times the input, a 6 dB attenuation means that the output voltage is half of the input, a 10 dB attenuation means that the output is 0.3 of the input, a 20 dB attenuation means that the output is 0.1 of the input, and so on.

association with insertion of pedicle screws (*16, 17*). Estimates regarding operations in the cerebellopontine angle also show evidence that intraoperative monitoring is cost effective (*46*).

The most extensive cost-benefit analysis of intraoperative neurophysiological monitoring has been presented in connection with operations that may affect the spinal cord. Corrective operations for scoliosis and other back operations have a low rate of occurrence of complications even without monitoring, but the complications of such operations, which are in the form of paraplegia or quadriplegia, are so severe and often affect young people who can be expected to live for a long time that the consequences of even a very few occurrences of such complications are enormous (see Chap. 10). Even the very conservative estimates of the advantages of intraoperative monitoring that have been conducted show substantial economic benefit from monitoring.

While it is relatively easy to accurately determine the costs of implementing intraoperative neurophysiological monitoring, it is much more difficult to estimate the costs associated with postoperative neurological deficits, which is one reason why it is difficult to estimate the economic benefit from intraoperative neurophysiological monitoring. Estimates of the economic costs of postoperative neurological deficits are usually restricted to estimates of cost of care, but such estimates should include an estimate of the economic value of human suffering and loss of quality of life, not only the actual cost of care for an individual. The value of human suffering has been conspicuously neglected in past discussions of the cost/benefit ratio of implementing any new addition to health care including intraoperative neurophysiological monitoring.

It is not possible to place a monetary value on every specific type of neurological deficit, and even if this were possible, the monetary values on specific deficits would vary from person to person. US courts of law grant monetary compensation to patients who have lost neural function due to injuries that were regarded as caused by negligence or other forms of malpractice. Compensation for suffering that is often granted when losses of body functions are considered in connection with such lawsuits far exceeds the cost of care. If the amounts granted in malpractice suits were used as guidelines for estimating the value of loss of neural functions, the economic costs of iatrogenic injuries would be enormous and would dwarf the costs of the kind of intraoperative monitoring that could reduce the incidence of postoperative neurological deficits. This would be a strong argument to justify the use of intraoperative monitoring in many operations.

Toleikis (*16*) has reported that his service had monitored more than 1,000 patients during placement of more than 5,000 pedicle screws. Postoperative assessment showed that only one patient had acquired postoperative neurological deficits caused by a misplaced pedicle screw. This patient had a threshold for stimulation of the pedicle screw that exceeded the established "warning threshold", but the surgeon elected to leave the screw in place. The patient's problems were resolved after removal of the screws and no permanent deficits remained.

Without monitoring, it has been reported that from 2% to 10% of operations have complications in connection with placement of pedicle screws (*16*). This means that 20–100 patients of every 1,000 would have some problems that were related to placement of pedicle screws. The use of monitoring has substantially decreased the risks in connection with placement of pedicle screws and therefore, reduced complications.

The estimated cost of monitoring 1,000 patients is $1,000,000. If monitoring were implemented, it would have prevented complications in 20 patients (using the lowest estimate of 2%). The direct cost of such complications was estimated to be $50,000 for each patient, but this figure is conservative and the costs of medical treatment for complications from nerve root injuries and rehabilitation can easily exceed $50,000. This means that the direct economic saving from monitoring would be at least $50,000 x 20=$1,000,000 for each 1,000 patients who are operated upon, which means that monitoring is economically sound.

Everyone would agree that complications from pedicle screw misplacement means a substantial decrease in quality of life, which cannot be measured in money. Also, consider that the estimates of direct costs outlined above are conservative using the lowest reported rate of complications (2%) without monitoring. If the highest reported rate of complications is used (10%), the economic savings become substantially greater.

Operations in the cerebellopontine angle, such as those to remove vestibular schwannoma, carry a large risk of the patient losing facial function postoperatively before introduction of intraoperative neurophysiological monitoring. Before monitoring was available, many surgeons did not even try to save facial function in large tumors because they believed it was not possible. Introduction of intraoperative neurophysiological monitoring changed perception, and it became rare to lose facial function after operations for tumors smaller than 2.5 cm in diameter. Facial function was preserved routinely in patients with larger tumors.

Loss of facial function is not only a cosmetic handicap, but it also causes impairment of the vision because the ability to secrete tears is lost, and it makes it difficult for the patient to eat, both of which greatly affect quality of life. It was encouraging that the NIH Consensus Conference of Acoustic Tumors (old name for vestibular schwannoma) (1991) (*1*) early after general introduction of facial nerve monitoring found intraoperative monitoring of value in preventing the loss of facial function following removal of acoustic tumors in the cerebellopontine angle. However, to date, there have been no estimations published on the economic implications of losing facial function, and consequently, it has not been possible to estimate the benefits of preventing the loss of facial function in economic terms. Again, if loss of facial function would be compensated economically in a similar way as courts of law often compensate loss of function in malpractice lawsuits, the use of intraoperative monitoring of facial function would appear as a highly cost-effective preventative method. Similar reasoning would apply to intraoperatively monitoring of auditory function.

In evaluating human suffering in monetary terms, what are the implications of an elderly person losing facial function compared to a young person who could be expected to live for many years? What are the implications of a young musician suffering hearing loss compared with a person who is less dependent on hearing and does not have to communicate verbally in a noisy environment?

Several cranial nerves are at risk of injury in skull base operations, and the use of intraoperative monitoring can reduce the risk of losing function of cranial motor nerves postoperatively. Loss of function of either CN III or CN XII causes perhaps the most severe handicaps, but intraoperative neurophysiological monitoring can reduce the risks to these nerves. A cost-benefit analysis has not been applied to such aspects of intraoperative injuries.

Other Benefits from Neurophysiology in the Operating Room

The value of intraoperative neurophysiological monitoring is not limited to reducing the risk of postoperative deficits. For example, intraoperative neurophysiological monitoring can:

1. promote the development of better operating methods
2. improve the outcome of some operations by helping the surgeon reach the therapeutic goal of the operation (better results and fewer re-operations)
3. shorten the time required to carry out an operation (reduced costs, and the risk of infections is proportional to the time an operation lasts)
4. give the surgeon a feeling of security, thus making the operation less stressful (less risk of mistakes)

These advantages of monitoring are difficult to evaluate quantitatively (and impossible to assign monetary values), but they contribute noticeably to reducing the risk of postoperative neurological deficits and thereby, increase the quality of medical care in general. There is little doubt that in many situations those aspects of the use of monitoring also reduce the cost of medical care.

WHICH OPERATIONS SHOULD BE MONITORED?

It is important to know the benefits that intraoperative neurophysiological monitoring offers to both the patient and the surgeon when deciding which patients and/or operations should be monitored. Current pressure to increase control over the costs involved in medical care places great demands on health care providers to produce evidence that intraoperative monitoring is indeed cost effective. Thus, decisions relating to which patients should be monitored intraoperatively are not only based on the benefits to the patient that can be expected from such intraoperative monitoring, but also on the immediate cost of intraoperative neurophysiological monitoring in relation to the savings in costs that such monitoring represents regarding postoperative care.

Traditionally, additions to medical care have been introduced and used because of their improvements of the quality of medical care rather than for saving costs. For instance, when intraoperative monitoring of blood pressure was first introduced to the operating room regimen, the (only) question at the time was whether or not it contributed significantly to the promotion of good health care. Naturally, the goal of modern medicine should be to reduce the risks related to the occurrence of any postoperative deficit as much as possible and to utilize all possible means for that goal. Unfortunately, this goal is unrealistic due to present economical constraints on health care, limited availability of skilled personnel, and other factors that cause the quality of medical care to depend on non-scientific and technical capabilities. Since purely economic factors play important roles for decisions regarding the use of new additions to health care, economically based arguments for the implementation of intraoperative neurophysiological monitoring are important in each individual operation.

The question about which patients could (possibly) benefit from intraoperative neurophysiological monitoring depends on many factors that are not always easy to define. One such factor is the patient's preoperative condition. There is no reason to monitor hearing in a patient who is already deaf from the disease for which he or she is being treated or from other causes. Patients with total facial palsy cannot possibly benefit from intraoperative facial monitoring, nor can patients with peripheral neuropathies that prevent obtaining preoperative SSEP recordings. Decisions on whether a certain type of monitoring should be used in a certain patient must, therefore, rely on assessment of the patient's preoperative situation.

Naturally, systems that cannot be affected by the operation should not be monitored. Thus, it would seem unjustified to monitor ABR during an operation to remove a tumor in the frontal portion of the brain. However, it must be considered that ABR are a good indicator of general brainstem function, and therefore, patients who are in poor general condition may benefit from monitoring ABR even if the operations are performed far from the anatomical location of the neural territory covered by ABR monitoring. Again, a decision on whether to do intraoperative neurophysiological monitoring must be made on the basis of each individual patient, as is the case in medical treatment in general.

There may be legal ramifications pertaining to when intraoperative neurophysiological monitoring is, and is not, employed. A patient who acquires a postoperative deficit following an operation in which monitoring was not performed could claim that the likelihood of he or she acquiring the deficit might have been reduced if intraoperative monitoring had been completed. An interesting question arises as to whether a surgeon's choice of not to use intraoperative monitoring can result in a lawsuit against (and subsequent conviction of) the surgeon for negligence, because known techniques to achieve the best possible outcome of an operation were not utilized.

EFFICACY OF INTRAOPERATIVE MONITORING

The size of the decrease in the risk of postoperative neurological deficits through the use of intraoperative monitoring depends on the quality of monitoring and the expertise of the individuals who are doing the monitoring. If a change in neural function is not detected for one reason or another, then the monitoring is not useful. This is known as a false-negative result. There are many reasons why a false-negative result may occur. For example, the wrong system may be monitored, the person who is responsible for monitoring may not understand what the changes in the recorded electrical potentials mean or the changes could be obscured in one way or another. If the surgeon does not take action in response to detected changes in function, monitoring has no value. Alarming the surgeon when there is actually no surgically induced change in neural function (false-positive responses) may jeopardize the credibility of the monitoring team and cause the surgeon not to respond when real changes occur.

CONSEQUENCES OF FALSE-POSITIVE AND FALSE-NEGATIVE RESPONSES

In medical diagnostics or in screening for specific diseases, a false-negative response to a test may result in a disease condition being overlooked because the test (mistakenly) indicated an absence of disease. This may result in delay of treatment or no treatment at all. A false-positive response to a test (indicating the presence of a disease when in fact there is no disease present) is less harmful because the results only produce unnecessary additional tests and examinations and could possibly result in treating a disease that does not exist. False positive tests cause extra costs to health care.

False-negative results in intraoperative neurophysiological monitoring may result in a patient acquiring a postoperative neurologic deficit because the occurrence of neural injury was not detected intraoperatively. False-negative results in intraoperative monitoring are, therefore, serious and may result in a serious postoperative neurological deficit.

Some investigators have defined false-positive responses in intraoperative monitoring to include all changes in the recorded potentials that do not result in neurological deficits. That definition is unfortunate and reminds one of Russian roulette. The fact that changes can occur with a minimal risk of neurological deficits is the very basis of intraoperative monitoring that makes it possible to detect changes in function before these changes are associated with injuries that cause permanent deficits. Intraoperative neurophysiological monitoring is used not as a warning of an imminent disaster, but rather to provide information that indicates when a particular portion of the nervous system has been affected in a way that may imply a certain risk for postoperative neurological deficit.

Equipment failures that could cause the impression of a major change in function of the system being monitored are very rare now with modern equipment. Unexpected, dramatic events in the recorded potentials, such as total loss of the (waveform) potentials, are instead often signs of a serious condition in the patient's status that must be addressed immediately to avoid the risk of a catastrophic operative outcome rather than false positive results of monitoring. Therefore, a delay in reporting such a change to the surgeon to check equipment or some other possible technical difficulties will most likely reduce the surgeon's chances to reverse the manipulation that caused the change and thereby, increase the risk of the patient's acquiring a permanent postoperative neurological deficit. Such unusual events should, therefore, be promptly reported to the surgeon. If, in fact, the change in the recorded neuroelectrical potentials is caused by a technical problem, the cost of alerting the surgeon unnecessarily is small – simply resulting in a few minutes of lost operating time.

The number of false-negative responses should be kept to an absolute minimum by all available means, while conversely, false-positive responses (according to the strict definition mentioned immediately above) should be tolerated, and in fact may be used to respond to changes in neural function before the likelihood of postoperative permanent deficits become noticeable.

There may be another type of false-positive response in connection with intraoperative monitoring that deserves attention, namely, the situation where the results of intraoperative monitoring show a change in the function of a specific part of the nervous system, while in fact, the observed change in function was caused by harmless events such as irrigation with solutions below body temperature.

EVALUATION OF BENEFITS FROM ELECTROPHYSIOLOGIC GUIDANCE OF THE SURGEON IN AN OPERATION

The value of advantages from guidance of the surgeon in operations is more difficult to evaluate than the benefit from reducing the risk of postoperative deficits. Neurophysiological guidance has made repair of peripheral nerves, and treatment for some disorders of cranial nerves, more efficient. Additionally, it is the impression that neurophysiological guidance has increased the precision with which therapeutical lesions in specific structures of the CNS can be made. Neurophysiological guidance has made precise implantations of electrodes for permanent stimulation possible and has increased the efficacy of treatments of many forms of movement disorders and pain, the values for which are difficult to quantify. However, reviews of articles published regarding a

specific operation, pallidotomy, and implantation of electrodes for DBS has not shown advantages of neurophysiological guidance regarding precision nor in regard to complication (13). The results of such studies of the literature may not be representative because it seems more likely that surgeons who use complex procedures will publish their results than surgeons who use less sophisticated methods.

BENEFITS FROM RESEARCH IN THE OPERATING ROOM

Even more difficult to evaluate than the advantages noted above are the advantages from basic and applied research that are conducted in connection with the use of electrophysiological techniques in the operating room. However, research in the operating room has contributed to development of better treatment and better operating methods with less risk of postoperative deficits, and it has contributed to basic understanding of the function of the normal nervous system and the pathological nervous system. Some of these benefits have immediate impact while others have long-term benefit. In fact, this kind of research has been responsible for much progress in surgical and medical treatments of many different disorders. Most people will, therefore, agree that this aspect of bringing neurophysiological techniques and expertise into the operating room can produce enormous progress in treatment of disorders of the nervous system. However, converting these benefits into monetary values is impossible, and it is even difficult to estimate the extent of the contribution to better patient care from research.

REFERENCES

1. Anonymous (1991) Acoustic neuroma, NIH consensus development program. Online 1991 Dec 11–13 9:1–24.
2. Sala F, MJ Krzan and V Deletis (2002) Intraoperative neurophysiological monitoring in

pediatric neurosurgery: why, when, how? Childs Nerv Syst 18:264–87.

3. Angelo R and AR Møller (1996) Contralateral evoked brainstem auditory potentials as an indicator of intraoperative brainstem manipulation in cerebellopontine angle tumors. Neurol Res 18:528–40.

4. Legatt AD (2002) Current practice of motor evoked potential monitoring: results of a survey. J Clin Neurophysiol 19:454–60.

5. Møller AR and MB Møller (1989) Does intraoperative monitoring of auditory evoked potentials reduce incidence of hearing loss as a complication of microvascular decompression of cranial nerves? Neurosurgery 24:257–63.

6. Bose B, AK Sestokas and DM Schwartz (2004) Neurophysiological monitoring of spinal cord function during instrumented anterior cervical fusion. J Neursosurg Spine 4:202–7.

7. Langeloo DD, A Lelivelt, H Louis Journee et al (2003) Transcranial electrical motor-evoked potential monitoring during surgery for spinal deformity: a study of 145 patients. Spine 28:1043–50.

8. Happel L and D Kline (2002) Intraoperative Neurophysiology of the Peripheral Nervous System, in *Neurophysiology in Neurosurgery*, V Deletis and JL Shils, Editors. 2002, Academic Press: Amsterdam. 169–95.

9. Haines SJ and F Torres (1991) Intraoperative monitoring of the facial nerve during decompressive surgery for hemifacial spasm. J Neurosurg 74:254–7.

10. Møller AR and PJ Jannetta (1987) Monitoring facial EMG during microvascular decompression operations for hemifacial spasm. J Neurosurg 66:681–5.

11. Hatem J, M Sindou and C Vial (2001) Intraoperative monitoring of facial EMG responses during microvascular decompression for hemifacial spasm. Prognostic value for long-term outcome: a study in a 33-patient series. Br J Neurosurg 15:496–9.

12. Arle JE and JL Shils (2007) Neurosurgical decision-making with IOM: DBS surgery. Neurophysiol Clin 37:449–55.

13. Hariz MI and H Fodstad (1999) Do microelectrode techniques increase accuracy or decrease risks in pallidotomy and deep brain stimulation? A critical review of the literature. Stereotact Funct Neurosurg 72:157–69.

14. Lopez JR (2004) The use of evoked potentials in intraoperative neurophysiologic monitoring. Phys Med Rehabil Clin North Am 15:63–84.

15. Radtke RA, W Erwin and RH Wilkins (1989) Intraoperative brainstem auditory evoked potentials: significant decrease in post-operative morbidity. Neurology 39:187–91.

16. Toleikis JR, (2002) Neurophysiological monitoring during pedicle screw placement, in *Neurophysiology in Neurosurgrey*, V Deletis and JL Shils, Editors. Elsevier: Amsterdam. 231–64.

17. Toleikis JR, JP Skelly, AO Carlvin et al (2000) The usefulness of electrical stimulation for assessing pedicle screw placements. J Spin Disord 13:283–9.

18. Linden R, C Tator, C Benedict et al (1988) Electro-physiological monitoring during acoutic neuroma and other posterior fossa surgery. Le Journal des Sciences Neurologiques 15:73–81.

19. Polo G, C Fischer, MP Sindou et al (2004) Brainstem auditory evoked potential monitoring during microvascular decompression for hemifacial spasm: intraoperative brainstem auditory evoked potential changes and warning values to prevent hearing loss – prospective study in a consecutive series of 84 patients. Neurosurgery 54:104–6.

20. Kveton JF (1990) The efficacy of brainstem auditory evoked potentials in acoustic tumor surgery. Laryngoscope 100:1171–3.

21. Haupt WF and S Horsch (1992) Evoked potential monitoring in carotid surgery: a review of 994 cases. Neurology 42:835–8.

22. Dinkel M, H Schweiger and P Goerlitz (1992) Monitoring during carotid surgery: somatosensory evoked potentials vs. carotid stump pressure. J Neurosurg Anesthesiol 4:167–75.

23. Nash CL, RA Lorig, LA Schatzinger et al (1977) Spinal cord monitoring during operative treatment of the spine. Clin Orthop 126:100–5.

24. Brown RH and CL Nash (1979) Current status of spinal cord monitoring. Spine 4:466–78.

25. Deletis V (2002) Intraoperative neurophysiology and methodologies used to monitor the functional integrity of the motor system, in *Neurophysiology in Neurosurgery*, V Deletis and JL Shils, Editors. Academic Press: Amsterdam. 25–51.

26. Nuwer MR, EG Dawson, LG Carlson et al (1995) Somatosensory evoked potential spinal cord monitoring reduces neurologic deficits after

scoliosis surgery: results of a large multicenter study. Electroenceph Clin Neurophys 96:6–11.

27. Kothbauer KF (2002) Motor evoked potential monitoring for intramedullary spinal cord tumor surgery, in *Neurophysiology in Neurosurgery*, V Deletis and JL Shils, Editors. Academic Press: Amsterdam. 73–92.

28. Nuwer MR (1988) Use of somatosensory evoked potentials for intraoperative monitoring of cerebral and spinal cord function. Neurologic Clin 6:881–97.

29. Nuwer MR, J Daube, C Fischer et al (1993) Neuromonitroing during surgery. Report of an IFCN committee. Electroenceph Clin Neurophysiol 87:263–76.

30. Tsirikos AI, J Aderinto, SK Tucker et al (2004) Spinal cord monitoring using intraoperative somatosensory evoked potentials for spinal trauma. J Spinal Disord Tech 17:385–94.

31. Wilson L, E Lin and A Lalwani (2003) Cost-effectiveness of intraoperative facial nerve monitoring in middle ear or mastoid surgery. Laryngoscope 113:1736–45.

32. Terrell JE, PR Kileny, C Yian et al (1997) Clinical outcome of continuous facial nerve monitoring during primary parotidectomy. Arch Otolaryngol Head Neck Surg 123:1081–7.

33. Bejjani GK, PC Nora, PL Vera et al (1998) The predictive value of intraoperative somatosensory evoked potential monitoring: review of 244 procedures. Neurosurgery 43:498–500.

34. Fischer RS, P Raudzens and M Nunemacher (1995) Efficacy of intraoperative neurophysiological monitoring. J Clin Neurophysiol 12:97–109.

35. Møller AR (1995) Intraoperative neurophysiologic monitoring in neurosurgery: benefits, efficacy, and cost-effectiveness, in *Clinical Neurosurgery, Proceedings of the Congress of Neurological Surgeons' 1994 Meeting*. Williams & Wilkins: Baltimore. 171–9.

36. Cedzich C, J Schramm, CF Mengedoht et al (1988) Factors that limit the use of flash visual evoked potentials for surgical monitoring. Electroenceph Clin Neurophysiol 71:142–5.

37. Pratt H, WH Martin, N Bleich et al (1994) A high-intensity, goggle-mounted flash stimulator for short-latency visual evoked potentials. Electroenceph Clin Neurophysiol 92:469–72.

38. Happel L and D Kline (1991) Nerve lesions in continuity, in *Operative nerve repair and reconstruction 1st ed vol 1*, RH Gelberman, Editor. J.B. Lippincott: Philadelphia. 601–16.

39. Shils JL, M Tagliati and RL Alterman (2002) Neurophysiological monitoring during neurosurgery for movement disorders, in *Neurophysiology in Neurosurgery*, V Deletis and JL Shils, Editors. Academic Press: Amsterdam. 405–48.

40. Starr PA, RS Turner, G Rau et al (2004) Microelectrode-guided implantation of deep brain stimulators into the globus pallidus internus for dystonia: techniques, electrode locations, and outcomes. Neurosurg Focus 17:20–31.

41. House J and D Brackmann (1985) Facial nerve grading system. Otolaryngol Head Neck Surg 93:146–67.

42. Brach JS, JM Van Swearingen, J Lenert et al (1997) Facial Neuromuscular Retraining for Oral Synkinesis. Plast Reconstr Surg 99:1922–31.

43. Johnson PC, H Brown, WM Kuzon et al (1994) Simultaneous quantitation of facial movements: the maximal static response assay of facial nerve function. Ann Plast Surg 32:171–9.

44. Kato BM, MJ LaRouere, DI Bojrab et al (2004) Evaluating quality of life after endolymphatic Sac Surgery: the Ménière's Disease Outcomes Questionnaire. Otol Neurotol 25:339–44.

45. Nikolopoulos TP, I Johnson and GM O'Donoghue (1998) Quality of life after acoustic neuroma surgery. Laryngoscope 108:1382–5.

46. Kombos T, O Suess and M Brock (2002) Cost analysis of intraoperative neurophysiological monitoring (IOM). Zentralbl Neurochir 63:141–5.

Appendix

APPENDIX A BRODMANN'S AREAS (SEE FIGS. A.1 AND A.2)

Areas 1, 2, and 3	Primary somatosensory cortex (frequently referred to as areas 3, 1, 2 by convention)	Area 23	Ventral posterior cingulate cortex
Area 4	Primary motor cortex	Area 24	Ventral anterior cingulate cortex
Area 5	Somatosensory association cortex	Area 25	Subgenual cortex
		Area 26	Ectosplenial area
Area 6	Premotor and supplementary motor cortex (secondary motor cortex)	Area 28	Posterior entorhinal cortex
		Area 29	Retrosplenial cingular cortex
Area 7	Somatosensory association cortex	Area 30	Part of cingular cortex
Area 8	Includes frontal eye fields	Area 31	Dorsal posterior cingular cortex
Area 9	Dorsolateral prefrontal cortex	Area 32	Dorsal anterior cingulate cortex
Area 10	Frontopolar area (most rostral part of superior and middle frontal gyri)	Area 34	Anterior entorhinal cortex (on the parahippocampal gyrus)
Area 11	Orbitofrontal area (orbital and rectus gyri, plus part of the rostral part of the superior frontal gyrus)	Area 35	Perirhinal cortex (on the parahippocampal gyrus)
		Area 36	Parahippocampal cortex (on the parahippocampal gyrus)
Area 12	Orbitofrontal area (used to be part of BA11, refers to the area between the superior frontal gyrus and the inferior rostral sulcus)	Area 37	Fusiform gyrus
		Area 38	Temporopolar area (most rostral part of the superior and middle temporal gyri)
Areas 13 and 14	Insular cortex	Area 39	Angular gyrus, part of Wernicke's area
Area 15	Anterior temporal lobe	Area 40	Supramarginal gyrus part of Wernicke's area
Area 17	Primary visual cortex (V1)		
Area 18	Visual association cortex (V2)	Areas 41 and 42	Primary and auditory association cortex
Area 19	V3	Area 43	Subcentral area (between insula and post/precentral gyrus)
Area 20	Inferior temporal gyrus		
Area 21	Middle temporal gyrus		
Area 22	Superior temporal gyrus, of which the rostral part participates to Wernicke's area	Area 44	Pars opercularis, part of Broca's area
		Area 45	Pars triangularis Broca's area
		Area 46	Dorsolateral prefrontal cortex
		Area 47	Inferior prefrontal gyrus

From: *Intraoperative Neurophysiological Monitoring: Third Edition*
By A.R. Møller, DOI 10.1007/978-1-4419-7436-5,
© Springer Science+Business Media, LLC 2011

| Area 48 | Retrosubicular area (a small part of the medial surface of the temporal lobe) | Area 52 | Parainsular area (at the junction of the temporal lobe and the insula) |

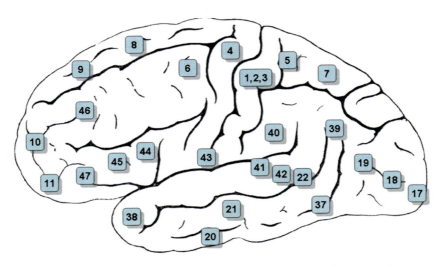

Figure A.1: Brodmann areas on the lateral surface of the brain (from Gray's Anatomy).

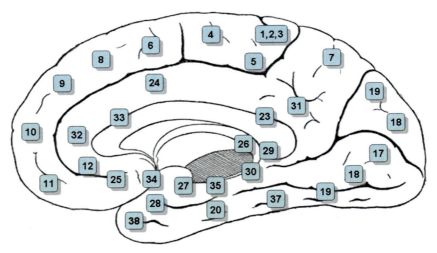

Figure A.2: Brodmann area on the medial surface of the brain.

APPENDIX B

Cranial Nerves: Anatomy and Physiology

We have 12 cranial nerves; some are sensory nerves, some are motor nerves, and some are part of the autonomic nervous system.

I. Olfactory nerve	Conscious sensory:	Smell
	Unconscious:	Pheromones
II. Optic nerve	Sensory:	Vision
III. Oculomotor nerve	Motor:	Eye Movements
		Innervates all extraocular muscles, except the superior oblique and lateral rectus muscles. Innervates the striated muscle of the eyelid.
	Autonomic:	Mediates pupillary constriction and accommodation for near vision.
IV. Trochlear nerve	Motor:	Eye Movements
		Innervates superior oblique muscle.
V. Trigeminal nerve	Sensory:	Mediates cutaneous and proprioceptive sensations from skin, muscles, and joints in the face and mouth, including the teeth and from the anterior 2/3 of the tongue.
	Motor:	Innervates muscles of mastication.
VI. Abducens nerve	Motor:	Eye Movements
		Innervates lateral rectus muscle.
VII. Facial nerve	Motor:	Innervates muscles of facial expression.
	Autonomic:	Lacrimal and salivary glands.
	Sensory:	Mediates taste and possible sensation from part of the face (behind the ear).
		Nervous intermedius
		Pain deep in the ear; possibly taste.
VIII. Vestibulocochlear nerve	Sensory:	Hearing
		Equilibrium, postural reflexes, orientation of the head in space.
IX. Glossopharyngeal nerve	Sensory:	Taste, innervates taste buds in the posterior third of tongue.
		Mediates visceral sensation from palate and posterior third of the tongue.
		Innervates the carotid body.
	Motor:	Muscles in posterior throat (stylopharyngeal muscle).
	Autonomic:	Parotid gland.

X. Vagus nerve	Sensory:	Mediates visceral sensation from the pharynx, larynx, thorax, and many organs in the abdomen.
		Innervates the skin in the ear canal and taste buds in the epiglottis
	Autonomic:	Contains autonomic fibers that innervate smooth muscle in heart, blood vessels, trachea, bronchi, esophagus, stomach, and intestine.
	Motor:	Innervates striated muscles in the soft palate, pharynx, and the larynx.
XI. Spinal accessory nerve	Motor:	Innervates the trapezius and sternocleidomastoid muscles.
XII. Hypoglossal nerve	Motor:	Innervates intrinsic muscles of the tongue.

FUNCTIONS OF THE CRANIAL NERVES

CN I. Olfactory Nerve: Sense of smell, communicates chemical airborne messages to the brain.

CN II. Optic Nerve: Sense of vision, communicates optic information. Variations in contrast are the most powerful stimulations of the visual system.

CN III. Oculomotor Nerve: Controls four of the six extraocular eye muscles: the superior, the inferior, the medial rectus muscles, and the inferior oblique muscles. The muscles innervated by CN III move the eye in all directions, and therefore, lesions to CN III affect essentially all eye movements and cause the eye to be deviated downward and outward. It also innervates the eyelid and can alone close the eye when lying down. Lesions to CN III cause ptosis (partial closure of the eyelid). CN III contains autonomic fibers that control the size of the pupil and stretches the lens to achieve accommodation. Lesions to CN III can essentially make the eye useless.

CN IV. Trochlear Nerve: Controls the trochlear muscle, and contraction of this muscle causes the eye to move downward and medially when it is in a position medial to the midline. Lesions of CN IV affect downward and medial movements of the eye.

CN V. Trigeminal Nerve: This nerve's sensory portion – the portio major – innervates the skin of the face, mucosa of the mouth and nasopharynx, and the cornea. This portion of CN V thereby communicates sensory information about touch and pain from the face and the mouth. CN V is the nerve that causes toothache and severe pain of trigeminal neuralgia. Lesions to the sensory portion of CN V cause a loss of sensation of the face. Loss of corneal sensation may result in corneal bruises.

The motor potion of CN V – the portio minor – controls the muscles of mastication. Lesions to the motor portion of CN V cause atrophy of the mastication muscles.

CN VI. Abducens Nerve: Controls eye movements from the midline to a lateral position. Lesions of CN VI prevent movements of the eye from the midline and outward.

CN VII. Facial Nerve: Controls the mimic muscles of the face. CN VII is often monitored intraoperatively because it is at risk in all operations to remove acoustic tumors, and it is involved in diseases such as hemifacial spasm. The autonomic fibers of CN VII control both tear glands and salivary glands. A loss of facial function is cosmetically devastating and makes it difficult to eat, and the lack of tears and the inability to close the eye may result in injures to the cornea.

Nervus Intermedius: Perhaps taste. Deep ear pain (geniculate neuralgia).

CN VIII. Vestibulocochlear Nerve: This nerve has two parts: one, the auditory nerve, that communicates auditory information and the other, the vestibular nerve, mediates information about head movements (balance). While the covering of the nerve fibers of most of the brainstem cranial nerves changes from peripheral myelin to central myelin a few millimeters from the brainstem, the transitional zone for CN VIII is in the internal auditory meatus, which means that CN VIII throughout its entire intracranial course (approximately 1 cm) is covered with central myelin and it has no epineurium, which causes CN VIII to have mechanical properties similar to those of the brain, making it more fragile than other cranial nerves.

In fact, we can do quite well without the vestibular part of the inner ear or the vestibular part of CN VIII being functioning, but if injured suddenly or on one side only severe balance disturbances can result. The success of adapting to such disequilibrium depends on one's age (better when younger than when older).

CN IX. Glossopharyngeal Nerve: Communicates sensory information from the throat to the brain and information about blood pressure to the cardiovascular centers. The motor portion of CN IX controls the stylopharyngeal muscle. Lesions of CN IX cause a loss of gag reflex on the affected side, and a risk of choking on food. Lesions on one side likely have little effect on cardiovascular function, but a loss of CN IX on both sides is fatal.

CN X. Vagus Nerve: This nerve's name means the "vagabondering" nerve, descriptive in that it travels around in a large portion of the body. This nerve conveys parasympathetic input to the entire chest and abdomen, and it controls the vocal cords, the heart, and the diaphragm. The most noticeable effect of unilateral lesions to CN X is hoarseness because the vocal cords on the affected side cannot close. CN X also has a large afferent portion (about 80% of the fibers) that carries information to the brain from the heart and viscera. The vagus nerve may carry more complex sensory information from the lower body, such as from genitalia. The vagus nerve is asymmetric, and it is the right vagus that controls the heart. Consequently, lesions of CN X on the left side or electrical stimulation of the left CN X has little effect on the cardiovascular system. Bilateral severance of the vagal nerve is fatal.

CN XI. Spinal Accessory Nerve: Controls muscles in the neck and shoulder (sternocleidomastoid and trapezoid muscles). Lesions of CN XI cause atrophy of the muscles that are innervated by that nerve.

CN XII. Hypoglossal Nerve: Controls movements of the tongue. Unilateral lesions to CN XII cause deviation of the tongue and atrophy of the tongue on the affected side. Bilateral lesions make it almost impossible to speak and swallow.

Abbreviations

A1	Primary auditory cortex	DNLL	Dorsal nucleus of the lateral lemniscus
A2	Secondary auditory cortex		
AAF	Anterior auditory field	DPV	Disabling positional vertigo
AAMI	Association for the Advancement of Medical Instrumentation	DRG	Dorsal root ganglia
		ECoG	Electrocochleography
ABI	Auditory brainstem implants	EEG	Electroencephalography
ABR	Auditory brainstem responses	EKG	Electrocardiogram
AC	Alternating current	EMG	Electromyography
Ach	Acetylcholine	EP	Erb's point
AEP	Auditory evoked potentials	EPSP	Excitatory postsynaptic potentials
AI	Anterior insula	fMRI	Functional magnetic resonance imaging
AN	Auditory nerve		
AP	Action potentials	FN	Facial nerve
APB	Abductor pollicis brevis	GABA	Gamma-amino butyric acid
ARM	Arteria radicularis magna	GABA$_A$	GABA receptor type A
ASA	Anterior spinal artery	GN	Gracilis nucleus
AVCN	Anterior ventral cochlear nucleus	GPe	Globus pallidus external part
AVF	Arteriovenous fistula	GPi	Globus pallidus internal part
AVM	Arteriovenous malformations	GPN	Glossopharyngeal neuralgia
BAEP	Brainstem auditory evoked potentials	HA	Habenula perforate
		HFS	Hemifacial spasm
BDNF	Brain-derived neurotrophic factor	HGPPS	Horizontal gaze palsy and progressive scoliosis
CAP	Compound action potentials		
CCT	Central conduction time	HIV	Human immunodeficiency virus
CEA	Carotid endarterectomy	HL	Hearing level
cm	Centimeter	I	Electrical current
CM	Cochlear microphonics	IC	Inferior colliculus
CMAP	Compound muscle action potentials	ICC	Central nucleus of the inferior colliculus
CMN	Centromedian nucleus	IEC	International Electrotechnical Commission
CMRR	Common-mode rejection ratio		
CN	Cranial nerve	IH	Inner hair cells
CNAP	Compound nerve action potentials	IPL	Interpeak latency
CNS	Central nervous system	ISI	Inter stimulus interval
CoN	Cochlear nerve	IVN	Inferior vestibular nerve
CPA	Cerebellopontine angle	kohm	Kilo ohm
CPG	Central pattern generator	LED	Light-emitting diodes
CT	Corticospinal tract	LGN	Lateral geniculate nucleus
DAS	Dorsal acoustic stria	LL	Lateral lemniscus
dB	Decibel	LLR	Long latency response
DBS	Deep brain stimulation	LR	Lateral rectus muscle
DC	Direct current	LSO	Lateral superior olive
DCN	Dorsal cochlear nucleus	LV	Lateral ventricle
DCS	Direct cortical stimulation	m/s	Meter per second

M1	Primary motor area
M2	Alternative designation for the supplementary motor area
M3	Alternative designation for the premotor area
mA	Milliampere
MA	Masseter muscles
MAC	Minimal alveolar concentration
MCA	Middle cerebral artery
MEP	Motor evoked potentials
MGB	Medial geniculate body
MGP	Medial segment of globus pallidus
MI	Middle insula
mm	Millimeter
Mohm	Megaohm
MR	Medial rectus muscles
MRI	Magnetic resonance imaging
MRSCA	Motor speech related cortical areas
ms	Millisecond
MSO	Medial superior olivary nucleus
mV	Millivolt
MVD	Microvascular decompression
NA	Noradrenaline
NC	Noncephalic
NF2	Neurofibromatosis type 2
NIHL	Noise-induced hearing loss
NMDA	N-Methyl-d-aspartic acid (receptor)
NMEP	Neurogenic motor evoked potentials
NTB	Nucleus of the trapezoidal body
OC	Optic chiasm
PA	Pial arteries
PAF	Posterior auditory field
PD	Parkinson's disease
PeSPL	Peak equivalent sound pressure level
PFC	Prefrontal cortices
PFMC	Prefrontal motor cortex
PI	Posterior insula
PICA	Posterior inferior cerebellar arteries
PI-VN	Posteriolateral ventral nucleus of the thalamus
PMA	Premotor area
PMd	Dorsal premotor area
PMv	Ventral premotor area
pps	Pulses per second
PSA	Posterior spinal artery
PVCN	Posterior ventral cochlear nucleus
R	Resistance
REM	Rapid eye movement (sleep)

REZ	Root exit zone
RMS	Root mean square
S1	Primary somatosensory cortex
SA	Sulcal arteries
SC	Superior colliculus
SL	Sensation level
SLR	Short latency response
SM	Stria of Monakow (dorsal stria)
SMA	Supplementary motor area
SN	Substantia nigra
SNc	Substantia nigra pars compacta
SNR	Signal-to-noise ratio
SNr	Substantia nigra pars reticulata
SOC	Superior olivary complex
SP	Summating potential
SpES	Spinal cord electrical stimulation
SSEP	Somatosensory evoked potentials
STN	Subthalamic nucleus
SVN	Superior vestibular nerve
TB	Trapezoidal body
Tc-MEP	Transcranial motor evoked potentials
tEMG	Triggered EMG
TEP	Trigeminal evoked potentials
TES	Transcranial electric stimulation
TGN	Trigeminal neuralgia
TIVA	Total intravenous anesthesia
TMS	Transcranial magnetic stimulation
UL	Underwriters laboratories
V	Volt
V1	Primary visual cortex
VAS	Ventral acoustic stria
VB	Ventrobasal nucleus of the thalamus
VEP	Visual evoked potentials
VN	Vestibular nerve
VNLL	Ventral nucleus of the lateral lemniscus
VPL	Ventral posterior lateral nucleus of the thalamus
VPM	Ventral posterior medial nucleus of the thalamus
VPN	Ventral posterior nucleus of the thalamus
μA	Microampere
μm	Micrometer
μs	Microsecond
μV	Microvolt

Index